Behavioral Aspects of AIDS

Behavioral Aspects of AIDS

Edited by
David G. Ostrow
University of Michigan
Ann Arbor, Michigan

Plenum Medical Book Company
New York and London

Library of Congress Cataloging-in-Publication Data

Behavioral aspects of AIDS / edited by David G. Ostrow.
p. cm.
Includes bibliographical references.
Includes index.
ISBN 0-306-43452-0
1. AIDS (Disease)--Psychological aspects. 2. AIDS (Disease)--Pevention. 3. AIDS (Disease)--Patients--Mental health services. I. Ostrow, David G., 1947-
[DNLM: 1. Acquired Immunodeficiency Syndrome--psychology. 2. Behavior. 3. Delivery of Health Care. 4. Mental Disorders--etiology. WD 308 B419]
RC607.A26B44 1990
616.97'92--dc20
DNLM/DLC
for Library of Congress
90-7242
CIP

233 Spring Street, New York, N.Y. 10013

Plenum Medical Book Company is an imprint of Plenum Publishing Corporation

Printed in the United States of America

Contributors

JAMES ASHE • Department of Neurology, The Johns Hopkins University School of Medicine, Baltimore, Maryland 21205

J. HAMPTON ATKINSON III • Psychiatry Service, San Diego Veterans Administration Medical Center, San Diego, California 92161; Department of Psychiatry, University of California, San Diego School of Medicine, La Jolla, California 92093

JAY BAER • Department of Psychiatry, Tufts University School of Medicine, Boston, Massachusetts 02111

T. PETER BRIDGE • Intramural Research Program, National Institute of Mental Health, Bethesda, Maryland 20892

KATIE A. BUSCH • Department of Psychiatry, Rush–Presbyterian–St. Luke's Medical Center, Chicago, Illinois 60612

LARRY L. BYE • Communication Technologies, San Francisco, California 94111

CAROLE A. CAMPBELL • Department of Sociology, California State University, Long Beach, California 90840

DANIEL DEFERT • AIDES Federation Nationale, Paris Cedex 75010, France

DON C. DES JARLAIS • Beth Israel Medical Center, New York, New York 10013; Narcotic Drug and Research, Inc., New York, New York 10013

JAMES W. DILLEY • Department of Psychiatry, University of California, San Francisco, California 94105; and University of California, San Francisco–AIDS Health Project, San Francisco, California 94193-0884

FRANCISCO FERNANDEZ • St. Luke's Episcopal Hospital, Houston, Texas 77030; Department of Psychiatry and Behavioral Sciences, Baylor College of Medicine, Houston, Texas 77030

SAMUEL R. FRIEDMAN • Narcotic and Drug Research, Inc., New York, New York 10013

GEORGE FULOP • Division of Behavioral Medicine and Consultation Psychiatry, Department of Psychiatry, Mount Sinai School of Medicine, New York, New York 10029

IGOR GRANT • Psychiatry Service, San Diego Veterans Administration Medical Center, San Diego, California 92161; Department of Psychiatry, University of California, San Diego School of Medicine, La Jolla, California 92093

JOHN R. HESSELINK • Psychiatry Service, San Diego Veterans Administration Medical Center, San Diego, California 92161; Department of Radiology, University of California, San Diego School of Medicine, La Jolla, California 92093

LORING J. INGRAHAM • Intramural Research Program, National Institute of Mental Health, Bethesda, Maryland 20892

DOUGLAS JABS • Department of Ophthalmology, The Johns Hopkins University School of Medicine, Baltimore, Maryland 21205

ROBB W. JOHNSON • Fenway Community Health Center, Boston, Massachusetts 02115

JILL JOSEPH • Department of Epidemiology, University of Michigan School of Public Health, Ann Arbor, Michigan 48109

CAROLINE J. KENNEDY • Psychiatry Service, San Diego Veterans Administration Medical Center, San Diego, California 92161; Department of Medicine, University of California, San Diego School of Medicine, La Jolla, California 92093

RAND E. LENHART • Formerly, Psychological Services, Cornell University, Ithaca, New York 14853–4401

JOEL K. LEVY • Department of Psychiatry and Behavioral Sciences, Baylor College of Medicine, Houston, Texas

SARZ MAXWELL • Department of Psychiatry, Rush–Presbyterian–St. Luke's Medical Center, Chicago, Illinois 60612

JUSTIN C. McARTHUR • Department of Neurology, The Johns Hopkins University School of Medicine, Baltimore, Maryland 21205

DAVID MILLER • Academic Department of Genitourinary Medicine, The Middlesex Hospital Medical School, London W1N 8AA, England

DAVID G. OSTROW • Midwest AIDS Biobehavioral Research Center, Institute for Social Research; Department of Psychiatry, University of Michigan School of Medicine, Ann Arbor, Michigan 48109

MICHAEL W. ROSS • Albion Street AIDS Centre, The Sydney Hospital, Surry Hills, NSW 2010, Australia

CAITLIN C. RYAN • AIDS Policy Center, Intergovernmental Health Policy Project, George Washington University, Washington, D.C. 20007

RITCH C. SAVIN-WILLIAMS • Department of Human Development and Family Studies, Cornell University, Ithaca, New York 14853-4401

BERTRAM SCHAFFNER • William Alanson White Institute of Psychoanalysis and Psychology, New York, New York 10023

JAMES J. STRAIN • Mount Sinai Medical Center, New York, New York 10029-6577

JEFF STRYKER • Department of Public Health Policy and Administration, University of Michigan, School of Public Health, Ann Arbor, Michigan 48109-2029

MICHAEL TRAUGOTT • Center for Political Studies, Institute for Social Research, University of Michigan, Ann Arbor, Michigan 48106

JOYCELYN SUE WOODS • Narcotic Drug Research, Inc., New York, New York 10013

DOOLEY WORTH • Montefiore Medical Center and Department of Epidemiology and Social Medicine, The Women's Center, Bronx, New York 10467

Preface

As we enter the last decade of the twentieth century, the AIDS epidemic looms ever larger and threatening. The specter of upwards of a million deaths in the United States and perhaps many millions worldwide from a sexually transmitted virus shakes our belief in modern medical science, while challenging the foundations of democratic society. Almost ten years into the epidemic, and with an enormous body of basic science research on the Human Immunodeficiency Virus (HIV), we still do not know why AIDS emerged when it did or how to stop its spread. A very humbling experience for scientists, clinicians, public health experts, politicians, and the general public.

Yet there are signs that a well coordinated multidisciplinary research program can conquer the epidemic and, perhaps, provide the basis for preventing future epidemics. The HIV family of viruses is now better understood, both in terms of structure and function, than any other virus. Genetically engineered peptides and nucleic acids are being tested as specific treatments or vaccines against HIV infection/disease. Most promising are the strides which have been made in understanding those aspects of human behavior which have contributed to the spread of HIV infection and which must be substantially modified if AIDS is to be controlled and eventually eradicated. The basis of that understanding has roots in a diverse set of disciplines which have converged in the work presented in this book. Psychiatry, epidemiology, sociology, anthropology, and the neurosciences have all contributed individually and in combination to the behavioral understanding of AIDS. This is perhaps a new and unique approach to the understanding and control of an infectious disease, at least in the twentieth century.

The emergence of the behavioral approach to understanding AIDS has its roots in several earlier periods of study, epitomized by studies of the sexual transmission of hepatitis B in the 1970s and earlier work on the ethnography of intravenous drug use. Each of those, in turn, was facilitated by social changes which demystified and permitted the study of previously "hidden" populations. And each contributed to the development of biological therapies—opiate antagonists for heroin addiction and a vaccine against hepatitis B. Whether or not we are on the verge of similar biological breakthroughs in the treatment or prevention of HIV infection is debatable. What is clear is that the future course of the AIDS epidemic is being shaped by human behavior and increasingly by interventions which seek to modify behavior.

The individual chapters in this book summarize the available behavioral information, describe its application to clinical problems, and, to a varying extent, discuss the research challenges which lie ahead. It is hoped that taken as a whole they contribute to our understanding of HIV infection and disease more than do the individual parts. In any rapidly growing field, new developments make books obsolete even before they appear. While all of the contributors to this volume have had the opportunity to update their chapters just prior to publication, there are undoubtedly gaps in information which editing and updating cannot fill. There is no way that this collection can be totally comprehensive in such an expanding field, where new areas of research and intervention appear daily. Several chapters are devoted to providing information and guidance for persons working in the field of AIDS so that they can be aware of the clinical, ethical, and public health policy implications of new behavioral research findings as they emerge.

I am especially grateful to all of the contributors to this book, who took the time out from their own research or clinical work to write their chapters. Most of the contributors have also participated in several of the symposia, courses, and workshops on behavioral aspects of AIDS which contributed to the conceptualization and organization of the book. I have had the pleasure to work with several editors at Plenum, beginning with Hilary Evans, who shepherded the first book on sexual behavior and sexually transmitted diseases, *Homosexuality and STDs: Diagnosis, Treatment and Research,* and began the discussions which lead to the proposal for the current publication. Janice Stern was most helpful in the difficult process of realizing the project, especially in helping to find the best contributors for each chapter and support their efforts. And finally, Mr. Eliot Werner took over the project for the final editing and production work. Many thanks to them and to all the scientists and clinicians working to find better ways to stop this epidemic.

David G. Ostrow

Ann Arbor, Michigan

Contents

II. PREVENTION: HIV RISK REDUCTION

IV. HEALTH CARE DELIVERY ISSUES

Introduction

A New Social Reformer

The Patient

DANIEL DEFERT

INTRODUCTION

Until 1981, we believed that in our societies any ill person could at any moment present himself to the world—to the family, to doctors and nurses, to work colleagues, to the church, to the school, to the government—and receive from each the same attention, the same treatment, and the same solicitude. We believed that a homogeneous space had been created around disease, and that this concerned only medical treatment. With the coming of acquired immune deficiency syndrome (AIDS), this social space has been fragmented. The person carrying human immunodeficiency syndrome (HIV) does not any longer concern everybody. He is no longer the bearer of universal symbols. Is it not true that those who care for him are only those who share his existential choices, his age, his sentiments, and the same risk? It is in the fragmentation of this social space that the community movements organized themselves. Their functions and their services serve as analyzers of social deficiencies, backwardness, and needs.

Community action saw its first model as early as January, 1982 with the formation of the New York Gay Men's Health Crisis. This was then followed in nearly all the metropolitan areas of the developed world and nearly always on the initiative of homosexual men and women. We should render particular homage to the role of homosexual doctors. The Fifth International AIDS Conference has taught us that this method of help has become internationalized from Soweto to Bangkok, but in Cuba seropositive individuals remain in quarantine.

Coming as I do from France, I have probably not met the unlimited violence of discrimination, injustice in meeting the financial burden of illness (AZT treatment is currently financed by the state and the hospitals are not profit making organizations in France), and government indifference which people affected with HIV or AIDS meet in greater or lesser degree throughout the world. Nevertheless, having started in 1984 in Paris a nongovernment organization of help and information, called AIDES, which in French also means "support," and which has now spread throughout the whole of France, I will recount our collective experience and also use some analytical instruments in the hope of

DANIEL DEFERT • AIDES Federation Nationale, Paris Cedex 75010, France.

trying to understand medical institutions, the human body and sexuality. These concepts are shared widely in the world today and were left to us by the philosopher and my personal friend Michel Foucault, in whose memory I founded AIDES. I will not give an account of all the justified bitterness which has been provoked by the denial of rights and discrimination against these individuals, because after so many years and so much effort it is now time to take stock of the examples of cases where patients suffering from AIDS or HIV have managed to change their environment by working through their community organizations.

First of all, our environment starts inside us, in our body on which it acts. But HIV cuts our body in two, into the physiological body, which is in the end threatened, and the socially menacing body. Or as Alain Emmanuel Dreuilhe wrote in the autobiography of his combat against the virus, into "wounds and shells."

Two different semiologies, one medical and one social; two different forms of fear, divide the body. In support groups, one often hears the refrain: "I am another." To be able to find a point of support inside oneself, a familiarity with oneself when the body and the social relationship have been damaged, is one of the first and most complex functions of community help.

By rapidly producing the notion of sexuality without risk or safer sex, community action invented a notion whose philosophical significance goes far beyond the preventive efficacy which we all recognize. In this idea are combined the vital spirit of desire and a number of behavior patterns which integrate it socially. Our educational strategies, which are all derived from this concept, have not explored the full force of this idea. The Western notion of sexuality related to procreation is thus officially dissociated, and the pleasure of our patients, whom we used to love for their suffering, is now officially taken into account. These notions completely overthrow our traditional social and moral conventions. The medical institution establishes with its patients a specific proximity and a specific violence, due to the discipline of its organization, its techniques of investigation, and the limits of its relational and therapeutic possibilities. *It is this violence that had to be reduced.*

MODIFICATION OF THE DOCTOR–PATIENT RELATIONSHIP

In 1985 it became technically possible to test the blood of donors for HIV antibodies. The medical profession debated whether it was justified to inform the blood donor of his/her serological status. The decision was made to inform the patient, to put an end to the epidemic. The medical institution feared that a donor may one day attack the blood bank legally for not having informed him of the risk he was carrying.

Between a medical technique that allows a diagnosis to be known and hidden from the patient, and a legal approach that obliges the institution to inform the seropositive subject because he is responsible for the health of others, community pressure imposed that the psychological identity of the individual also be taken into account, including his capacity to receive the diagnosis, to cope with it over time, and to ensure that he will not be discriminated against socially. This community action confirmed a tendency which is to be seen in modern law: the judicial subject and the psychological subject have equal value from the point of view of the composition of the social identity.

In the nineteenth century, it was not uncommon to ask those suffering from contagious diseases to denounce their partners. The modern state can no longer so easily impose something of such a private nature on an individual. Community pressure has contributed to the opening up of anonymous and free screening centers. The notion of screening has shifted, from the often mythical protective fears of societies, towards the capacity of an individual to cope with a medical phenomenon, a phenomenon without any immediate therapeutic perspective. Screening without the knowledge of the patient is still conducted. But these silent practices are no longer inscribed in the relationship that society officially entertains with patients.

Four structural elements in the doctor–patient relationship have been transformed: the position of death and the revealing of the intimacy of life have intensified the emotional aspect of this relationship, while the sharing of medical knowledge and the insertion of the doctor in a network of other health workers (because of the variety of manifestations and therapies available) have relativized the technical aspect of the relationship.

The clinical relationship must be supported by a relationship of speech and listening: the doctor must know how the patient represents his own illness to himself, to gain a knowledge of the patient's degree of acceptance and compliance with the therapeutic strategy proposed. In this context, where the patient is ceaselessly thrown back to other patients, is the doctor–patient relationship still this singular dialogue of medical humanism? It is becoming decentered, towards the autonomy of the patient and his free choice. These four transformations mean that medical practice is much less normative today and can be more easily challenged by other approaches.

TRANSFORMATIONS IN HOSPITAL ORGANIZATION

These changes also affect the relationship between the patient and the hospital team. The symbolic force of the diagnosis felt by every patient intensifies his emotional relationships with the whole of the medical team, regardless of the professional hierarchy. A nurse once said to me: "In two years, the spread of AIDS has changed the hospital hierarchical system as much as the events of May 1968." In previous AIDS Congresses, studies of the hospital context reported a reduction in the time passed by staff in patient rooms and in physical contact with them. Today, it would appear that the hospital staff try to read, through the needs of the patients and the community organizations that have come into place, their own need to express their anxiety, their emotions, and their professional mourning. The treating staff formulate the same demand to be heard and to be informed as the patients themselves.

The hospital organization itself is obliged to take into account in its organization and its discipline, the rhythms of the economic life of patients if it does not wish to increase their professional exclusion. So we have outpatient departments which open in the evening, and there is increasing cooperation between hospital doctors and general practitioners in the community to increase the medical follow-up of patients without interfering with the rhythms of their social lives.

Modern societies have delegated to medicine complete sovereignty over death, which is treated like a disease. Bristling with tubes, the patient slowly withers away physiologically, in the middle of a medical team which has replaced the social community. In the case of AIDS, where death is not only announced long in advance, but also befriended, an increasing number of patients prefer to die at home, surrounded by their friends. The quality of life in the last few days is more highly prized than an assisted longevity. The rituals of bereavement are often divided in two: first, a family ceremony around a death without a cause, and a second ceremony between friends where the choices of lifestyle are reaffirmed. Mourning had lost its social visibility. More forbidden still are the tears shed for a homosexual lover or a drug-addicted child.

There is a tendency for these mournings to be resocialized within supporting community organizations, as if a society which disapproved too strongly of emotions suddenly found it was itself pathological. And although it is quite true that all these new attitudes concerning death appeared under the pressure of a paramedical environment, in which one can detect certain landmarks such as *The Meaning of Death* by H. Feifel, in 1959, *On Death and Dying* by Elizabeth Kübler–Ross in 1969, this action of the human sciences on medicine was considerably relayed and amplified by community action.

THE SHARING AND CONTROL OF MEDICAL KNOWLEDGE

But perhaps the greatest change that HIV-positive individuals have effected in an effort to control their environment is their appropriation of medical knowledge. An increasing literature, written by patients and destined to be read by patients and doctors, keeps them regularly informed of both conventional and alternative treatments. The international circulation of persons undergoing treatment, to investigate pharmacological developments, has become one of the standard forms of scientific traveling, and as such requires the same freedom. In Paris these organizations campaigned to reinforce the guarantees of confidentiality in epidemiological studies and the free access of PWAs to information and treatment resources. Microbiologists, clinicians, and volunteers are organizing themselves to experiment with compounds without the constraints and norms of administrations, professional organizations, or private companies.

One can recall that the commercial license for azidothymidine (Retrovir®) in Phase II was obtained due to the emotional pressure of patients and their organizations. We are already in a state of crisis regarding therapeutic trials. And poor trials can jeopardize the future of patients. The urgency of the matter makes it increasingly intolerable to highly motivated patients to await the results of long trials against placebo. This is especially so when these studies create constraints before patients can have access to a given treatment.

Is it completely unrealistic to develop new methods of evaluating drugs which do not involve placebo studies as at present? And if these placebo studies are absolutely essential, should they not include more patients so as to demonstrate clearly that it is not the economic vested interests of private companies, or professions or countries which are against the extension of these clinical trials? Ethical questions are not only an internal matter of methodology, but they have become a worldwide demand for openness.

In actual fact, the hospital institution, hospital staff, and patients are feeling the effects of a structural change in our systems of treatment. The history of the modern hospital is that of an increasing dissociation of the assistance and the therapeutic functions. The therapeutic function has become separated in its own right and gradually more tailored into highly specialized medical acts, nullifying any global approach to the individual. Medicine has become one of the most advanced forms of technology. And in this context, if we have been able to reduce the time required to accomplish a given technical act, we cannot reduce the time required for relational activities. For this reason, these relational activities have gradually been removed from the sphere of the hospital. They are sometimes reintroduced into the hospital in the form of a technical relationship ensured by a psychotherapist, or abandoned to charity. In actual fact, as Michel Foucault analyzed, the modern medical system could not have developed without the support of an external factor, the family. And the specificity of this epidemic has been that it has damaged people in their family relationships. This is why the self-help organizations of patients, substituting for the family circle, take on all their significance.

The community movements into which HIV-positive individuals organize themselves had to reintroduce the relational factor into the structure of treatment. They had to collect money to ensure food and housing for those who were left homeless, because in our societies young people have become the category which is least protected socially. Patients have become the educators of medical, paramedical, social, and educational workers. Their experiences, relayed by the media, have become one of the essential sources of our collective experience of this disease. Their function becomes more political everyday.

TRANSFORMATION OF THE RELATIONSHIP BETWEEN SOCIETY AND THE DISEASE

In a long process that started some 200 years ago, it was the doctor who was associated with all the major social reforms. It was he who instigated the architecture and the hierarchy of hospitals, the cleaning up of cities. He drew attention to the development of demography, industrial hygiene, military conscription, and so forth. The new revealer of needs, of medical and social emergencies, is now the person with HIV and AIDS. As a mediator between hidden social currents and one of our most central institutions, the medical one, the HIV patient is a bridge between the experts who make the dividing lines between health and disease, life and death, the pluralism of private life and the right to solidarity. The patient not only represents the connection between pauperism and health as in the nineteenth century, but between liberty and health. He has become the new social reformer.

The very word "patient" has become technically and socially problematic. Technically who is ill? The person who belongs to group IV, group III, group II, or group I of the CDC classification? The asymptomatic person who is offered pretreatment? Very early the American gay community groups opposed using such terms as "ill" or "patient" or "victim" which imply a relationship with the doctor, and suggested a more community-based expression in which the personal confrontation with the disease of AIDS was highlighted: person with AIDS (PWA), a term that reflects considerable mobilization and effort. By all these changes, persons with AIDS are surely making an effort with which we can all identify: are they not in the process of reconstituting the figure of the patient in a way which is accepted and supported by all of us, with a universal significance? Until now, the patient was a figure of pain, in which Christianity long recognized the reflection of its agonizing god. Is not all this changing?

Even so, we can see already two limits to this tendency: one comes from the movement of the epidemic itself, the other comes from the logic of state intervention.

FUTURE OF COMMUNITY ACTION

First, there is not one, but several epidemics, somewhat spread in time, and which are different from each other not only in their modes of transmission, but also in the sanitary conditions surrounding each epidemic, and in the economic, cultural, medical, and political resources available to cope with it. Now, a community organization constitutes itself around three elements: a sociological element, a geographical element, and a political element.

Sociological Element

The mobilization of people, for the most part working free, who are close in their life-style, their age, their culture, their social or ethnic origin, to the persons requiring their services. Beyond a certain limit of marginalization, the will to associate into a group cannot exist. The criminalization, when it exists, of the homosexual, the drug addict, and the prostitute makes them inaccessible to this form of expression.

Geographical Element

The proximity of supply and demand ensures the optimization of community services. They depend, therefore, on the human resources available in each territory: women's organizations, social workers, or paramedical workers, religious groups, militant groups already attached to other forms of survival.

Political Element

The political direction of a community organization is under the control of those who use its services. This is what distinguishes them radically from the traditional health care organizations. Are all the human resources available in this disease ready to accept or to share the leadership of the campaign with those who were up to now always legally and economically excluded? It is precisely the mastery of one's life which gives it sense, and in our experience, it is this which prolongs it.

As regards the logic of state intervention, this consists in addressing the individual in his juridical abstraction, the family in its moral and demographic individuality, or society in general. Here is a net with a very large mesh to seize these regional figures of the epidemic with which we are concerned: few states recognized these groups, which needed to be recognized. Few states from early in the epidemic helped them by giving them the means of carrying out their tasks of information, organization, and prophylaxis. This would no doubt have tarnished the image of state power.

Today, however, the credibility of the state depends very much on its concern for AIDS, at least for the fraction of society which has the legitimate means of reprimanding it. How will states manage to combine their concern for their own image and their responsibility towards the different regions of society where the virus has now penetrated? The idea that states have of their own image is unfortunately part and parcel of the environment of infected persons. Which economist will calculate one day how many human lives have to pay for this concern of the state for its own image?

I

AIDS

Contributions of the Behavioral Sciences

1

Psychiatric Aspects of AIDS

An Overview

DAVID G. OSTROW

INTRODUCTION

The pace of the new acquired immune deficiency syndrome (AIDS) discoveries and clinical complications is such that those actively involved in AIDS clinical research might feel caught in a vortex of events, many of which appear to be out of control. During the past 9 years, since the syndrome called AIDS was first described, I have attempted to observe and understand the response of the general public and various groups to the AIDS epidemic. The experimental work on which many of these observations is based is an ongoing study of approximately 1000 gay and bisexual men at high risk of AIDS. These men comprise the Chicago cohort of a Multicenter AIDS Cohort Study (MACS), which is funded by the National Institute of Allergic and Infectious Diseases (NIAID) and the National Cancer Institute (NCI). The aim of the MACS is to describe the natural history and epidemiology of AIDS and human immunodeficiency virus (HIV), formerly known as HTLV-III or LAV-related disease. In Chicago, 95% of the MACS cohort is also participating in a National Institute of Mental Health (NIMH)-funded study of the psychosocial consequences of being at high risk of AIDS. In this chapter I present some models incorporating organizing principles to help us understand the context in which AIDS impacts on behavior. They are presented here in the hope that such organizing concepts may help us to impact in a constructive fashion on the psychological and social consequences of AIDS.

The epidemic curve of new AIDS cases (Fig. 1) combined with the well-known fate of any single person with AIDS is enough to explain the magnitude, if not the form, of these responses. No other medical event in recent history has caused the degree of public fear and private response that the AIDS epidemic has produced. With the recognition that perhaps 30–100 times as many persons with AIDS are already infected with a virus that

This chapter originally appeared as Ostrow D: Models for understanding the psychiatric consequences of AIDS, in Bridge TP, Mirsky AF, Goodwin FK (eds): *Psychological, Neuropsychiatric, and Substance Abuse Aspects of AIDS*. New York, Raven Press, 1988, pp 85–94. It is reprinted here with permission.

DAVID G. OSTROW • Midwest AIDS Biobehavioral Research Center, Institute for Social Research, and Department of Psychiatry, University of Michigan School of Medicine, Ann Arbor, Michigan 48109.

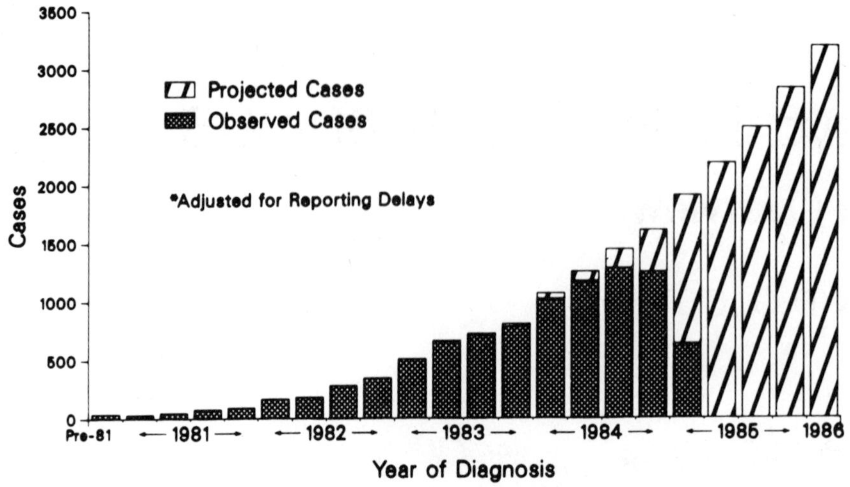

FIGURE 1. Incidence of AIDS in the United States as reported to the Centers of Disease Control (CDC) as of April 15, 1985 (cross-hatched bars) and projected through mid-1986 (striped bars). (From Curan.[1])

represents a ticking time bomb,[1] there has been a dramatic increase in the second epidemic, the epidemic of fear. This fear, whether it be of death, contamination, or just passivity in the face of a mortal threat, may well be the driving force behind all behavioral responses to AIDS. Certainly the fear of AIDS is the encouragement for various other campaigns that seek to exploit the public's fears for political ends and that in turn are the source of a growing sense in the affected communities that America is rapidly moving toward adoption of extreme measures such as mandatory HIV testing and quarantining of positive persons.

In our Chicago cohort we have seen a recent increase in fearful and angry responses to the question: "Is there anything else about AIDS and how it has affected you that you would like to tell us?" These expressions of fear and anger at the reaction of general society to AIDS have shown a dramatic increase in parallel with increased media coverage of AIDS quarantine and mass HIV screening proposals.[2] This observation leads to the conclusion that "fear of quarantine" is indeed a very real part of the psychiatric picture of AIDS in the United States. Whether or not such measures as quarantine are ultimately undertaken, the increasing discussion of quarantine proposals indicates the potential for negative social change and totalitarian responses to AIDS in our society.

Many positive behavioral responses to AIDS are taking place both in so-called high-risk individuals and members of that elusive group, "the general population." As early as 1983, we were seeing a dramatic reversal in direction of sexual behavioral change in prospectively examined gay men.[3] These observed reductions in numbers of partners or specific sexual activities illustrate what amounts to a "sexual counterrevolution" but do not tell us anything about individual behavioral responses, which are actually quite heterogeneous. When we examined a particular sexual activity, such as receptive anal intercourse, and the change in individual frequency of this behavior at two points of observation, we saw several different behavioral responses. These ranged from adoption of abstinence to reduction in frequency and/or partner numbers to some men who did not change their behavior at all between 1982 and 1983.

In 1984 we began to ask men who were having sexual activities that were generally considered high risk why they continued such activity. The reasons given included gratification overcoming judgment, peer or partner pressure, and various rationalizations of minimal risk.[4] These observations, which parallel explanations given for other types of unhealthy behavior, lead to a relatively simple model for understanding some of the psychiatric consequences of AIDS (Fig. 2). This structural model of barriers to behavioral change is simply the one first proposed by Freud and elaborated by many other proponents of psychoanalytical theory. Not only does it attempt to explain why behaviors that are known to be unhealthy do continue, it predicts a significant amount of psychological distress in persons who consciously recognize the risk involved in those behaviors but find themselves unable to reduce or stop their behavior. This helps us to understand the magnitude of the anxiety and stress being generated by the AIDS epidemic and the significant psychopathology that may result.

A PSYCHOSOCIAL MODEL OF THE BEHAVIORAL CONSEQUENCES OF AIDS

A more complex but realistic model goes beyond the intrapsychic realm to incorporate the role of social forces in shaping our responses to AIDS (Fig. 3). In this model, social responses are characterized as being "positive" if they lead to containment of the

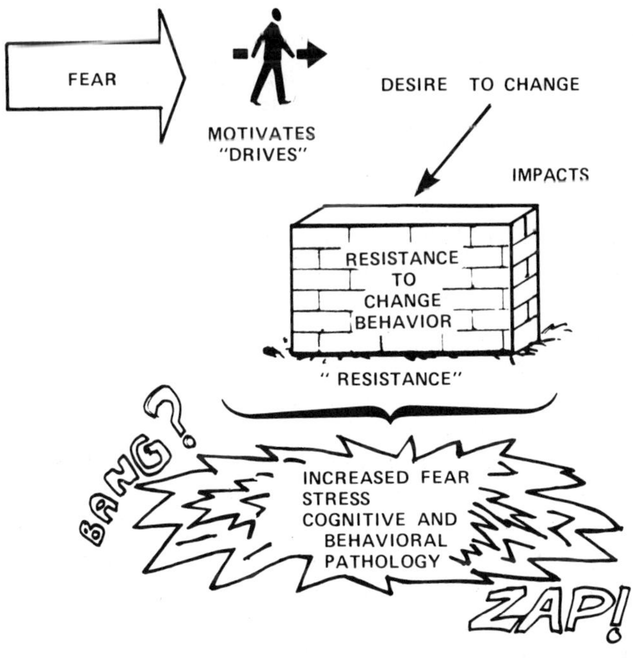

FIGURE 2. A structural model of the psychiatric effects of AIDS.

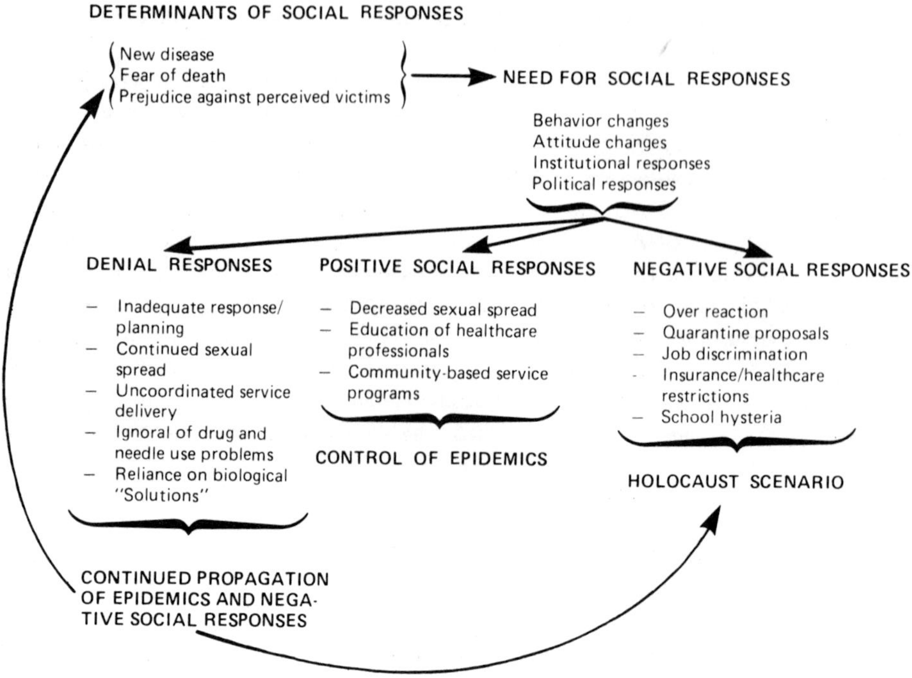

FIGURE 3. A psychosocial model of the psychiatric effects of AIDS.

physical and emotional causes of the epidemics, as "negative" if they contribute toward the negative social outcomes, and as "denial" if they continue to propagate the underlying causes of the dual epidemics of AIDS and AIDS fear through denial of their long-term consequences.

When looked at from the broader psychosocial perspective, some very basic aspects of behavioral change motivation are seen as important potential determinants of the behavioral responses to AIDS. These include an individual's belief in the efficacy of behavioral change to alter his risk of developing AIDS, his knowledge about and skills in maintaining behavioral change, perceived peer and societal support for those changes, and the availability of services that provide support for behavioral change. Recently presented cross-sectional findings in the psychosocial study indicate that knowledge about AIDS and belief in the efficacy of one's behavioral changes are strong retrospective predictors of reported sexual behavior change from "unsafe" to "safe" practices.[5] We need to keep this finding and its implications in mind when considering the setting up of programs to test at-risk individuals for HIV antibodies and use those results to motivate risk reduction. According to findings from the Baltimore MACS, persons receiving a negative antibody test result may, in fact, experience a negative impact on their ability to maintain behavioral changes that reduce risk of exposure of their sexual partners or themselves.[6] The importance of the vigorous pursuit of information regarding both cofactors for disease progression and possible therapeutic interventions is also underlined by these findings.

THE SPECTRUM OF AIDS-RELATED PSYCHIATRIC ILLNESS

In addition to the fear of developing AIDS and a feeling of inefficacy in those behavioral changes already taken, persons in AIDS risk groups may have a number of other sources of chronic stress. These include the social isolation and stigmatization that being in an AIDS risk group or having prodromal symptoms produces; the sense of helplessness one has in dealing with the disease for which there is no cure and for which there are at present no available interventions to prevent its development once infected; the significant loss of friends, lovers, and others to the disease; the giving up of sexual or drug-use behaviors and the loss of pleasure and anxiety reduction that these behavioral changes may entail; the related loss of intimacy when major forms of close social interaction are deemed "unsafe"; and the significant fear of quarantine and expectations of a "holocaust scenario" reported by many of our subjects. Given the number and magnitude of sources of chronic stress that are present in persons at high risk of AIDS, it is not surprising that we see an enormous range of psychiatric morbidity in our study population. We and others have observed a continuum of AIDS-related psychiatric problems ranging from anxiety and dysphoria to full-blown immobilization, psychosis, and even suicide[7] (Fig. 4).

A BIOLOGICAL MODEL OF THE PSYCHIATRIC CONSEQUENCES OF AIDS

The psychological and social stresses produced by AIDS and AIDS fear are not the entire story of this epidemic and its psychiatric consequences. As other contributions to this volume describe, there is a growing recognition that HIV can directly infect the

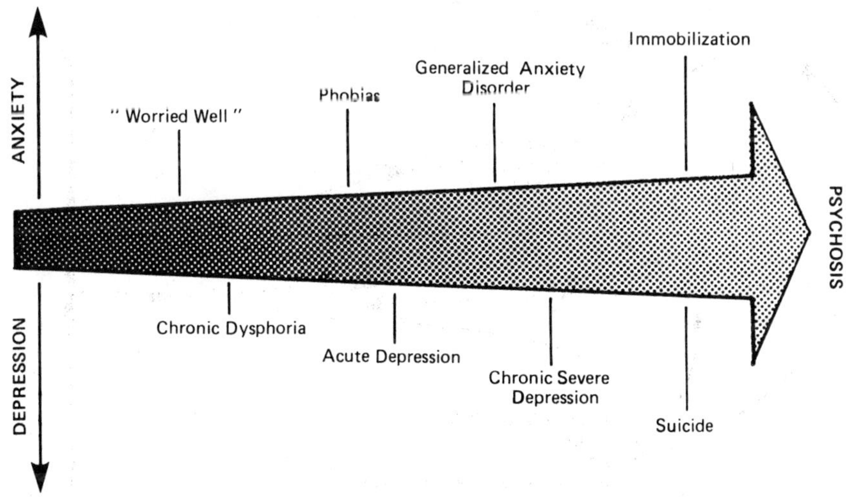

FIGURE 4. The continuum of AIDS-related psychiatric problems. Problems manifesting themselves primarily in anxiety symptoms are shown above, whereas those predominantly affective are shown below the *arrow*. (From Ostrow.)

central nervous system (CNS), producing a variety of serious neurological and psychiatric complications. A biological model for the psychiatric implications of AIDS must therefore include both direct and indirect effects on behavior (Fig. 5). This model recognizes not only that the virus is a biological contributor to various psychological problems but that serologic tests for antibodies to HIV embody many psychosocial implications themselves.

Among the psychiatric problems embodied in the HIV antibody test are its ambiguities. Although developed as a test for exposure to AIDS and not AIDS itself, the test is viewed by many and used in ever increasing frequency as a "test for AIDS." There is enormous anxiety about being tested, with some persons seriously decompensating when given a positive test result. There is also denial present in the belief that a negative test result definitively indicates that one has not been exposed or will not develop AIDS. Conversely, a positive test result embodies many of the aspects of isolation and stigmatization that were discussed for the disease itself. Our subjects fear discrimination based on testing and are angry at the misuse of the test to deny them insurance, employment, and other rights. No wonder, therefore, that individuals can develop major depression as a result of the helplessness and stress involved with the disease of AIDS and programs to test them for exposure to the virus believed necessary to produce AIDS.

THE VIRUS OF FEAR MODEL

Another model for the psychiatric effects of AIDS considers the fear of AIDS as the major vector and individual susceptibility to that fear as determining its psychiatric consequences, in a fashion analogous to the postulated effects of HIV infection on T cells (Fig. 6).

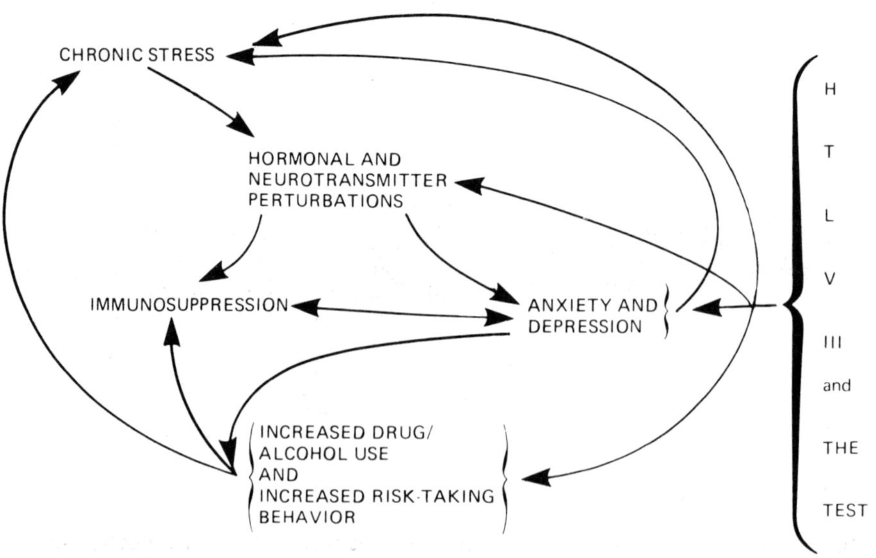

FIGURE 5. A biological model for the psychiatric effects of AIDS.

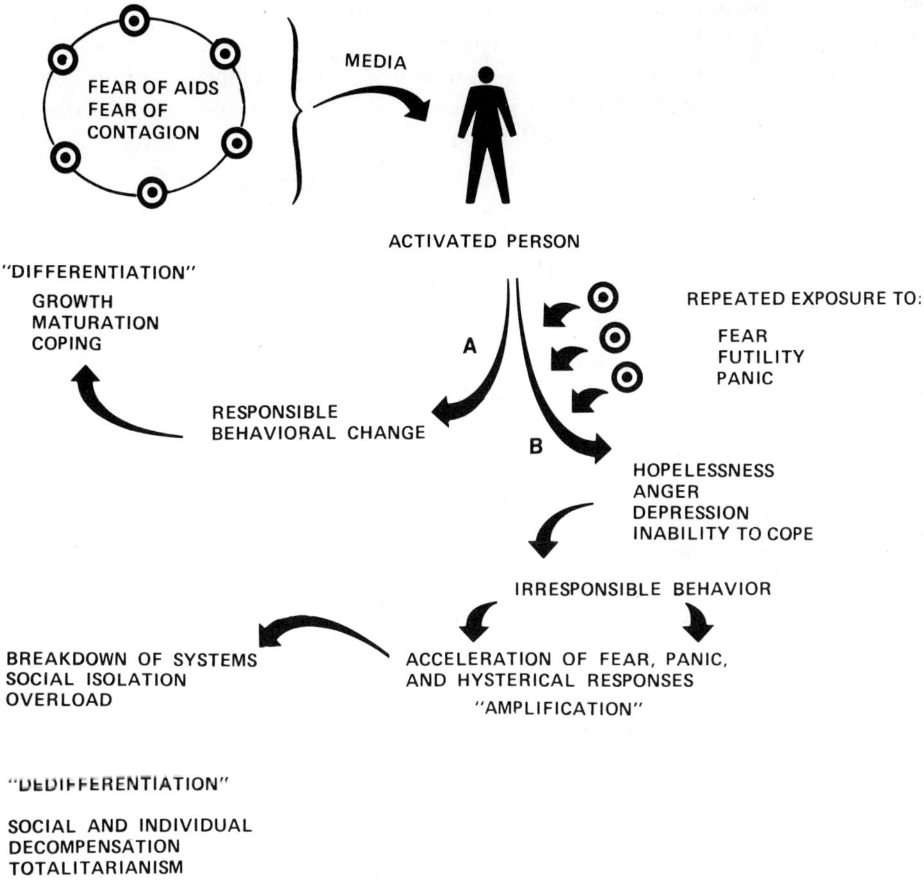

FIGURE 6. A model for the potential outcomes of exposure of susceptible persons to the fear of AIDS.

By substituting the fear of AIDS for the virus itself and the media as the carrier of that agent, we see that a person can either respond positively to exposure to the various elements of AIDS and AIDS fear by developing maturing responses or develop a dedifferentiation response leading to individual decompensation and, ultimately, social totalitarianism. The determinants of those responses must be a variety of individual characteristics as well as the psychosocial milieu and the way in which the information is conveyed to the individual. This model is analogous to how we currently view the vulnerability to depression in persons with a positive family history of affective disorders and who have been exposed to environmental or other stressors. We do not yet know the biological, characterological, psychosocial, or other factors that determine an individual's vulnerability to decompensate given repeated exposures to AIDS fear. However, given the enormous negative implications of individual and social dedifferentiation, it is extremely important that we study, understand, and intervene to prevent such outcomes.[8]

An example of the ways in which fear of AIDS can produce significant psychological distress and impair functioning in a vulnerable individual is illustrated with data obtained from the larger MACS cohort from all four cities participating in the study. We have recently reported[9] significantly increased scores on several subscales and total symptom scores of the Center for Epidemiological Studies—Depression (CES-D) questionnaire in men who see themselves as being at high risk for developing AIDS. This perceived high risk is manifested by individuals who report themselves as having enlarged lymph nodes or other symptoms of ARC, whether or not they actually have those symptoms on physical examination. The significant effect of perception of lymphadenopathy on psychological functioning was present in both the HIV antibody-negative and -positive men. Since we can limit the analysis to men who have remained antibody negative for 6–12 months and are thus extremely unlikely to be infected with the virus, we cannot ascribe this psychological distress to the neurological or psychological effects of "hidden" viral infection. We see it instead as residing in one's perceived risk of developing AIDS and the resulting stress that produces in vulnerable individuals.

This finding was confirmed when we performed a multiple repression analysis on the CES-D factors, showing that the number of perceived AIDS-related complex (ARC) symptoms, including self-reported "glands," were highly correlated with elevated scores on all subscales and the total (CES-D) score (Table 1). In conformation of our psychosocial model was the finding that a negative response to the question "Is there anyone you can talk to about important problems?" was a significant independent predictor of increased psychological distress.

CONCLUSIONS

The various models for psychiatric effects of AIDS presented here each have implications that need to be integrated into a unified psychiatric model in order to be most useful (Fig. 7). Behavior change, whether it be on an individual, group, societal, or institutional basis, is motivated by both fear and force, but also by gratification and altruism. This

TABLE 1. Relative Ranking of MRA determinants of CES-D Scores

	CES-D factor				
Significant MRA correlates	Total	Depression	Enervation	Positive affect	Interpersonal sensitivities
Total number of self-reported ARC symptoms	1	1	1	1	1
No one to talk to	2	2	2	2	3
Perceived glands	3	3	4	4	—
Education level[a]	4	—	3	3	5
Perceived glands—serostatus interaction[a]	5	4	8	5	—
Number anonymous partners	6	8	6	6	4
Age[a]	7	5	5	—	2
AIDS sex partner	—	6	—	—	—

[a]These are negative correlates; i.e., increased education level, age, and positive serostatus all decreased CES-D scores.

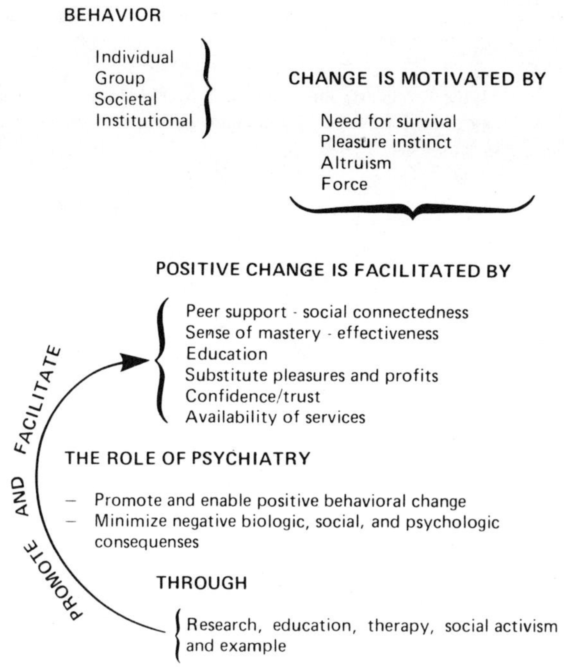

FIGURE 7. An integrated model for psychiatry's positive potential roles in meeting the mental health challenges of AIDS.

motivation is not sufficient in and of itself to produce positive change, which must also be facilitated by a variety of psychosocial, educational, and institutional supports and resources. The role of psychiatry in this model is to promote and enable positive behavioral change while minimizing the negative biological, social, and psychological consequences of that change. As psychiatrists we can accomplish this through research, education, therapy, social activism, and even by example. The responsibilities of such a role are enormous. But the potential risks were we not to mobilize the mental health professions to pursue actively positive behavioral change in response to AIDS are unthinkable.

REFERENCES

1. Curran JW: The epidemiology and prevention of AIDS. *Ann Intern Med* 103:657–662, 1985.
2. Ostrow DG, Eller M, Joseph JG: Epidemic control measures for AIDS: A psychosocial and historical discussion of policy alternatives, in Carliss IB and Pittman-Lindeman M. (eds.): *AIDS: Principles, Practices and Politics*. New York: Hemisphere Publishing, 1988, pp. 19–31.
3. Ostrow DG, Altman NL, Wallemark C-B, et al: Patterns of homosexual behavior, 1979–1983, in *Proceedings of the conjoint STD Meeting*. Montreal, International STD Research Society, 1984, p 12.
4. Ostrow DG, Emmons CA, Altman NL, et al: Sexual behavior change and persistence in homosexual men, in *Proceedings of the First International AIDS Conference*. Atlanta, U.S. Public Health Service, 1985, p 71.
5. Joseph JG, Montgomery SB, Emmons CA, et al: Magnitude and determinants of behavioral risk reduction: Longitudinal analysis of a cohort at risk of AIDS. *Psychology and Health* 7:73–96, 1987.

6. Fox R, Odaka N, Brookmeyer, et al: Effect of HIV antibody disclosure on subsequent sexual activity in homosexual men. *AIDS* 1:241–246, 1987.
7. Ostrow DJ: A psychiatric overview of AIDS. *Int J Neurosci* 32:647–659, 1987.
8. Ostrow DG: Issues and analysis: Psychiatric implications of AIDS. *Masters Psychiatry* 1:21–23, 1985.
9. Ostrow DG, Monjan A, Joseph J, et al: HIV-related symptoms and psychological functioning in a cohort of homosexual men. *Am. J. Psychiatry* 146:737–742, 1989.

2

Psychovenereology

Psychological Aspects of AIDS and Other Sexually Transmissible Diseases

MICHAEL W. ROSS

INTRODUCTION

Psychological variables are intimately associated with sexually transmissible diseases (STDs) in both immediate and more distant senses. The immediate associations involve the social psychology of demand characteristics of situations that may lead to higher risk of infection or of the environment itself or the actors in it. The more distant psychological determinants involve personality styles or attitudes to sex and sexuality, which may put an individual at greater risk of STD infection. There will also be person–situation interactions in which these two sets of psychological variables interact. Very little is known, however, about the decision-making process as it concerns decisions to have sex, the safety of that sex, or decisions to use prophylaxis. Indeed, little is known of how individual actors in sexual encounters conceptualize their interaction[1]: Ross[2] noted that as many as 15 different meanings may be associated with sexual encounters, ranging from the emotional to the ritual (Table 1). Clearly, what we have to date regarded as the psychology of the sexual encounter is itself a complex field and it may ultimately be demonstrated that the psychological concommitants of sexual encounters will differ with different meanings being associated with such encounters.

A third area of psychology associated with acquired immune deficiency syndrome (AIDS) and other STDs is that of clinical psychology or psychiatry, in which maladaptive or pathological responses to infection (or fear of infection) may occur. This area is of more immediate importance to the clinician in dealing with the presenting patient, and has been brought into prominance by the range of marked psychological traumas associated with AIDS.

This chapter reviews in turn the psychological variables associated with STDs (including AIDS) by examining the specific situations which may lead to increased risk of STD infection. These include as a general measure personality and attitudinal variables

MICHAEL W. ROSS • Albion Street AIDS Centre, The Sydney Hospital, Surry Hills, NSW 2010, Australia.

TABLE 1. Theoretical Aspects and Meanings of Sexual Relationships

Aspects	Meanings
Reproduction	Continuation of species
Religious	Symbolic of union
Emotional	Extension of love for partner
Release of sexual urge	Release of frustration or libido
Financial	Prostitution
Duty	Socially expected, as in some marriages
Antisocial statement	Rejection of parental/social values
Ritual	During particular ceremonies; symbolic
Hedonistic (recreational)	Enjoyment
Experimental	Exploration of sexual feelings and behaviors
Relational	As part of wider social and attitudinal affinities
Dominance	Rape; expression of difference in relative power
Peer-sanctioned	Normative; status oriented
Forbidden or taboo	Associated with guilt or punishment
Dynastic	Cementing relations between families or groups
Mentor	Teaching sexuality to younger individuals

associated with increased STD infections and possible models of how they may produce increased risk behavior. More specific behaviors that may be directly related to increased risk of infection include the psychological concomitants of high partner numbers, of particular places of sexual contact, and of particular sexual practices. Following on from this, normal and abnormal reactions and illness behaviors related to STD infections are reviewed and presented as schemata of the psychological processes of STD infection. At the outset, it must be noted that there is often little available research to draw on, and that a significant proportion of this work is on homosexual men and Western societies and may not be generalizable to other populations.

PSYCHOLOGICAL VARIABLES ASSOCIATED WITH RISK OF STD INFECTION

The variables associated with increased risk of contracting STDs include those associated with those behaviors that carry an increased risk of infection. In addition to specific behaviors such as high partner numbers, specific sexual practices, and the place in which the sexual behavior occurs, this includes a more general review of the variables associated with STD infection. This section concentrates on the host and environmental aspects of the host–environment–agent triad in terms of associations of psychological and sociocultural variables with known risks and review some of the data and schemata used to explain the contribution of psychological variables to the variance associated with STD infection. When psychosocial factors can be associated with risk of STD infection, this provides a possibility of modifying such factors to decrease the probability of infection as well as information on which educational strategies may be based.

PERSONALITY AND ATTITUDINAL VARIABLES

Hart[3] argued not only that there is "increasing recognition of venereal disease as a behavioral disease," but also that all the sociological variables implicated in venereal disease are primarily related to the personality of the individual. He reported for his heterosexual sample that an increase in extraversion, and to a lesser extent neuroticism as measured by the Eysenck Personality Inventory,[4] were associated with increased STD infection and appeared to underlie many of the sociological variables he found to differentiate his infected and noninfected groups. Similar peaks on neuroticism for both heterosexual and homosexual men were noted by Wells and Schofield,[5] although they found their homosexual patients to be more introverted that the heterosexuals, and by Fulford et al.,[6] who found significant and positive correlations between neuroticism and syphilis and gonorrhea infection in their total homosexual and heterosexual sample. They also reported that clinic patients scored higher on psychoticism, extraversion, and neuroticism when compared with Eysenck's norms and that bisexuals had the highest elevations of neuroticism and psychoticism compared to homosexual and heterosexual men. Measured on Eysenck's Sexual Attitudes Inventory, Fulford et al. found clinic subjects generally to be less interested than Eysenck's controls in physical sex and pornography, to have less sexual excitement, and greater prudishness, sexual disgust, and neurotic sexual attitudes. Homosexual patients did not differ from heterosexual patients, but surprisingly the bisexual patients accounted for most of these differences between clinic patients and controls. They also found bisexual men to be the only group with evidence of psychological disorder.

While there is some evidence of increased scores on personality traits such as neuroticism and extraversion for those individuals with STD infections, most studies took patients presenting at STD clinics and failed to discriminate between those with a single infection and those with multiple infections. Further difficulties in interpretation arise from use of test norms as control groups without establishing the degree of comparability. Although some studies have established that some 40% of heterosexual patients at STD clinics are likely psychiatric cases based on screening questionnaires such as the GHQ,[7,8] there has been little evidence of actual disorder but considerable speculation about the possible underlying psychodynamics of individuals who contract STDs. However, this may be biassed by the type of individual who seeks treatment at public clinics as opposed to private practitioners: Ross[9] found that those attending private practitioners tended to be older and more conservative.

In 1964, Hooker[10] suggested that the homosexual man who "seeks escape from loneliness and guilt in 'compulsive cruising' . . . is more likely to be infected with an STD." Oriel[11] also suggested that compulsive promiscuity is due to emotional insecurity or personality disorders. Parental relationships have also been suggested as a contributing factor in STD infections. Morton[12] saw the "lack of an intelligent and affectionate approach by parents" as a causative factor, and Fluker[13] wrote of unhappy homes, parental indifference, overcrowding, and parental severity as further contributors. It is of particular interest that Hart[14] reported that soldiers coming from large (four or more children) families are at significantly greater risk of STD infection, and Ross[15,16] reported that parental relationships are among the significant predictors of multiple STD infections in the four Western countries he studied.

Other psychological factors may have both direct and indirect effects on infection rates, particularly environmental stresses. Hart[14] noted in his classic studies of STDs in troops in Vietnam that "the environmental stresses of war produced behaviour patterns which many would not otherwise experience." The stresses of immigration are similarly acknowledged by Armytage,[17] who comments that one half of the men with gonorrhea in the United Kingdom during the 1960s were immigrants; Oriel[11] also noted that single migrants frequently have numerous sexual encounters until they settle into their new cultural background. This apparently holds for nonwestern societies, as Hart[18] reported that in single laborers and married immigrants in Papua New Guinea, recourse to prostitutes and, to a lesser extent, homosexual behavior, are more common outlets, of which venereal disease is a prominent sequel. There is some very convincing evidence in the numerous studies in which STD incidence rates in immigrants and soldiers are increased markedly (in comparison with baseline rates prior to immigration or war) that instability and insecurity resulting from a change to an alien culture or environment is associated with lack of discrimination in, or increase in frequency of, sexual contacts. However, it is unclear whether it is stress itself or the social disruption associated with immigration or war and that reduces opportunities for marriage that is responsible.

It could be argued that in most Western societies, a homosexual orientation is one that both produces stress and removes individuals from the seemingly stable and secure heterosexual culture they have been brought up in; thus they become *sexual immigrants* within their own society. The association of stress with STD infection as a test of this hypothesis would provide some indication of whether the stress of a homosexual orientation is a contributor to the increased incidence of STDs in homosexual men.

By contrast, a little-cited but important study by Kelus[19] in Poland took random samples of STD clinic attenders and inhabitants in a town near Warsaw and found no differences between inhabitants and patients apart from a tendency for patients to be more urbanized and less religious. However, Kelus provided two models to describe how neuroticism or psychological problems might lead to different sequelae in terms of STDs, which can be schematically represented:

Neuroticism→Promiscuity→STDs
Neuroticism→Sexual inhibition→STDs

This model, however, sees the influence on STD incidence as occurring through partner numbers alone. Kelus suggests that in more permissive societies, neuroticism would lead to promiscuity, while in the more restrictive society, neuroticism would lead to sexual inhibition. Thus, how individuals cope with their psyche in relation to their sexuality depends on the psychological and cultural context of that individual. It is of interest that Ross[16] found that there was a lower level of STDs in homosexual men in the two smallest and most agrarian countries studied, Finland and Ireland, and the highest in the two largest and most industrialized and cosmopolitan societies, Sweden and Australia, providing indirect support for the hypothesis put forward by Kelus that cultural factors may influence STD incidence rates. The model does not indicate what intervening variables between neuroticism and sexual activity occur, however, and also assumes that neuroticism is associated with partner numbers. This latter assumption is not consistently supported by the available evidence reviewed in the section on psychological concomitants of partner numbers. By contrast, Hooker[10] suggested that "for some, the seeking of sexual contacts with other males is an activity which is isolated from all other aspects of their lives." We cannot assume that psychological factors that influence partner contacts will be obvious in other areas of the individual's life, but perhaps only in specifically sexual attitudes, unless any denial that may mark isolated sexual behavior is evident in different forms in other aspects of the individual's behavior.

Further personality variables associated with increased risk of STD infection in homosexual men by Ross[20] include their views of the meaning of their sexual orientation. Ross identified three attitudinal factors, which he labeled Consensus—Order—Conflict, and —Anarchy factors. Swedish homosexual men who scored high on the Consensus—Order factor saw their sexual relationships as being based on a heterosexual model and had more conservative attitudes toward them. Sexual expression was not seen as a factor setting heterosexuals apart from others, proportion in relationships was high, and partner numbers were low. Those who scored high on the second (Conflict) factor, in contrast, saw their homosexuality as being an expression of challenge to conventional norms and thus as a more highly psychologically cathected act. Such individuals were more likely to have high partner numbers (presumable because they saw homosexual encounters as a politically significant act) and not believe in homosexual relationships. For such individuals, clearly the risk of STD infection is higher. The third dimension, labeled Anarchy, measures the attitude that individuals should be controlled by their own beliefs and values, and that sexual behavior will depend on the individuals, time, place, and situation. Not surprisingly, such individuals' beliefs are unrelated to any behaviors that might put them at greater or lesser risk for STD infection. Thus, belief systems about the meaning of one's sexual behavior do have clear implications for risk of STD contraction, at least in homosexual men. However, it is difficult to see how such attitudinal factors may be extrapolated to heterosexual men, who generally do not question their sexual orientation. By contrast, these dimensions may have some clinical value in the case of heterosexual women, for whom sexual behavior may have political implications.

Other attitudes to sex may be clearly and consistently associated with behaviors that place individuals at greater risk of STD infection. Eysenck's Sexual Attitudes Inventory,[21] which yields 13 interpretable dimensions in heterosexual men and women (Table 2), raises a number of questions as to their applicability to sexual, and particularly homosexual, behavior. In his initial study on the sexual attitudes of university students, Eysenck found that high psychoticism scorers also tended to score higher on sexual curiosity, attitudes to premarital sex, promiscuity, and hostility scales, being more sexually curious, more accepting of premarital sex, more promiscuous, and more hostile. Extroverts tended to score high on the promiscuity scales and low on the nervousness scale (more promiscuous and less sexually nervous), while high scorers on the neuroticism scale had significantly lower scores on sexual satisfaction and significantly higher scores on excitement, nervousness, sexual hostility, sexual guilt, and sexual inhibition. As well as having high construct validity, these results fit in surprisingly well with those of Hart.[3,22] Hart found that extroversion was a marked feature of those with STD infection in his study of Australian soldiers in Vietnam, and that high neuroticism scores were closely associated with venereoneurosis (preoccupation with bodily processes which individuals imagine are associated with onset or incomplete cure of STDs or irrational concern and obsessive behaviors designed to confirm or negate these fears). Clearly, Hart's data, along with those of Wells,[23] parallel those of Eysenck[21] in finding a close association between

TABLE 2. Sexual Attitudes in Heterosexual Individuals

Permissiveness	Prudishness
Satisfaction with sex	Dominance–submission
Neurotic sex	Sexual disgust
Impersonal sex	Sexual excitement
Pornography	Physical sex
Sexual shyness	Aggressive sex

extroversion and STD infections. Hart[3] went so far as to comment that "certain sociological parameters to venereal infection may be of a secondary nature, in that all are primarily related to the personality of the individual." In this regard, Hart's model is the antithesis of Kelus's model in stressing the primary importance of personality rather than culture.

More recently, Fulford et al.[24] used Eysenck's personality measures of psychoticism, extroversion, neuroticism, and their associated Lie scale; he found that whereas neuroticism correlated positively with syphilis and gonorrhea infections, extroversion correlated negatively with the diagnosis of syphilis. These findings are somewhat confusing and in the opposite direction to what might be expected from previous research. However, Fulford et al.[24] also used the second (adult) versions of Eysenck's[21] sexual attitudes questionnaire in the sample of 180 male STD clinic attenders and found that their total samples scored lower than Eysenck's adult male sample on the factors measuring interest in pornography, sexual excitement, interest in physical sex, interest in aggressive sex, and displayed greater prudishness and sexual disgust. These results are also in the opposite direction to that expected. The only difference between small subsamples of heterosexual and homosexual men was that homosexual clinic attenders had a lower interest in physical sex, again contrary to what might be expected. Bisexual men, however, scored significantly higher than heterosexuals for neurotic sex, impersonal sex, prudishness, and sexual disgust, and lower on sexual excitement, which suggests that their bisexual respondents had atypically abnormal sexual attitudes. Fulford et al.[24] reported that the differences between the total clinic sample and Eysenck's adult sample were mainly due to the contribution of the bisexual men. They did not, however, examine the links between the sexual attitudes in the sample and STD infections. Given that their respondents were all from an STD clinic, however, the lack of significant differences between their sample and Eysenck's adult males may be a function of inadequate variance.

However, Ross[20] refactored the Eysenck Sexual Attitudes Inventory after rewording it to make it appropriate for homosexual men and derived nine interpretable dimensions from an Australian sample; a replication in a Californian sample yielded 11 interpretable dimensions. Those scales that were consistent across cultures measured degree of libido and control; interest in, and arousal by, pornography; comfort with women; sexual permissiveness; sexual prudishness; and fear of sexual relationships. Using the Australian data, Ross (Table 3) found that, as anticipated, sexual attitudes did underlie sexual behaviors. In fact, six of the nine scales were predictors of partner numbers, five were predictors of particular sexual practices, and six were predictors of places of partner contact. The scales predicting partner numbers were those measuring fear of sexual

TABLE 3. Sexual Attitudes in Homosexual Individuals

Fear of sexual relationships	Importance of affect and relationship
Interest in pornography	Prudishness
Sexual excitement	Permissiveness
Comfort with women	Libido and control
Acceptance of sexuality	

relationships, interest in pornography, level of sexual excitability, sexual prudishness, sexual permissiveness, and degree of control of libido. Of particular interest, however, is the fact that all these scales were related in a curvilinear, rather than a linear, fashion to partner numbers, with those with zero and high partner numbers having greater fear of sexual relationships and sexual prudishness and lower interest in pornography, degree of sexual excitability, and sexual permissiveness. Those with higher partner numbers are highest on the degree of control of libido scale, suggesting that a combination of fear of closeness to partners in sexual relationships and lower libido leads to zero or few partners, and that fear of closeness to partners in sexual relationships and high libido and lack of control of libido to high numbers of partners. Intuitively, this makes psychodynamic as well as psychometric sense. This is of considerable importance for further research, as it also implies the existence of intervening cofactors that may determine the differences between those with high or low partner numbers.

Ross found that for particular sexual activities, higher scale scores were associated with high frequency of preferring specific practices, with the exception of mutual masturbation, where this trend was reversed. Places of partner contact also followed a similar pattern, with those making contact through friends the exception. It would thus appear that personality factors influencing sexual behaviors are of central importance in determining the existence of at-risk behaviors for AIDS and other STDs, despite the relative paucity of research on them. There is to date little if any research on the etiology of sexual attitudes or modification of them.

PSYCHOLOGICAL CONCOMITANTS OF PARTNER NUMBERS

Partner numbers may be an important determinant of STD infection, as greater numbers may increase the probability of infection with a pathogen. However, it is important to note that if sexual practices that do not transfer body fluids are used, partner numbers are immaterial. Similarly, if all partners are monogamous, there is no risk. Thus, the association of partner numbers with STD infection is dependent on other risks, which may explain why Ross[20] found that partner numbers were not invariably associated with risk of STD infection in homosexual men. Unfortunately, little work has been carried out on the concomitants of partner numbers in heterosexual individuals. Schofield[25] reported that there is little if any evidence that individuals with high numbers of partners have personality defects, are emotionally damaged, or come from a less than adequate social milieu. Looking at homosexual men in the United States, Goode and Troiden[26] found that those with higher partner numbers tended to prefer emotionally superficial sex and also tended to be less well educated. Ross[20] found that, as with attitudes toward sexuality, those with no or multiple partners had very similar responses on many variables, and it was those with moderate partner numbers who were significantly different on a number of variables, including relations with parents during childhood and adolescence.

While negative experiences predispose to higher partner numbers, the most negative parental rearing pattern tends to decrease the partner numbers within the one-to-multiple partners group. It is therefore of particular interest to look at other factors that may covary with parental rearing patterns to influence partner numbers. Three variables relate to mood state and external contributors: confusion, fatigue [as measured by the Profile of Mood States (POMS)], and stress. In each of these, the pattern is for the highest levels to occur in the no-partner group, and the lowest in the multiple-partner group. It seems fairly clear from these data that dysphoric mood state has the effect of depressing partner numbers. Alternative explanations include suggesting that high partner numbers protect against stress, confusion, and fatigue through their effect on increasing self-esteem, or that the association is not causal but produced by covariance with some unknown factor. Nevertheless, it has been noted[27] that depression increased in homosexual men who reduced their risk of contracting human immunodeficiency virus (HIV), which does suggest that there is some association between mood state and partner numbers.

It is apparent that homosexual men with higher numbers of partners differ from those with lower partner numbers on a number of indices. The most consistent of these include parental rearing patterns, stressors, expectations of negative reactions to their homosexuality by significant others and by society in general, masculinity in terms of self-perception and preference for a more feminine partner, and alcohol consumption. The picture that emerges for the high-partner individual is of a male who is conventionally masculine and who believes that there is little negative reaction to his homosexuality. He will have had a more negative parental rearing pattern and be under less stress than will low-partner numbers men, tend to binge-drink alcohol more frequently, be more involved in the homosexual subculture and see his homosexuality as more central to his life-style, and have had more STD infections. These data illustrate the multifactorial nature of the variables associated with high partner numbers, ranging from negative parental rearing patterns suggestive of a need to compensate through higher partner numbers, a belief that homosexuality is not perceived negatively by society and by significant others, lack of stressors or dysphoric mood states, and adherence to conventional norms of masculinity including dominance and a perception of the male role as incorporating multiple sexual contracts. This picture appears to be internally consistent across white Western cultures.

PSYCHOLOGICAL CONCOMITANTS OF PARTICULAR SEXUAL PRACTICES

The importance of particular sexual practices on STD transmission has been highlighted by the AIDS epidemic. Particular sexual practices involving the transmission of body fluids, including unprotected anal or vaginal intercourse, brachioproctic activities, and (possibly) fellatio, are now discouraged, and any information that may assist in the understanding of the processes underlying choice of particular sexual activities is important. There is little previous research on the psychological variables associated with preferences for particular sexual practices in homosexual men and none on heterosexual individuals, although Haist and Hewitt[28] noted that homosexual men who preferred the anal insertee role also tended to prefer the oral insertee role in fellatio. However, Hooker found no relationship between sexual activity preferences and gender role. Ross[20] found that homosexual men who preferred oral activities, including both fellatio and analingus, appear to be differentiated from those with no such preference by negative maternal rearing patterns and by mood states, suggesting that they may be related both to gratification of oral dependency needs and to hedonism. Preference for insertor and insertee roles in both fellatio and anal intercourse appeared to be strongly related to conventional masculine and feminine sex roles, and activities such as full-body contact and mutual masturbation appear to be non-role related. It would appear that these last two activities occur when there is emphasis on emotional as well as physical closeness and that they lead, as expected, to decreased frequencies of STD infection. Ross's data also suggest that sexual socialization into homosexual subcultures and, to a lesser extent, parental and peer models, have a major influence on the type of sexual activities indulged in; that is, increased time and degree of socialization into the homosexual subculture increases preference for specific roles, as does degree of organization (in terms of differentiation and specialization) of the homosexual subculture within which that socialization occurs. In terms of modifying sexual practices to reduce risk of STD infection, it will clearly be most difficult to modify the specific behaviors of those who have been socialized early and for some time in the more specialized homosexual subcultures such as occur in major metropolitan area, and easiest to alter the practices of those who are in smaller areas and have been in gay subcultures for a shorter time. Preference for particular practices do appear to be more a function of the crystallization of tastes rather than of psychological imperatives, although the influence of masculine and feminine sex roles does appear to be associated with the most "risky" behaviors.

PSYCHOLOGICAL CONCOMITANTS OF PARTNER ANONYMITY AND PLACES OF SEXUAL CONTACT

Partner anonymity and place of sexual contact play an important part in STD infection. The links are threefold: (1) the possibility of contact tracing anonymous partners is virtually impossible; (2) in some places of anonymous contact, such as gay bathhouses, there are opportunities for multiple contacts with multiple partners within a short time span; and (3) such places have their own demand characteristics, which may lead to person–situation interactions in which the situation effect is significant. Apart from the classic study conducted by Humphreys,[29] which classified those using public conveniences as places for sexual gratification into four groups: *trade,* ambisexuals, gays, and *closet queens,* there are few data on places of sexual contact. Humphreys's *trade* group comprised married men who worked as truck drivers, machine operators, or clerical workers; in 63% of those marriages, both husband and wife were Roman Catholic. In this group, two thirds took an insertor role in fellatio in sexual encounters. Ambisexuals were married men with double the median income of the *trade* group, and usually Protestants. Two thirds of this group were insertees in fellatio. Such individuals saw themselves as bisexual but were able to compartmentalize their sexual orientations into heterosexual and homosexual without much interaction or conflict between the two. The gay group were individuals who were unmarried and had no preference for sexual roles and who had independent occupations, while the *closet queens* were also unmarried but in lower-middle-class occupations in which they were dependent on others for employment. They avoided homosexual contacts in other places in the homosexual subculture, of which they are not a part. Humphreys found that most of these individuals preferred to play the insertor role, at least until they lost their attractiveness, and one half of this group were also Roman Catholic, suggesting that religion might have some influence on sexual expression in terms of anonymity. While the *closet queens* would appear to embody those who avoid emotional contact, they clearly have little or no contact with the homosexual subculture and therefore do not appear in samples.

Ross[20] demonstrated some marked differences between those preferring particular places of meeting sexual partners. Those meeting in bars tended to prefer social as well as emotional contacts but had overinvolved parents who may have made extended interaction difficult, and those making contacts through friends preferred homosocial as well as homosexual contacts to an even greater degree. Contrary to expectations, those meeting partners through cruising have more positive mood states and higher self-esteem than others and were markedly different to those who frequented bathhouses. These latter individuals appear to be more depressed and more avoiding of close emotional contacts, probably as a result of having experienced much more negative parental rearing practices, which may have provided negative relationship models. These findings again cast some light on the potential dynamics of those involved in meeting partners at particular venues and particularly in terms of those who attend homosexual bath houses. It would appear that psychological variables, particularly mood states, may be strongly associated with the drive for partners as well as the context in which they are sought, and the relationship between mood and partner-seeking suggested above would seem to be substantiated by these data. Clearly, future research must concentrate on whether such underlying psychodynamics can be modified: it is doubtful that education alone will have any effect for such individuals.

THE PSYCHOLOGY OF STD INFECTIONS

The second area of importance in considering psychological aspects of STDs is the psychological aspects of infection, including the reactions of those infected and the abnormal behavior, including illness behavior and venereoneuroses, in those infected. This section considers the presentation and management of the psychosocial manifestations and psychopathology in STDs.

Reactions to STD Infection

Little of a scientific nature has been written about the meaning of STD infection to the individual, and little empirical research carried out on this area. Ross[20] postulated a model of the meaning of STDs to the individual, but attempts to quantify this and assess the psychological variables associated with these conceptualizations of STD infections have not been carried out. The importance of this model lies in its attempt to explain the beliefs underlying psychological reactions to STDs and the reasons for psychopathology when it occurs.

In discussion the meaning of STDs to the individual, we have identified at least five separate attributions.

1. STDs are a deserved outcome of indiscriminate sexual behavior and punishment for sexual sins.
2. STDs are a consequence of individual inadequacy that leads to sexually indiscriminate behavior.
3. STDs are a consequence of a breakdown in traditional social values and rapid social change.
4. STDs are the result of an individual coming into intimate contact with a virulent pathogen.
5. STDs are a sign of being sexually active and are a matter of pride.

Note that there is a hierarchy of blame from attribution 1 to attribution 5. The hierarchy of blame is a concomitant of a similar hierarchy of the degree to which the individual is responsible for the infection. It is almost impossible to investigate social and psychological associations with STD infection and not have an implicit model underlying one's hypotheses. One must also recognize that different models will apply in different cultures, and will depend on the degree to which sexual behavior is cathected (i.e., the degree to which there is a psychological investment in it).

More important, the meaning of STDs to the patient and to a lesser degree the attending health professional will affect not only the compliance with treatment, but also the psychological sequelae and the subsequent risks of exposure to STDs the individual takes. These may be examined by reference to the five attributions proposed.

STD as Punishment

When the individual sees the STD as punishment, a particularly religious background or have never having come to terms with sexuality is not uncommon In the case of the homosexual man, the individual will probably be at one of the first three stages of homosexual adjustment described by Cass,[30] in which their sexual orientation is not usually publicly acknowledged and almost invariably not accepted. Cass's stages are (1) identity confusion, (2) identity comparison, (3) identity tolerance, (4) identity acceptance, (5) identity pride, and (6) identity synthesis. The combination of the stigma of STD along with the stigma of homosexuality is an extremely powerful one, and the homosexual STD patient who sees his infection as an indication that he is being punished will need careful attention. The result of infection is likely to include remorse or sometimes clinical or subclinical depression as the individual is faced with the evidence of a sexual behavior that he has probably compartmentalized or denied. In such cases, the anxiety or embarrassment may lead to defaulting from treatment or to denial of a homosexual orientation in the first place. Ross[9] noted that some 20% of STD clinic attenders who are homosexual deny their real sexual orientation to the attending physician and that these individuals are most likely to expect the most negative reactions to their sexuality from others. Such individuals are also most likely to be first attenders; when they also attend private physicians rather than public clinics, they may tend to deny their sexuality to a greater extent. It is important that the attending physician does not accept or reinforce the patient's negative view of his sexuality, particularly as this may be one of the first times the patient has admitted his sexual orientation to anyone outside of a small circle. Sometimes patients have apparently accepted their sexuality in the past but return to attribution 1 when they contract one of the more severe STDs. For example, some people with AIDS who have been living openly homosexual lives have seen their disease as a "punishment from God" and blamed it on their homosexuality. In some cases, this may also be associated with an increase in religiosity in a person with AIDS. The combination of sexuality and STDs is a psychologically powerful one, and for the patient's mental well-being, if it is apparent that they see their STD infection as a "punishment," assessment of the need for reassurance or correction must be made. The situation is more difficult if this is part of the patient's "acceptance" of either AIDS or death, or both. In such cases, it is helpful to have access to accepting clergy for referral.

This first category of the meaning of infection to the individual is most notable for its mental health consequences, which in many cases require more attention than the STD. Venereophobia, in which there is no evidence of STD infection but the patient is convinced that infection has occurred, most commonly occurs in patients who see it as punishment for some real or imagined misdeed, usually of a sexual nature. The prominence given to AIDS during the past few years has made AIDS phobias a reasonably common clinical phenomenon in venereology, with the individuals presenting usually being concerned over sexual contact outside of primary relationships and experiencing stress at work or in relationships that often acts as a trigger.[31] Brief insight-oriented counselling is the treatment of choice, provided there is no evidence of psychosis, but it is important not to perform repeated HIV testing, which may only reinforce the patient's conviction of infection.

STD as Evidence of Maladjustment

This second category has much in common with the first category in which STDs are seen as a punishment. While the reason for the individual's dysphoria on realizing that he has an STD is a result of lack of acceptance of his sexual orientation, the basis is not religious, and the dysphoria not so pronounced. Nevertheless, the major sequelae are also likely to be in mental status, but denial through compartmentalization of sexual orientation may also be present. Married men frequently fall into this category, and their homosexual activities are thus likely to occur in public toilets to avoid the need for emotional contact with a partner. (Humphreys[29] found that 54% of men who had sex in public toilets were married.) As a result, the contacts are often likely to be unknown, and there is the added complication that the patient's wife may have been infected, and be unaware of her spouse's bisexuality. Since a sizable proportion of homosexual men (10–20%) marry and, since those who marry are usually those less accepting of their homosexuality,[32,33] such individuals may be frequently represented in those with sexual orientation dysphorias. In contrast to situations in which individuals are unhappy at being homosexual, however, such patients become disturbed by their sexuality only when it produces negative consequences such as STD infection. The advent of AIDS has also produced a marked increase in patients falling into this category during the past few years.

A second group within this category are those with mild dysphoria with a treatable STD infection and who recognize that there is nothing they can do about their sexual orientation but feel that it might be easier to be heterosexual. They rarely present a problem in terms of either compliance with treatment or mental state. By contrast, too great a degree of dysphoria may result in anonymous sexual contacts, since having known partners and affective contact could be too guilt engendering. Contact tracing is thus likely to be difficult, although returning for proof of cure is usually not a problem. Treatment of this attributional group is similar to that of the first group if AIDS phobias arise, and may require psychotherapy.

STD as the Fault of a Sick Society

In this group, the blame for STD infection is likely to be projected rather than introjected, and the individual is most likely to be at Cass's[30] fifth stage of homosexual development. The fifth stage, according to Cass, is the period in which the individual accepts his homosexuality and defines his entire life-style in terms of it. Thus, to the extent to which he allocates blame for STD infection, it cannot lie with his sexual orientation, which is so centrally important to him, but must lie elsewhere. Elsewhere is usually the society that so stigmatizes homosexuals that they are forced to meet in secluded places and have impersonal sexual contacts. Stigmatization may also affect the number of sexual partners by lowering self-esteem to the point where relationships are not possible, and either multiple partners or no partners may be the adjustment sought to assuage a negative self-image. While these arguments are based on reality in countries in which sexuality is severely stigmatized and legal penalties are severe, they appear to apply seldom to those whose sexuality (particularly homosexuality) is the central defining construct of their life-style. Essentially, those who believe that STDs are the fault of a discriminatory society are unable to accept that any fault lies with them and are therefore unresponsive to suggestions about cutting down at-risk practices. In some cases, such a suggestions will be construed as a condemnation of their homosexuality, and the medical interaction will be terminated. In others, STD infection becomes a red badge of courage, indicating emancipation from the perceived restrictive and bourgeois sexual habits of monogamy and possession of sexual partners. Where sexual behavior is seen as a political or social statement, it is most unlikely that it will be open to modification.

Similarly, where an individual has *come out* recently as a homosexual, it is most likely that there will be more frequent sexual contacts both in response to a previous deficit of sexual contact in most cases, and because one mode of understanding of homosexuality centers on its sexual component rather than its affective or social component. In such cases, sexual activity may be higher than it would otherwise be, because of an affirmation of the individual's core identity. If this is the case, suggestions that attempt to modify sexual behavior could be seen as a rejection of their homosexuality: thus, the point should be cautiously broached. Usually individuals move on the Cass's stage 6, and the issue is not so fraught with danger. If, however, this does not appear to be occurring after a lapse of several years, it may be advisable to raise the issue by ascertaining the meaning of sexual behavior to the patient and by attempting to identify any personal difficulties that may be driving their sexual behavior. Generally, this stage is the opposite of the STD as Punishment group, in that the latter see their sexuality as inviting retribution, while the former see their sexuality as a central and positive aspect of their life-style.

STD as Just Another Infection

For some individuals, STD infection is not highly cathected and carries no investment in psychic energy. Such individuals are likely to be in Cass's stage 5 or stage 6, in which a homosexual orientation is seen as being only one of many identifications the individual has, and not central to identity or life-style. STD infection (AIDS excepted) is medically just another infection with varying risks associated, but few people are able to see it that way. In terms of dealing with individuals at this stage of STD perception, there is little problem in making suggestions of modification of at-risk behaviors; on the other hand, if infection is not cathected, there is little reason to do so unless the risk is a major one (e.g., with hepatitis B or AIDS).

People who fall into this category tend to have identified themselves as actively heterosexual or as homosexual for longer and to approach sexuality in a fairly hedonistic way. Thus, if modification to partner numbers as a response to AIDS is necessary, partner numbers may be cut down without great psychological trauma. However, if partner numbers are important to the person to maintain self-esteem, then that individual probably falls into the category of seeing STDs as the "fault of a sick society."

STD as a Source of Pride

In some situations, particularly with adolescents who are eager to demonstrate their maturity by demonstrating sexual conquest or desirability, STDs may be a source or pride. In such a situation, it will be difficult to suggest preventive measures since they may diminish the individual's identity as adult or sexually desirable and threaten one of their sources of self-esteem. Such individuals may also fall into the fifth stage, "identity pride," of Cass's[30] model, and may see attempts to reduce the chances of recurrence (although not cure of individual episodes) as diminishing what may be seen as a mark of prestige among peers. With the advent of AIDS, it is to be hoped that this attitude will become less common. It may be possible to invest condom use with some of the positive properties of STDs in this attribution as a preventive strategy.

While the aim of venereologists should be to remove the psychological involvement to the point where STDs are just another infectious disease, the attendant consequence is to also remove the pressures, positive and negative, on individuals to modify their behaviors. Pressure to modify behavior will thus be a consequence of the risks carried by STDs (e.g., high risk of AIDS, low for gonorrhea). However, by now it will have been recognized that patients are not the only ones with beliefs about STDs.

Medical Reactions to STD

Each of the five stages described can also be used to describe medical attitudes to STD infection. Those who have read widely on the subject will be able to classify various authorities on a continuum from seeing gonococci as "God's little helpers" through to approaching them as just a part of infectious disease management. The important thing to note is that our attitudes as health-care professionals will affect not only our approach to our patients but that our own attitudes will interact with those of our patients. The consequence of this for behavior modification of risky behaviors is enormous. To give two examples, the physician whose attributions of STDs are at the first level will discourage avoidance of risks because the "punishment" is preordained and presumably unavoidable. Nor will any distinction be made between safe and unsafe sexual acts because the "punishment" is seen as being for sexual activity, not particular specific sexual acts! On the other hand, the physician who subscribes to attribution 4—that sexuality is important and that STDs are just another infection—may well have removed the pressures on individuals to modify their behaviors. This is particularly dangerous when physicians see sexual contact in political terms and feel that to urge patients to decrease sexual partner numbers is tantamount to rejection of a particular mode of sexual expression.

The interaction between patients and physicians who hold conflicting attributions for STDs may also lead to tension, anger, transference, and countertransference issues and resistance to taking advice or treatment, particularly when more divergent attributions are held. It is critical to ascertain one's own position and make some estimate of the position of ones patient before seeing to educate or to modify risky behaviors.

Psychological Reactions to HIV Seropositivity

Just as there are stages of reaction to attributions for STD infection, there are stages through which individuals may pass when infected with AIDS or other STDs. The case of AIDS is the most clearly defined, given the major traumas associated with a potentially fatal sexually transmissible infection. In many ways, these are similar to the model of stages of coming to terms with terminal illness described by Kübler-Ross[34] but also differ in some important respects, since the trauma is often the stigmatization rather than the possibility of death. These reactions are more marked the lower one goes down the attributional scale. It is important to realize that the emotional impact of telling an individual that they have HIV infection is not significantly different from that of telling them they have full AIDS. In a two-country study of homosexual men, Rosser and Ross[35] found that the emotional distress of being informed one was anti HIV positive, had AIDS-related complex, or had full AIDS was judged to be of the same emotional magnitude, although the amount of life change judged to be associated with these diagnoses was significantly different.

Ross et al.[36] described the reactions of homosexual men to asymptomatic HIV infection. These psychological stages and the clinical issues associated with such stages are summarized in Table 4. They point out that infection with the AIDS virus may not lead to death for a high proportion of individuals; thus, the Kübler-Ross model of acceptance of terminal illness is frequently inappropriate, particularly if, as is believed, cofactors may influence progression of HIV infection. There is, in addition, like a homosexual orientation, considerable stigma attached to infection and the stigmatized status is not usually visible or identifiable. For this reason, their model contains some similarities to models of homosexual identity formation. This is to be expected, since a significant proportion of individuals carrying antibodies to HIV in the Western world are homosexual or bisexual men. In many cases, they will use a previously appropriate and successful model to manage a second stigmatized status such as HIV infection. Ross et al.[36] stress that the degree of clinical value of the model must, however, be determined by further research. They note that this model, while staged, is fluid (allowing for regression as well as

TABLE 4. Stages of AIDS Antibody-Positive Status Congruency in Homosexual Men

Reaction	Psychological processes	Common presenting issues
Stages 1 and 2: Shock, denial, anger	Guilt, powerlessness, anger	Anxiety, frustration, distress, acting out
Stage 3: Withdrawal	Recognition of stigma, isolation	Fear of infecting others, depression
Stage 4: Bargaining		
Substage 4a: "Coming out" to significant others	Testing of other's reactions and bargaining, stress displacement, need to be loved	Rejection, stress, confrontation
Substage 4b: Looking for other antibody-positives	Sharing, recognition, trust positive reinforcement, social support	Dependency, overinvolvement, loss of anonymity
Substage 4c: Special status	Turning alienation into a unique advantage, difference becomes special, needed by others	Dependency, "us and them" dichotomy overidentification
Substage 4d: Altruistic behavior	Group commitment and cohesiveness, desire to give and share, feeling of community	Burnout, overreaction, over compensation
Stage 5: Acceptance	Integrated antibody positive status with self-identity; balance between altruism and self; coming to terms with one's condition.	Apathy, resistance to change

progression) and that some individuals may neither experience every stage nor progress beyond particular stages.

Stages 1 and 2: Shock, Denial, and Anger

The initial stage describes the common reactions to major unanticipated trauma. Denial may operate as defense to prevent decompensation, but the psychological processes operating commonly include guilt at being responsible for infection, anger at self or at those perceived as responsible for infection, and powerlessness associated with lack of control or knowledge of outcome. This is exacerbated by associated minority status (further stigmatization within and beyond an already stigmatized group).

Stage 3: Withdrawal

Stage 3 describes the response to recognition that one has an infection that could lead to isolation, either imposed or self-imposed, sexual or social. Recognition of the associated stigma activates previously useful stigma management models, particularly those in use in groups such as homosexuals and intravenous drug users whose status, like that of the HIV antibody-positive individuals, is concealable. Individuals in this stage tend to keep to themselves as part of their uncertainty about the reactions of others. A significant component of this keeping to themselves may be related to fear of infecting others and to depression.

Stage 4: Bargaining

Stage 4A: "Coming Out" to Significant Others: Stage 4A follows at this point not the Kübler-Ross[34] model of terminal illness but more closely the Cass[30] model of stages of homosexual identity formation. Disclosing one's HIV antibody-positive status to certain carefully selected individuals follows the process of disclosure of sexual orientation or drug usage, with a careful disclosure to those who are most likely to be accepting or who are family or significant others. Psychological processes include bargaining with society (through those disclosed to) over acceptance, expression of the need to still be loved, and displacement of stress on to others. The form of the reaction of others will determine the presenting problems, but these commonly include coping with stress related to disclosure, rejection, and confrontation. If those disclosed to were unaware of the previous stigmatized status, reactions tend to be more consistently negative.

State 4B: Looking for Others. This stage also has elements in common with acceptance of a stigmatized identity as described by Cass,[30] particularly the seeking out of others in a similar situation. Processes involved include seeking positive reinforcement and the social and psychological support of others with whom one shares a common difficulty. Peer support provides confidence which comes with recognition of one's antibody-positive status and sharing of problems and reactions with those in a similar position. Difficulties which may emerge include dependency on antibody-positive peers, antibody-positive status becoming one's dominant identification to the exclusion of others, and loss of anonymity if one is identified with a stigmatized group.

Stage 4C: Special Status. This stage of antibody-positive status acceptance is one we have noted is common in those who have previously lacked a strong sense of identity. Those who have had no ambivalence about a previous stigmatized status such as a homosexual orientation may often proceed direct to stage 4D. State 4C turns alienation into an advantage (similar to the identity pride stage of Cass's[30] model of homosexual identity formation), in which individuals see themselves as something different and special, needed by others. Psychodynamically, this stage may also represent reaction formation or a sense of guilt or self-blame over becoming infected, leading to action in stage 4D. Problems associated with this stage include overidentification with, and dependency on, one's "special" status and splitting the world into an "us and them" dichotomy.

Stage 4D: Altruistic Behavior. Altruistic behavior connects the issues in stages 4B and 4C into action. There is a feeling of community and belonging within the stigmatized subgroup, and beyond this a desire to affirm that identity. The strong desire to give and share with others may be a part of the process of "making friends with one's disease" taken to the point of acceptance of a stigmatized status and denial of its stigma. The need to serve and in many cases to "go public," though, can lead to problems of burnout and overreaction. However, this is balanced by provision of a purpose in a life that may have been disrupted by a diagnosis of HIV antibody-positive status, as well as provision of a mechanism with which to cope with this status. Whether most of such individuals burn out, move to stage 6, or regress remains to be seen.

Stage 5: Acceptance

Most models, including those of Kübler-Ross[34] and Cass,[30] have a final acceptance of a perceived negative status or negative situation as their resolution. Logically, integration of antibody-positive status as part of one's identity should follow, although we have seen few cases to date. This stage appears to be a balance between the altruism of stage 4D and attention to self. Problems that tend to present are resistance to further change of those behaviors that may place self or others at risk, and a degree of apathy over health status.

These stages are a first approximation of the psychological processes operating in individuals who are HIV antibody positive. However, they do raise the issue of the normal progression of illness behaviors in individuals with STDs, and particularly the role of illness behaviors, given that there is no possibility of secondary gain, except as exhibited in factitious illness, such as factitious AIDS.[37,38] For treatable STDs, only one study has investigated the effect of illness behaviors in STDs.

Illness Behaviors in STD

Few data are available on illness behavior in STDs. To date, it has been assumed that illness behaviors in STDs were identical to those in other comparable illnesses. However, it has important implications for treatment. In the case of individuals with an erroneous conviction that they have an STD, which Hart[3] refers to as venereoneurosis, there is abnormal illness behavior in terms of both general hypochondriasis and a strong disease conviction without demonstrable pathology. There may also be an indication that the patient believes he "deserves" the infection. In the case of other individuals, and perhaps more common, is the refusal to see STD as an illness but perhaps only as a minor nonsignificant risk of a particular life-style. Clinical observation has tended to suggest that in the case of the absence of illness behavior, patients may frequently compromise treatment by discontinuing medication after symptoms have resolved, continuing sexual activity after symptom resolution but before clearance, or not returning for proof of cure. Thus, both abnormal illness behavior and lack of illness behavior may have implications for the management of STDs.

Ross[39] looked at illness behaviors in STD clinic attenders and found that, contrary to expectations, it was the repeated attenders rather than the first attenders who displayed the greatest anxiety and hypochondriasis over STD infection. Those with higher previous numbers of infections also tended to deny life stresses more, attributing their problems to the episode of illness. Such individuals also displayed significantly higher disease conviction and symptom preoccupation and higher levels of symptom exaggeration. In comparison, first attenders tended to deny that an STD was an illness, which would appear, in some cases, to be a denial of the contraction of an often stigmatizing illness. Compared with other illness behaviors, in which there may be substantial secondary gain, STD infection would appear to be quite different in manifestation in STDs and to be developed as a function of repeated infections. In such cases, it would appear that STD infection tends to be seen as a chance event until after several infections, when it is then seen not only as an illness but also as a result of particular behaviors.

In the same study, Ross also found that there were few differences in illness behavior with STD infections between heterosexual and homosexual men, apart from the fact that there is a less negative reaction to STD infection (probably given the greater awareness of

STDs in gay subcultures and the greater self-definition of homosexual men in sexual terms). Ross also noted, using non-STD controls attending general practice and psychiatric outpatients, that the STD clinic population was closer to the psychiatric population than the general practice one. This tends to confirm the finding of Catalan et al.[7] that 40% of a British STD clinic population had some degree of psychological disturbance on a screening test. It is unclear whether the disturbance was a function of having a stigmatized illness such as an STD or inherent in STD clinic attenders. The issue of the difference between public and private clinics, and of the accuracy of admissions at STD clinics, is an important one.

In a separate study, Ross[9] also found that admission of homosexuality in STD clinics varied significantly between countries (20–52% did not admit to being homosexual) although not between public and private clinics. Characteristics of individuals who did not admit to their sexuality included sex-role conservatism, number of previous STD infections, position on the Kinsey Scale, number of individuals from whom the respondent conceals his homosexuality, expected societal reaction to homosexuality, relationship with mother, and masculinity and femininity. The data also showed that those who deny homosexual contact consistently expect more negative reaction to their homosexuality and appear to be less accepting of their sexual orientation. This confirms the hypothesis that psychosocial factors account for a significant proportion of the variance in denial of homosexual orientation; up to 79% of the variance was accounted for by attitudinal variables. A second hypothesis, that there are common variables implicated cross-culturally, was also confirmed.

The picture that emerges of the variables predictive of whether the respondent reveals his homosexual orientation when presenting to a STD clinic or medical practitioner in each of the four countries is a coherent one. Nonadmitters are likely to conceal their homosexuality from most people, to expect the most negative social reaction to their homosexuality from significant others and society in general, and to believe in much more rigid and conservative sex roles for men and women. As compared with those who admit to homosexual contact, nonadmitters are more likely to report themselves as being more bisexual than exclusively homosexual, to have had no previous STD, and, interestingly, to have had poor relationships with their mother during adolescence. They are also more likely to be high scorers on "femininity" (passive, gentle, and empathic) and low on "masculinity" (not assertive or dominant). The nonadmitter thus emerges as an individual who expects particularly negative reactions to revealing his homosexuality and must probably therefore describe himself on questionnaires as bisexual. Such individuals also tend to accept common sex-role conservatism, which contributes to their lack of acceptance of their orientation, rather than vice-versa. MacDonald and Games[40] noted that homophobic heterosexuals believe that homosexuality violates sex-role stereotypes. Those individuals who denied a homosexual contact expected an extremely negative reaction to their homosexuality from others. Three items suggest that the nonadmitter feels that he is a failure, tends to have mild depressive episodes, and believes that he may be able to change his homosexual orientation. He also believes that he has a harder time than most in gaining friends, possibly a function of the avoidance of homosexual friends. These additional data amply confirm that the individual who does not admit to homosexual contact does not accept his own homosexuality and expects a strongly homophobic reaction from others.

These data have a number of practical applications. A lack of previous sexually transmitted infections in nonadmitters suggests that the clinic situation will be a new and potentially frightening one, in which condemnation is expected. In subsequent visits to a clinic, the patient will tend not to be too apprehensive if the clinician's approach has been nonjudgmental. In this context, the finding of a negative relationship with the mother in adolescence may be important. Respondents who had a less satisfactory relationship with a normally nurturant figure may transfer this to clinicians who are also seen as normally nurturant authority figures. Finally, the apparent passivity and lack of assertion that are also predictors of failure to reveal orientation suggest that nonadmitters have trouble expressing what is construed as negative information that may elicit a negative response. It may also be that when clinicians take histories in a manner that implies that any sexual contact was a heterosexual one, the patient may not have the courage to make a correction. These data suggest that there are significant and consistent psychological factors operating to prevent some homosexual men from revealing same-sex contacts in the context of STD clinics. However, these psychological factors will clearly operate in interaction with environmental factors such as the clinic, the clinician, and the legal and social climate regarding homosexuality. Individual practitioners can do little more than to be aware of the factors operating and seek to mitigate them actively through their interaction with patients, particularly emphasizing genuineness and empathy as well as specifically dealing with their therapeutic acceptance of what patients may consider shameful or abnormal practices. The imposition of shame and guilt upon sexual interactions by religious and other traditional moralities is the single most important cause of psychological problems in STD treatment and, if the physician is able to assess and deal with this early in the treatment process, many difficulties may be prevented or minimized. Lack of consideration may even introduce or reinforce shame or guilt and produce an iatrogenically strengthened psychopathology. A high index of suspicion for psychosocial problems attendant on STD infection or reported infection is mandatory to ensure maximal compliance with treatment, contact tracing, prevention and preventive education, and the possible contribution of psychosocial factors to relapse or reinfection should not be underestimated.

CONCLUSIONS

It can be demonstrated that psychological aspects of STDs play a central part in understanding their incidence, presentation, treatment, and prevention. It must also be recognized, however, that such studies are in their infancy and that psychovenereology as an important subdiscipline in the study of STDs has only recently emerged. There is clearly a need for further and detailed research, particularly on the social, societal, and situational determinants of at-risk behaviors, as well as studies on the characteristics of those who will use prophylaxis and respond to education to reduce risk.

Evidence to date suggests that while some psychological characteristics may predispose to those behaviors that may in turn lead to STD infection (through partner numbers, particular sexual practices, prophylactic behaviors, or places of partner contact), including extraversion and instrumental personality, particular attitudes to sexuality, and some variance will occur in person–situation interactions or with significant interactions with cofactors. It is hoped that it is in such areas that future exploration and research of psychosocial factors in venereology will emerge.

REFERENCES

1. Gagnon J, Simon W: *Sexual Conduct: The Social Sources of Human Sexuality*. London, Hutchinson, 1973.
2. Ross MW: A theory of normal homosexuality, in Diamant L (ed): *Male and Female Homosexuality: Psychological Approaches*. New York, Hemisphere, 1987, pp 237–259.
3. Hart G: *Sexual Maladjustment and Disease: An Introduction to Modern Venereology*. Chicago, Nelson-Hall, 1977.
4. Eysenck HJ, Eysenck SBG: *Manual of the EPI*. London, London University Press, 1964.
5. Wells BWP, Schofield CBS: Personality characteristics of homosexual men suffering from sexually transmitted diseases. *Br J Vener Dis* 48:75–78, 1972.
6. Fulford KWM, Catterall RD, Hoinville E, et al: Social and psychological factors in the distribution of STD in male clinic attenders. II. Personality disorders, psychiatric illness and abnormal sexual attitudes. *Br J Vener Dis* 59:381–385, 1983.
7. Catalan J, Bradley M, Gallwey J, et al: Sexual dysfunction and psychiatric morbidity in patients attending a clinic for sexually transmitted diseases. *Br J Psychiatry* 138:292–296, 1981.
8. Fitzpatrick R, Frost D, Ikkos G: Survey of psychological disturbance in patients attending a sexually transmitted diseases clinic. *Genitourinary Med* 62:111–115, 1986.
9. Ross MW: Psychosocial factors in admitting to homosexuality in sexually transmitted disease clinics. *Sexually Transm Dis* 12:83–86, 1985.
10. Hooker E: Male homosexual lifestyles and venereal disease, in *Proceedings of the World Forum on Syphilis and Other Trepanemotoses*. Public Health Service Publication 977. Washington DC, USGPO, 1964.
11. Oriel JD: The global pattern of sexually transmitted diseases. *South Afr Med J* 61:993–998, 1982.
12. Morton RS: *Venereal Diseases*. Harmondsworth, Middlesex, Penguin, 1966.
13. Fluker JL: The perils of promiscuity. *J Psychosomat Res* 27:153–156, 1983.
14. Hart G: Factors influencing venereal infection in a war environment. *Br J Vener Dis* 50:68–72, 1974.
15. Ross MW: Sexually transmitted diseases in homosexual men: A study of four societies. *Br J Vener Dis* 60:52–55, 1984.
16. Ross MW: Sociological and psychological predictors of STD infection in homosexual men. *Br J Vener Dis* 60:110–113, 1984.
17. Armytage WHG: Changing incidence and patterns of sexually transmitted diseases, in *Proceedings of the Fifteenth Annual Symposium of the Eugenics Society*, 1980, pp 159–170.
18. Hart G: Social and psychological aspects of venereal disease in Papua New Guinea. *Br J Vener Dis* 50:453–458, 1974.
19. Kelus J: Social and behavioural aspects of venereal disease. *Br J Vener Dis* 49:167–170, 1973.
20. Ross MW. *Psychovenereology: Personality and Lifestyle Factors in Sexually Transmitted Diseases in Homosexual Men*. New York, Praeger, 1986.
21. Eysenck HJ: *Sex and Personality*. London, Abacus, 1978.
22. Hart G: Psychological aspects of venereal disease in a war environment. *Soc Sci Med* 7:455–467, 1973.
23. Wells BWP: Personality characteristics of VD patients. *Br J Soc Clin Psychol* 8:246–252, 1969.
24. Fulford KWM, Catterall RD, Hoinville E, et al: Social and psychological factors in the distribution of STD in male clinic attenders. I. Demographic and social factors. *Br J Vener Dis* 59:376–380, 1983.
25. Schofield M: *Promiscuity*. London, Victor Gollancz, 1976.
26. Goode E, Troiden RR: Correlates and accompaniments of promiscuous sex among male homosexuals. *Psychiatry* 43:51–59, 1980.
27. McKusick L, Coates TJ, Wiley JA, et al: Prevention of HIV infection among gay and bisexual men: Two longitudinal studies. in *Second International Conference on AIDS*. Washington DC, USGPO, 1987, p 213.
28. Haist M, Hewitt J: The Butch–fem dichotomy in male homosexual behavior. *J Sex Res* 10:68–75, 1974.
29. Humphreys RAL: *Tearoom Trade: A Study of Impersonal Sex in Public Places*. London, Duckworth, 1970.
30. Cass VC: Homosexual identity formation: A theoretical model. *J Homosex* 4:219–235, 1979.
31. Ross MW: AIDS phobias: A report of four cases. *Psychopathology* 21:26–30, 1988.
32. Ross MW: *The Married Homosexual Man: A Psychological Study*. London, Routledge & Kegan Paul, 1983.
33. Ross MW: Heterosexual marriage of homosexual males: Some associated factors. *J Sex Marital Ther* 5:142–151, 1979.
34. Kübler-Ross E: *On Death and Dying*. London, Tavistock, 1969.
35. Rosser BRS, Ross MW: Emotional and life change impact of AIDS on homosexual men in two countries. *Psychol Health* 2:301–317, 1988.

36. Ross MW, Tebble WEM, Viliunas D: Staging of reactions to AIDS virus infection in asymptomatic homosexual men. *J Psychol Hum Sex* 2:93–104, 1989.
37. Miller F, Weiden P, Sacks M, et al: Two cases of factitious Acquired Immune Deficiency Syndrome. *Am J Psychiatry* 143:1483, 1986.
38. Robinson EN, Latham RH: A factitious case of Acquired Immune Deficiency Syndrome. *Sex Transm Dis* 14:54–57, 1987.
39. Ross MW: Illness behavior among patients attending a sexually transmitted disease clinic. *Sex Transm Dis* 14:174–179, 1987.
40. MacDonald AP, Games RG: Some characteristics of those who hold positive and negative attitudes toward homosexuals. *J Homosexual* 1:9–27, 1974.

II

Prevention

HIV Risk Reduction

3

Educational Strategies for Prevention of Sexual Transmission of HIV

ROBB W. JOHNSON, DAVID G. OSTROW, and JILL JOSEPH

INTRODUCTION

During the past few years, an impressive array of educational materials and programs have been produced with the aim of preventing further spread of human immunodeficiency virus (HIV) infection. However, due to the immediacy and gravity of the epidemic threat, many educational interventions have been initiated without adequate attention to their likely specific impact and without proper means of evaluating their effectiveness. This type of response may be justified by legitimate immediate concern with human life and suffering. However, it is imperative that preventive educational programs be carefully assessed for their actual impact on HIV transmission, as well as more proximate effects on knowledge, attitudes, or specific behavior.

The purpose of this chapter is to provide both the theoretical and practical bases for the development of educational programs designed to prevent further HIV transmission. As the various factors that combine to determine health behavior are discussed, it will become clear that acquired immune deficiency syndrome (AIDS) education programs neglect numerous crucial issues if they focus solely on correcting knowledge deficiencies.

Next, we outline several important practical considerations in the design, implementation, and evaluation of AIDS education programs. Examples of educational intervention are examined for their relationship to the theory previously discussed and to their known or presumed impacts. Future research directions are also discussed, with particular emphasis on the need for more rigorous evaluation of current and future programs.

ROBB W. JOHNSON • Fenway Community Health Center, Boston, Masachussetts 02115. DAVID G. OSTROW • Midwest AIDS Biobehavioral Research Center, Institute for Social Research, and Department of Psychiatry, University of Michigan School of Medicine, Ann Arbor, Michigan 48109. JILL JOSEPH • Department of Epidemiology, University of Michigan School of Public Health, Ann Arbor, Michigan 48109.

THE HEALTH BELIEF MODEL

Research on the determinants of health behaviors has revealed several unifying principles regarding behavioral decision-making. Recent studies on behavior modification in response to AIDS, thus far primarily conducted among gay men, have supported and added to our understanding of health behavior. A useful model for organizing this knowledge has been termed the *health belief model.* This model focuses on behaviors under an individual's control and presumes that people act in order to maximize net benefits of their actions. In making health decisions, individuals consider both health-related and non-health-related (e.g., social or economic) consequences of their actions. Concern with the immediate or short-term benefits of certain behaviors may lead people to disregard the negative long-term consequences of those behaviors.[1,2] For example, an individual's concern about possible sexual transmission of HIV may be obscured by immediate needs for sexual release, social approval from a romantic partner, or money received for prostitution.

According to the health belief model, a number of factors operate to either promote or retard desired behavior change:

- Knowledge of health risks and health-promoting behaviors
- Perception of oneself as being at risk and relating risk to one's actions
- Perceived effectiveness of behavior change and response efficacy
- Belief in the power of technological cures or preventions (e.g., faith that a vaccine to prevent HIV infection will soon be discovered)
- Sociodemographic variables
- Social network affiliation and group norms

The model places strong emphasis on cognitive processes in behavioral change. Prospective studies of cohorts of gay men at risk of AIDS and HIV infection have validated the relevance of the health belief model of behavioral change to the sexual transmission of HIV and have also identified more effective components significantly related to risk reduction efforts in this group, including

- Personality factors and the presence of certain cognitive cues
- Perceived ability to control sexual impulses
- Alcohol or drug use

Research on each of these factors as it relates to health-promoting behavior change is discussed here, as both research findings and resulting theory are certain to have important implications for the design and evaluation of preventive education interventions.

Knowledge

Knowledge of what constitutes risk is obviously an essential prerequisite to voluntary health-promoting behavior change. Knowledge about AIDS has been seen to play a role in motivating initial behavioral change, particularly in persons who see themselves as being at relatively low risk and are initially less informed about the disease and the routes of HIV transmission. Knowledge alone, however, does not ensure long-term sexual behavior change.[3–5] A study of the self-reported behaviors of Chicago gay men who were rated to be relatively well informed about AIDS showed that level of knowledge was related to several behavioral outcomes when analyzed cross-sectionally.[3] However, a later longitudinal analysis of the same cohort failed to show any such significant relationships. Furthermore, an analysis of recidivism concluded that, while average change was in the healthy direction, some individuals who initially adopted risk-reducing behaviors later reverted to risky practices in spite of being well informed.[4] A similar lack of predictive value has been reported regarding the relationship of knowledge levels to contraceptive use[6] and teenage pregnancy incidence.[7] Education that aims solely to increase knowledge would appear to be limited in its ability to induce and maintain alterations in sexual behavior.

Perception of Personal Risk

Perception of personal risk appears to be more important than objective knowledge in motivating behavioral change.[7] It has been noted that individuals tend to underestimate their own vulnerability, operating under an "optimistic bias" regarding their health.[8] Teenagers, for example, may have difficulty applying biological knowledge of sex and pregnancy to their behavior, believing as they characteristically do that "It (pregnancy) won't happen to me."[6] For sexually transmitted diseases, risk perception may be related to individuals' views of their partners. Some gay male participants in the Chicago cohort study expressed confidence that they could, and did, choose safe sexual partners. This study revealed a correlation between level of risk perception and several measures of risk reduction.[3,4]

It is important to note, however, that perception of risk was not shown to be sufficient for predicting behavior change in the Chicago study. Similarly, a nationwide telephone survey revealed that while 45% of adults perceiving themselves to be at risk of genital herpes had modified their behavior in response, risk perception alone was not a good predictor of change. Levels of behavior change were similar in men and women in spite of a significantly higher perception of risk among men.[9]

Perceived Effectiveness of Change and Response Efficacy

Individuals who are knowledgeable of behavioral risks and who feel they are personally at risk must also feel that they are capable of making recommended behavioral changes (response efficacy) and that those changes will actually make a difference for them (perceived effectiveness). It has been recognized that the behaviors important in HIV transmission may be marked by "low changeability" because of their centrality to the self-identity and daily functioning of at-risk individuals.[4,10,11] McKusick and colleagues suggest the possibility that, especially in a high incidence population such as the sexually active San Francisco gay community, individuals who have engaged in high-risk activities over many years may, in the belief that they are either already exposed or immune, see little point to changing their behavior now.[5] The Chicago research group indeed found a relationship between perceived effectiveness of behavior change and some behavior outcomes, except in groups perceiving themselves to be at highest risk.[3] This may suggest that highest-risk individuals recognize behavior change to be an effective means of risk reduction for others but perceive it to be "too late" in their own cases.

Because of the potentially long period of time between infection and development of disease and the lack of proof that life style changes will reduce chances of becoming ill, individuals at very high risk may not believe that behavior alterations will actually make a difference for them. Uncertainty about what impact discovery of positive serostatus may have on behavior contributes to the controversy over the usefulness of widespread HIV antibody testing in preventing AIDS. Some persons are likely to react to a positive test result with an increased sense of futility regarding behavioral risk reduction.[12] This major obstacle to prevention efforts may not be easily overcome until vigorous research efforts pinpoint potential life-style or psychosocial cofactors for disease progression in HIV-infected individuals. Preliminary findings indicate that immune challenge, such as that from repeated exposure to HIV or other infectious agents or from substance abuse, may precipitate disease in HIV-infected individuals.[13,14] Pending further research, these findings might be cited by educators (especially those addressing individuals who have tested antibody positive) to impress upon people the idea that it is never too late to benefit from changed behavior.

Careful attention must also be given to the importance of response efficacy in the design of educational messages. Insistence that celibacy or monogamy are the only appropriate protective responses may provide an example of a lack of attention to this factor in gay men. In addition to being seen as insensitive—coming as it does from a society that provides no support for even the stablest same-sex relationships—this recommendation may well be perceived by a large part of the target audience to be unrealistic.[15] McKusick reports from the San Francisco study of gay men that, although most subjects reported "a desire for more primary partnering in response to AIDS," there was not a significant increase in the number of such relationships over the first two years of the study. The researchers suggest that the complexities of forming and maintaining relationships may be "beyond the immediate scope of public health officials."[15]

Faith in Medical Technology

Because of stunning advances in modern medicine over recent decades, many Americans have come to expect that medicine will be there to take care of whatever health problems arise. Premature or inflated reports of vaccine or chemotherapy breakthroughs may contribute to an unrealistic expectation that a forthcoming cure will make bothersome behavior changes unnecessary.[16] This overconfidence in technological solutions to the control of AIDS and HIV transmission may reflect incorrect knowledge or be a form of denial of individual risk. Indeed, belief that science will provide a cure in the near future was found to be directly correlated with a continuing large number of partners and the persistence of high-risk sexual practices in both the Chicago and San Francisco cohort studies.[3,5]

Sociodemographic Variables

Sociodemographic variables that have been consistently related to various health behaviors include economic status, race, age, and access to health care. In the case of AIDS risk behaviors, geographical differences have been related to the degree of saturation of HIV positivity and likelihood of having a close friend or lover with AIDS. Such direct experience with the condition has been reported by some men to be motivational factors in behavioral change.[5]

Age is another variable likely to influence behaviors related to HIV transmission, though conflicting findings in the research to date indicate that the relationship is complex. Some researchers have found that increased age and years of homosexual activity are related to persistence of high-risk activity. Prior to the recognition of AIDS, this was also demonstrated for gay men at risk of hepatitis B infection[17] and suggests that sexual behavior patterns in this group may become increasingly resistant to change over time. Conversely, the Chicago Multicenter AIDS Cohort Study (MACS) of gay men found younger men to be at greater risk, suggesting that other variables may confound the relationship between age and behavior change. Among heterosexual women, it has been found that effective use of contraception is positively correlated not only with age and sexual experience, but also with involvement in a committed relationship.[18]

Little is known about racial and economic variables related to AIDS risk reduction in homosexual/bisexual men, as the vast majority of cohort study participants to date have been white, middle class, and well educated. Nonetheless, studies of other types of health behavior change have found education and income level to be positively related to the adoption of preventive health behaviors.[19] Certainly a lag in risk-reducing behavior change might be partly explained by lack of access to health care and information or by time and energy devoted to coping with crises more immediate than long-range health outcomes. There may also be other sociocultural factors involved as the few studies that have looked at racial differences in health-related behaviors have suggested the existence of significant differences not entirely explainable on the basis of economic or educational factors.[20] Specific minority issues in AIDS prevention education are discussed under Practical Considerations in this chapter.

Social Network Affiliation and Peer Norms

Social factors have repeatedly been reported to have a significant impact on health behavior. In their study of teenage health behaviors, Duryea and Okwumabua[21] found, in fact, that thoughts reported by teenagers responding to whether or not they would ride to a party with a drunk friend were four times more likely to be social in nature (e.g., "Who will be at the party that I like?") than specifically health related (e.g., "I might get killed"). An additional finding of their study supports other research that has suggested that an established social support network mediates against health-risky behavior.

Social reinforcement is especially important for behavior changes that require cooperation and social interaction.[22] Factors such as availability or desirability of partners, emotional needs for affection and contact, clarity of values, communication skills, and future plans are likely to influence sexual/reproductive health decisions.[23] The salience of social factors is clear when one considers that every sexual risk situation is a social transaction. For complete protection, risk reduction practices must be effectively employed every time there is such a transaction. Thus, the health decision-making process must be repeated over and over again, under varying social and environmental conditions. The Chicago cohort study recently demonstrated a significantly higher seroconversion rate for men using condoms for receptive anal intercourse in multiple partner situations compared to men using them in monogamous relationships.[24] Even in a monogamous relationship, however, chances of a lapse in protective behavior may rise with time, especially if one partner is more committed to risk reduction than the other (and thus bears sole responsibility for boundary setting). It is therefore important that issues of maintenance of safe behavior and risk of recidivism in a social context be addressed in educational interventions, no matter what the audience's apparent level of AIDS awareness may be.

The findings of the Chicago cohort study further suggest a complex relationship between social support, peer norms and behavioral risk reduction.[3,24] While membership in a gay social support network in itself was not predictive of behavioral change, the presence of peer norms supportive of risk reduction was the variable most consistently and positively associated with multiple measures of sexual risk reduction over time, including avoidance of anonymous partners and modification of receptive anal intercourse. These findings suggest that specific elements of peer support for "safer sex" practices need to be addressed in any community-based risk-reduction program. Similar findings are beginning to emerge in studies of intravenous (IV) drug use behaviors, such as those promoting the use of bleach to clean syringes.[25]

Personality Factors and Cognitive Cues

Although not part of the classic "health belief" model, certain personality factors and cognitive responses to external cues may need to be included in a modified health behavior model. Individuals of an oppositional character may view risk-reduction education as a struggle over control of their personal lives and therefore be resistant to change. Those who characteristically respond to anxiety with avoidance behavior as well as those with a strong sense of shame about sexual matters may fail to seek out frank and explicit information needed to institute changes (Gonsiorek JC: personal communication, 1988). Anecdotal reports of HIV infection have described individuals who habitually took sexual risks, and persisted even in the era of AIDS. Instances in which individuals exposed themselves or others in a fit of anger or depression have also been reported.

The study of Duryea and Okwumabua[21] supports the notion that some individuals are habitual risk-takers. They classified ninth graders as either health-risky decision makers or health-promoting decision-makers based on their responses to a drunk driving scenario. The two groups differed significantly on responses regarding various health-related decisions, as well as on degree of reflection when making health decisions. One third of the teens reported that stress (including depression, loneliness, and anger) would affect their decision.

Potentially distressing events or circumstances may be positively related to health promotion, in spite of their probable emotional costs. A study of a cohort of San Francisco gay men found that the ability to remember a "visual image of AIDS deterioration" was positively related to a reduction from many to a few partners per month.[5]

Sexual Impulse Control

Reported level of ability to control sexual impulses has also been found to be related to reduction in number of partners and the modification (via condom use or withdrawal) of anal intercourse.[3,4] Many of those who reported persistence in high-risk sexual behavior stated that the behaviors were too enjoyable for them to stop, even though they were aware of the risks involved.[26] Sexual impulse control is a complex behavioral characteristic which itself may be related to a broad set of biobehavioral factors including personality traits, environment, psychoactive substance use, partnership status, and affect. When individuals are sexually compulsive or "addicted," the immediate gratification or relief of tension resulting from a sexual encounter temporarily overshadows the potential negative consequences.

Alcohol or Drug Use

Behavioral research on AIDS that has considered substance abuse variables reveals a strong positive association between potential HIV-transmitting sexual behaviors and multiple measures of drug abuse, including use of drugs during sex, number of drugs used, and frequency of combining drugs and sex.[27] More than one half of those refraining from alcohol or drug use during sex were likely to have been at no risk of infection over the previous 6 months, while those who used alcohol or another drug even rarely during sex were 2–3½ times as likely as abstainers to be at high risk. Those who increased levels of risky behavior over a 6-month period were more likely to have used drugs, to have used multiple drugs, and to have had a high proportion of sexual encounters involving drugs, while "risk decreasers" were less likely to have done so. Results from the MACS studies have shown that reductions in high-risk sexual activities are significantly less likely if psychoactive substance use continues.[28,29]

These findings are of tremendous importance in helping direct AIDS prevention efforts, especially in light of the relatively high prevalence of alcohol and drug abuse in convenience samples of gay men, and the likelihood that IV drug users frequently have sexual encounters under the influence of drugs. These data reveal that, even in a highly sensitized cohort, some individuals are failing to adopt and maintain safer sex practices and indicate a need to focus more attention on the role of drugs and alcohol in behavioral change. Although the exact nature of the association between substance use and risky sex cannot yet be specified, the strength of the association warrants warnings against combining the two. In small groups or individual education/counseling, it is imperative that the role of substance use in impeding individual risk-reducing behavior change be explicitly explored for all those reporting drug or alcohol use.

The interaction of psychoactive substances and sexual risk-taking is likely to be of a complex nature.[30–32] The disinhibiting effects of alcohol are often cited as a primary factor. Wilson and Lawson[33] found that male college students who described themselves as entirely or primarily heterosexual were more likely to exhibit arousal to explicit homosexual films when they believed they had received enough alcohol to induce intoxication. The researchers speculated that a strong social reinforcer for heavy drinking may be that it provides a valid excuse for otherwise unacceptable behavior.

Factors other than disinhibition are probably important in the association. Zucker and colleagues,[34] in their analysis of a cohort of college women, found that those who had at any time been identified as heavy or heavy-escape drinkers initiated sex at an earlier age, used contraceptives less reliably, and engaged in sex more frequently than did those who had not. The nature of the relationship of alcohol to these behaviors remains unclear but, in this study, alcohol use may merely be indicative of a general *problem behavior syndrome* and thereby represent personal predisposition rather than disinhibition.

Much remains to be elucidated about the relationship of alcohol and drug use to sexual behavior and the ways in which social environment may modulate this relationship. Specific studies should more carefully explore the potentially multiple mechanisms by which substance use impacts behavior. In addition, until cofactors for the expression of HIV infection as disease are elucidated it may be necessary from a medical point of view to stress restraint in the use of drugs and alcohol, particularly for healthy seropositive individuals.

Summary

Each of the factors discussed above has significant implications for counseling and educational programs designed to prevent sexual transmission of HIV. Many of the observations cited were derived from research conducted either on health behaviors unrelated to AIDS or on relatively uniform samples of white gay men. It is possible, however, that similar factors will correlate with behavioral change in heterosexuals and in black and hispanic populations, and that a modified health belief model will serve as a useful heuristic tool in planning preventive interventions. What will differ is the way in which interventions are tailored to each of these populations in order to address those determinants of behavior individually and appropriately. Some of the practical considerations in designing and evaluating these interventions are discussed in the following section.

PRACTICAL CONSIDERATIONS

Setting Objectives

An important first step in any educational programming process is *needs assessment*. Many programs are misdirected because educators assume they understand what the audience does and does not know. It is particularly important in AIDS education that a baseline assessment be made both of knowledge and of what members of the target population feel they need in order to convert knowledge into action. This should be accompanied by an objective assessment of conscious and unconscious barriers to change. Educational objectives should then be set according to what is needed to increase the adoption and maintenance of risk-reducing behavior. An education program that produces AIDS experts but not behavioral risk reduction misses the point entirely.

Unfortunately, the primary goal of risk reduction, which is to interrupt the transmission of HIV, often becomes confounded by competing moralistic goals of the educating institutions. Such moralistic goals may include the elimination of IV drug use or same sex behavior, or the promotion of abstinence and monogamy (Gonsiorek JC: personal communication, 1988). It is generally advisable to focus on a limited set of behavioral changes that are perceived by target population members to be feasible, rather than confronting them with a broad-based health/moral agenda that is dehumanizing and that reduces response efficacy (the feeling that one is capable of adopting recommended behavior changes).

It is well recognized in health education that no single program is capable of targeting all identifiable needs of a population or likely to result in complete, persistent behavior change. For this reason, a combination of interventions, including the fostering of broad support in the target community, is likely to be most effective.

The Settings of the Intervention

Small Groups

While large lecture-type educational sessions may be efficient in addressing knowledge deficiencies, small group interventions provide better opportunities for addressing the unique concerns of individuals and the social aspects of health behavior such as the development of supportive networks and peer norms. Innovative small group interventions among gay men have included safer sex workshop "parties" in private homes, weekend workshops, and multisession groups meeting over a period of weeks. Similar group interventions have been initiated in drug treatment centers and in prison populations.[35] Researchers have demonstrated positive changes in attitudes regarding discussing condom use with partners and perceived peer acceptance of risk-reduction measures in gay men who participated in small group AIDS/safer sex education sessions.[36] Examples of specific educational activities conducted in these groups are discussed in the next section.

The dynamics of small group sessions will vary according to where they are conducted. Communication may be more honest, for example, in a group formed from individuals who did not previously know each other. On the other hand, the sensitive and personal nature of risk-reduction education may make some individuals uneasy about joining any group in which they do not know and trust everyone. Home parties, which use informal friendship circles to bring people together, have been used with success by community-based organizations such as the Houston KS/AIDS Foundation to reach gay men reluctant to participate in more open forums.[37]

Integrating AIDS Education into Social Settings

Additional barriers may keep individuals from joining in small group educational activities, including denial of risk behavior or of susceptibility to disease. Educators in the gay community have attempted to reach the less motivated segment of this population by educating in locations such as bars and bathhouses. These are common settings for both social and sexual contact and frequently provide tentative links to the community for closeted gays or those just coming out. In these relatively nonthreatening settings, at-risk individuals who may be less likely to seek out educational materials or attend formalized programs can receive vital preventive information. In addition, researchers at Gay Men's Health Crisis in New York have found that bar and bath program participants have tended to represent a wider range of racial, economic, and educational backgrounds than has been seen in other group interventions.[35]

Educational activities may have to be adapted for the informal atmosphere of bars and baths. Videos, informal discussions, and question-and-answer sessions may be more appropriate than the more structured activities possible in formal groups. Evaluation is also problematic in social settings. Innovative approaches to the evaluation of bathhouse or bar AIDS educational programs have included the use of "coupons" for acceptance into some structured ongoing programs, and measuring changes in condom sales or rectal gonorrhea incidence. It should be pointed out, however, that bar and particularly bathhouse owners may feel that AIDS prevention education programs are antithetical to their business interests and may not readily cooperate in the mounting of extensive educational programs on their premises. In addition, efforts to close bathhouses in several major U.S. cities, such as San Francisco and New York, have resulted in antagonistic relationships between public health officials and bathhouse owners and their clients, as detailed in Randy Shilts's book, *And the Band Played On.*[38]

Social-setting interventions in heterosexual communities have yet to be reported extensively in the literature. Where they have occurred, they have tended to focus on heterosexual women. In the Boston area, for example, the home party format has been utilized with women to disseminate safe sex information and offer a chance to discuss AIDS-related concerns.

Differences in risk perception are likely to create significant resistance to educators' efforts among owners and patrons of "singles" bars or other establishments popular for heterosexual socializing and sexual contact. In fact, precisely because there is strong denial in the community, there may be benefits to educating in these settings. Further efforts should be devoted to creating educational formats suitable for this audience and type of setting (including entertaining and informative videos) and to advocating their implementation.

The value of integrating AIDS information and discussion into diverse social and educational activities is stressed by educators at the Hetrick–Martin Institute for the Protection of Lesbian and Gay Youth (IPLGY) in New York.[39] It was found that early programs focusing on AIDS or safer sex (and so advertised) were poorly attended. It may be that denial or lack of motivation to learn about an unpleasant subject contributed to keeping youths away.[40] IPLGY educators believe, however, that the integration of AIDS education into other activities has important benefits above and beyond increasing attendance. One regular social activity at the Institute is the examination of film portrayals of gay life-styles. Educators have used the screening of the film, *Boys in the Band* for example, as a springboard for discussing gay stereotypes and the real prevalence of depression and maladaptive sexual or substance abuse behaviors in the gay community. Questions regarding the risks of such behaviors and possible risk-reducing adaptations are easily incorporated into such a discussion, and are lent a strong "real life" impact by the situations portrayed in the film.[39] Such an integrated approach addresses the fundamentally social nature of risk behavior more thoroughly than do isolated AIDS education sessions. A similar integrated approach would be valuable in all prevention programs, but especially so for school or youth audiences for whom socialization issues are likely to be prominent.

Individualized Education

Education/counseling on a confidential one-to-one basis offers a special opportunity to tailor communication to the individual's needs. Although skill and sensitivity is required in getting clients to discuss their full range of behavioral risk, this makes it possible for counselor and client to discuss specific problems in risk reduction and their possible solutions. A problem-solving approach that targets goals identified by the client and works toward behavioral changes the client feels are attainable may be more effective than group interventions in which concerns are addressed generally. This is particularly true if periodic follow-up contact is part of the intervention. Counseling should include an effort to help clients identify barriers to change or specific vulnerabilities to unsafe behavior, such as particular sexual partners, particular mood states, or particular social situations (Gonsiorek JC: personal communication, 1988).

Education in settings such as sexually transmitted disease (STD) clinics, pregnancy/contraception clinics, drug treatment centers or the offices of physicians or therapists may have an enhanced effect because of the increased sense of susceptibility that accompanies treatment or diagnosis, especially if the condition is one directly related to risk behavior (Chapter 2, this volume). It has also been suggested that advice in a medical setting carries for some people the weight of a medical prescription, increasing its impact. However, the commonly held assumption that medical "authorities" are judgmental concerning homosexuality and other forms of nontraditional sexual behavior can have a negative impact on the effectiveness of counseling given in a medical setting.[41]

Education in Conjunction with HIV Antibody Testing

For the above reasons, and also because people presenting for voluntary testing tend to be highly motivated and focused on the issue of their AIDS risk, the HIV antibody testing site is often viewed as an ideal site for AIDS education. Retention of information may be compromised, however, by anxiety, agitation, anger, or other emotions that often accompany testing. Attention must always be paid to how much information an individual can process at one time. Pamphlets or brief videos (which could be replayed at will) explaining the significance of the test and the meaning of results may be useful tools for the waiting room.

For those who are seropositive, it may be important to first focus on surviving immediate stresses. Since sex is often the last thing on the mind of such individuals at the time of receiving their results, a talk about risk reduction for future sexual activity may be more useful at a later time.[42] Thus, a one-time session with a test site counselor, without follow-up, may be less effective than an ongoing intervention. Referral to acceptable and accessible support and information sources becomes especially critical in situations in which follow-up by test site personnel is not possible.

Notification of the contacts of those known to be infected, with an attendant offer of education and testing, is seen by some as an important educational intervention. In describing the rationale behind notification of female contacts in San Francisco, Echenberg explains that mass education is efficient and effective for a population with a high prevalence of infection because the population members are likely to have a base level of awareness about their risk that encourages them to attend to AIDS-related messages.[43] For a relatively low-prevalence population such as sexually exposed women in San Francisco, however, attention to mass education messages may be low because of minimal risk perception; furthermore, the number of such women are still low enough to reach individually. Although no treatment is available for referred contacts (as is the case with other diseases for which tracing is employed), the opportunity afforded to provide education to individuals who do not perceive themselves to be at risk is believed by proponents to justify contact procedures. Requisites outlined by Echenberg for such a program include confidentiality for the index case, sensitive case counselors, voluntary participation in listing contacts and in receiving the intervention, and strict legal safeguards against subpoena of information. Even when such safeguards are "guaranteed," however, contact notification as an educational intervention remains controversial.

The Minnesota Department of Health has developed a series of interventions that include efforts to communicate with contact of infected or high-risk individuals (Gonsiorek JC: personal communication, 1988). The programs were developed in late 1986 and 1987 and have yet to be evaluated for their impact on HIV transmission. The first of these services, Partner Outreach Services (POS), is offered to all seropositive individuals. They are told of the free and confidential service at the time their blood is drawn and are immediately referred to a POS mental health professional after receiving their positive result. The goal of POS is to assist clients in informing their own contacts of their seropositive status; clients may choose to remain anonymous. Counselors assist clients in making decisions about who they wish to contact and making specific action plans for telling them. In the experience of the Department, clients are initially focused on medical concerns. Only after these and broader psychosocial concerns have been addressed are most amenable to partner outreach efforts. It has not been unusual for a number of sessions to be required before clients are ready for partner outreach discussions.

The Department also offers contact notification services for seropositive clients who do not wish to inform their partners themselves. Such clients may remain anonymous, though their contacts obviously do not. Clients give a list of contacts to a health department staff member, who subsequently contacts them by telephone only with the request that they meet with a staff member to receive important health information. No specifics are given over the phone. Contact lists are confidential, are protected by statute from subpoena, and are destroyed after 6 months.

Another program recently developed at the Minnesota Department of Health is Behavior Based Counseling and Outreach Services (BBCOS). For this program, any untested or known seronegative individual with a history of unsafe sex or needle use activity within the last year may participate. The program's goals are to help clients increase their repertoire of noninsertive sexual behaviors, and to engage in sexual behavior only when not under the influence of alcohol or drugs. Clients are also encouraged to refer partners with whom they have had previous unsafe behavior. BBCOS clients participate in a five- to six-session small group educational program in which preventive information is shared in an atmosphere providing support and feedback. Individual counseling sessions are held concurrently to help clients decide treatment goals and identify psychosocial issues that play a role in unsafe behavior. Follow-up to ascertain progress occurs at 1, 3, 6, and 12 months, and clients are encouraged to return whenever they have an unsafe experience or come close to having one.

Role of the Media

Surveys of AIDS knowledge and attitudes in diverse populations have revealed that radio and television have been the major sources of AIDS information for most people. Magazines and newspapers were generally the next most common source.[45,46] It is apparent from gaps in reported knowledge and the persistence of misconceptions, however, that the media may not have been used as effectively as it might be. AIDS information has emerged in fragmented, often conflicting news headlines over the years. Seldom have there been comprehensive educational presentations in the media and, until very recently, public service announcements have been virtually nonexistent in the United States, in contrast to the vigorous official responses of some other countries with fewer AIDS cases. Osborn has contrasted the marked absence of AIDS informational advertising to the omnipresent promotional campaigns for the armed services, deploring the government's relative silence on the epidemic.[46]

Meanwhile, media dramas only rarely deal with themes of AIDS risks, while the portrayal of sex without complications continues relatively unabated. This is particularly unfortunate because the potential of entertainment programs to portray health-promoting models and influence norms is large. Recently there have been encouraging signs of responsibility among the producers of some programs, as more characters are mentioning concern about sexually transmitted disease and condom use. In order to build and expand upon current educational efforts, both entertainment and news media representatives need to be targeted for education themselves, preferably well in advance of their treatment of any AIDS-related theme.

Where the media has been purposefully employed as an educational tool, mixed results have been obtained. Although mass media was judged to be effective in drawing attention to problems with cholesterol and intrauterine devices, for example, initial publicity about the 1964 Surgeon General's report on smoking appeared to have minimal effects on behavior.[47] It has been suggested that the media is most effective in changing health behaviors when substitutes are readily available, when health messages support prior inclinations, or when social support exists for the recommended change.[48] It is likely that the media alone will not be enough to change risk behaviors for AIDS, but it may be an important adjunct to other interventions.

Experience from the 1986 AIDS educational campaign in the United Kingdom highlights the importance of determining clear objectives and evaluating attainment of them. After a mass awareness campaign in the print media, it was observed that the general level of concern was raised in both high and low-risk individuals. People reported they felt they needed more information, and wanted to turn to the medical profession for answers. While some knowledge gaps were filled, there was no change in reports of several misconceptions. In addition, it was found that there were problems with the readability of the initial set of ads; changes were later made accordingly.[49] Careful consideration must be given to the objectives, to the likely public response, to the context of existing knowledge into which the information will be received, and to the resources available for handling the information and clarification needs that result from any mass campaign.

For programs or public service announcements to be optimally effective, they should be slotted for times in which members of the specific target population are most likely to be watching. For example, Ginzburg suggests that afternoon and late night slots may be best for reaching the majority of IV drug users, since traditional prime time is also prime time for drug transactions and therefore this audience may not be available during evening hours.[49]

Tailoring Interventions to Target Audiences

From the beginning, a problem in AIDS education has been getting people to accept the messages as being relevant to *them*. In many cases, messages have been couched in language or values that had little meaning for those who needed the information most. Since no single message will be able to address the complex determinants of health behavior for diverse populations, efforts must be made to individualize messages as much as possible. Principles of market research may be employed (as well as professional market researchers) to help clarify the true needs of target populations and their preferred modes of learning. Calling together focus groups of target population members in order to get their input in the early stages of program design is one useful strategy. Assumptions should never be made about what target audiences do or do not know, nor should they be made about their likelihood to respond to specific intervention styles.

Appropriate Language and Literacy Requirements

Once a target population for a program or specific material is determined, an assessment of that population's language, typical reading level, and terminology preferences must be made. Focus groups drawn from the target population will be valuable for their input in the drafting and evaluation of materials, although their representativeness of the target population must be considered. An effort should be made to design materials so as to exclude as few target population members as possible. When literacy may be an issue, for example, information should be conveyed pictorially wherever possible. Television and video may provide the most effective means for reaching illiterate or marginally literate individuals.

Where bilingual materials are developed in tandem, problems often arise from literal translation. Ideally, materials for Spanish and English speakers should be developed separately, each "from the ground up." Anglo educators must further avoid any tendency to lump all the members of any racial or cultural minority into one group, assuming they have similar language or information preferences. For example, the needs of Spanish speaking Cubans, Puerto Ricans, and Central Americans may be very dissimilar.

Credible Educators

Research in health education supports the commonly held belief that effectiveness of the message increases with similarity and trust between educator and target.[50,51] Those who are culturally sensitive, and therefore able to frame messages in meaningful language and a realistic social context, are most likely to make an impression on people. Thus, a current or former IV drug user who tells other users that it is both desirable and possible to stop sharing unclean needles will be vastly more convincing than the local health department professional educator. Some programs have been successful in training indigenous health workers, themselves former drug users, to provide educational outreach in high-risk areas.[49] Similarly, outreach education for gay and bisexual men by members of their own population are seen to be most effective in meaningfully addressing specific behaviors and issues of concern. Both populations, which are defined in part by the social stigma and illegality of behaviors in which their members take part, may be resistant to educators whom they perceive to be part of the mainstream society that has labeled them deviant. By the same token, educators from these populations may have difficulty in responding to the distinct issues faced by "mainstream" heterosexuals trying to reduce risk. Thus, if heterosexual audiences perceived an educator to be gay or lesbian, his or her credibility as a source of relevant information could suffer.

The reality of limited educational staffs in most organizations often means that educators have little choice but to try to be all things to all people. Arguably, some information from the wrong person is better than the right information from no one. Nevertheless, a broad commitment should be made by administrators to recruit educators credible within their organization's primary target audiences and to assign job responsibilities accordingly. In addition, efforts to mobilize members of at-risk communities to educate their peers can play an important role in spreading prevention information. To paraphrase Dr. Harvey Feldman of San Francisco's Mid-City Consortium to Combat AIDS, a pioneer in ethnographically-based education efforts for IV drug users, "It's easier to teach AIDS to street-wise ex-addicts than to teach jive to AIDS-wise persons with little or no street experience."

Considerations for Specific Targets

Homosexually Active Men Not Identifying Themselves as Gay or Bisexual. Since many men who have sex with other men do not define themselves as gay or bisexual, educational messages that focus on group labels rather than on specific behaviors may be disregarded by large numbers of persons at risk. Because labeling oneself as gay or bisexual may seem more threatening than engaging in same-sex sexual activity, such individuals may fail to apply those labels to themselves. While they are not available for study through voluntary research or testing programs, a suggestion of the importance of reaching at-risk men who do not see themselves as such is provided by the results of blood donation screening programs. When detailed epidemiological investigations have been possible there, a majority of persons found to be HIV antibody positive have turned out to have behavioral risk factors, even though they initially denied membership in an "AIDS high-risk group." These individuals can only be accessed for education as part of the "general population" target group. This is just one reason why it is essential to not make assumptions about the sexual orientation of a general audience and to speak frankly about the specific *behaviors* that put one at risk.

Heterosexuals. Early emphasis on a limited number of "risk groups" created the idea in the minds of those outside of these groups that AIDS was an affliction with which they need not be concerned. To many, AIDS seemed to be an epidemic of degenerates, remote from themselves. Persistence of this attitude is evidenced in the fact that most heterosexuals tend to interpret sexual information in education materials as pertaining only to people in "high-risk groups" and not to themselves.[52] Public doubt and confusion about risks to heterosexuals has, unfortunately, not been abated by conflicting reports and persistent controversy over the likelihood of HIV spreading into the "general population." There is no debate about whether heterosexuals are vulnerable to sexual transmission of HIV. Airing the debate over just how many are likely to be affected by the epidemic serves little educational purpose for individual at-risk heterosexuals. Rather than focusing on trends in the population, people should be encouraged to concentrate on their responsibility for risk reduction in their own lives. Many who deny or fail to perceive their sexual risk tend to focus on information regarding casual transmission. This displaces AIDS anxiety from internal issues which the individual may not be ready to confront to external circumstances for which others can be held accountable. For pamphlets and other materials to be effective, they must begin with a clear statement that it is sexual contact and needle use, not casual contact, that poses risk for heterosexuals.

Education aimed at heterosexually active persons will necessarily include not only cautions on the risks in vaginal intercourse, but also frank discussion of the risks in the full range of sexual activities, including anal intercourse and oral sex. Researchers have reported that as many as 10% of women may regularly practice receptive anal intercourse, albeit less frequently and with fewer partners on the average than gay men.[53] This is the most risky sexual activity for transmission of HIV, and there is as much (if not more) stigma attached to it for heterosexuals as for male homosexuals; therefore, it is extremely important that health professionals and educators adopt an equally thorough and nonjudgmental interviewing approach when making risk assessments for, and educating, both groups.

It is often suggested that, because the prevalence of HIV infection is currently low in the "general population," non-needle-using heterosexuals can be protected if educated to abstain from sex until a mutually monogamous relationship can be established. Although a comprehensive study of the adoption of monogamy among heterosexuals in response to AIDS has yet to be reported, results from such studies in gay men (who can be expected to be more highly motivated than U.S. heterosexuals to change because of the relatively high prevalence of AIDS in their population) remind us that the complete elimination of previously enjoyed behavior is not a simple matter. In a study evaluating the adoption of a range of changes believed to reduce risk in gay men, the adoption of monogamy was the least frequent behavioral change.[54]

Heterosexuals might expect to find more support in society for a move toward monogamy, but unless it is fully and mutually adopted, monogamy provides incomplete protection. All sexually active individuals must realize that, when mutual monogamy with uninfected individuals is not guaranteed, modification of sexual behavior to reduce risks is essential. Since we cannot afford to depend on full adoption of monogamy by all, heterosexuals, too, will require realistic and rational "safer sex" education in all its complexity.

An issue of growing significance for the education of heterosexuals is the role of HIV antibody testing in making decisions about sexual partners and activities. In general there is less resistance to testing among heterosexuals, as fewer of them are concerned about discrimination issues. In addition, fewer of them are likely to forego testing and alter their behavior under the assumption that they are already infected. It therefore appears that heterosexuals are more likely to consider HIV antibody testing as an appropriate way to proceed in a new relationship. Indeed, the emergence of antibody negative dating services for heterosexuals is evidence of growing interest in this approach. The proliferation of "AIDS Free" clubs using frequent and expensive antibody testing with promotion of sexual coupling among members, illustrates the strong desire of sexually active heterosexuals to find ways to protect themselves from AIDS without having to limit their sexual repertoires. It is essential that educators fully address with all sexually active audiences limitations of the test and the dangers of misinterpreting the results. Negative test status may give a false sense of security to those who fail to realize that exposure may have occurred in the months immediately preceding the test, and that infection could occur at any time in the future if one partner has unprotected sex with an infected individual.

People of Color. A disproportionate number of AIDS cases are seen among black and hispanic individuals. Through 1988, 70% of women and children with AIDS in the United States had been black or hispanic. The majority of these cases are related to IV drug use, either from direct needle use, from sexual contact with an IV drug user, or perinatal exposure from a mother infected in these ways. Black IV drug users may be at higher risk than are their white counterparts, as there are indications that blacks inject drugs and share needles more often than drug-using whites.[55] Cultural factors may make sharing of needles more accepted and expected among minority IV drug users, although it is also possible that new or sterile works are simply more readily available to whites.[56]

Blacks and hispanics have also tended to have worse prognoses and shorter survival after diagnosis than whites. In large measure, this difference may result from the high number of IV drug users (whose health status is likely to be poor) represented in the minority PWA population. However, other host and environmental factors may also be involved. Minority individuals with AIDS may have worse health status prior to infection and more frequent exposures to infectious agents. Alternatively, shorter survival periods may reflect poor access to care and relatively late diagnosis. More people of color than whites are faced with a lack of appropriate and sensitive providers, poor distribution of health services, and inadequate insurance. In addition, they themselves may have varying perceptions of the severity of illness and different cultural norms about help-seeking behavior.[57]

It is possible that blacks and hispanics are also at higher risk than whites due to differences in sexual behavior. There may, for example, be cultural differences in sex roles or other norms that influence communication and assertiveness in sexual relationships. Black youth tend to be more sexually active than their white counterparts, and to initiate sexual intercourse an average of two years earlier.[58] Some studies have revealed racial and ethnic differences in contraceptive behavior.[59]

Among males with AIDS whose risk factor was sexual contact, a significantly greater proportion of blacks and hispanics identified themselves as bisexual than did whites.[56] This has important ramifications for secondary transmission to women as well as for educational interventions. Homosexually active men not identifying themselves as homosexuals may be less inclined to consider themselves to be in a "risk group" and to seek out education offered for or by gay men. Even minority men who consider themselves gay may have weaker ties to an identifiable gay community than do many whites, making them more difficult to reach through predominantly white gay community organizations.

Discrepancies between whites and people of color in access to care have been paralleled by discrepancies in access to AIDS prevention interventions. Early education programs sponsored by the gay white community and later programs started by white-dominated public agencies were usually ill equipped and often disinclined to intervene appropriately in minority communities. In addition, the absence of significant numbers of minorities in research studies on AIDS knowledge, attitudes, and behavioral change has made it difficult to draw conclusions about what racial or ethnic differences might exist in the determinants of risk behavior and correspondingly appropriate educational interventions. There is presently an urgent need for more equitable involvement of minorities in both research and in those agencies which deliver AIDS health care and educational services. Traditional methods of service delivery may well prove inadequate. For services to be most effective, community members should collaborate on planning and assume leadership roles in implementing resulting programs.[60]

As the caseload in minority communities becomes conspicuously higher and the myth that AIDS is a disease of white gay males is debunked, the level of AIDS anxiety in these communities is likely to increase. The initial reaction of many in the black community, including community leaders, has often been to deny the extent of its present and probably future impact. Many have attempted to distance themselves from the epidemic because of the stigma attached to its most common modes of transmission. Historically, gay activism has been muted in minority communities, and homosexuality has been less visible and less accepted in them. Meanwhile, many are uncomfortable with the reinforcement of negative stereotypes resulting from the high percentage of minorities among IV drug use cases. Interwoven with this discomfort may be a fear of discrimination that may be imminent if race and ethnicity become any more closely associated with the AIDS epidemic.

In order to create truly effective educational interventions for minority communities, it is necessary that denial and distancing behaviors be overcome in order to mobilize community members at all levels. Broad-based community awareness and organizing efforts such as those seen in the gay community may be necessary. The creation of minority AIDS task forces in various parts of the country demonstrates that advocacy, networking, and educational efforts have begun. This community-based movement must continue and expand, utilizing indigenous educators and informal communication networks to challenge those who persist in risk behaviors. Churches, which have in the past played an important role in minority social movements, must come to terms with the value conflicts engendered by this epidemic and use their influence to help mobilize and educate their membership.[60]

Intravenous Drug Users. This chapter does not address specifics of education to promote needle-using behavior change. Needle users must also be targeted, however, for education regarding sexual risks. Some researchers have reported that awareness of sexual risks may be low among IV drug users, and that some users are under the misconception that an infection acquired through needle use is only passed on through needle use. Other evidence suggests that perception of heterosexual transmission risks, especially from female to male, may be limited in the general population. Overcoming such misconceptions is particularly urgent in this population, with its high prevalence of HIV infection. Seroprevalence studies of men and women entering detoxification centers in New York City showed that similar proportions (over 60%) of each were infected.[61] In a separate study, only 3% of heroin-addicted women in drug treatment programs reported asking their partners to use condoms.[62] Such findings highlight the urgent need for more proactive distribution of explicit information about sex and pregnancy risks to the IV drug-using population and their partners. In addition, it must be stressed that infectivity cannot be determined by appearance and that, under conditions of high seroprevalence, it is safest to presume that all intravenous drug-using sexual partners are infected.

Substance abuse treatment programs are settings in which AIDS education should be encouraged for several reasons, including the previously described association between substance use and high-risk sexual activity and the extremely high risk of HIV infection among IV drug users. However, substance abuse facilities also present special problems regarding acceptance of AIDS education by staff, potential disruption of the treatment milieu, and confidentiality if HIV antibody testing is performed. An additional barrier to effective AIDS prevention education in substance abuse treatment is the frequent absence, especially in nonurban communities, of appropriate peer role models for homosexual men or women in programs that rely heavily on peer role modeling, such as Alcoholics or Narcotics Anonymous.[32] Despite the obstacles, the high likelihood that participants in substance abuse treatment programs will be at increased risk for HIV transmission makes incorporation of preventive education and counseling into all such programs imperative.

One approach has been to set up programs within substance abuse treatment programs that use peer counselors, including homosexually identified staff, as contact persons. Alternatively, local gay community-based AIDS education organizations can be contracted to provide counseling within the facility. Recently established substance abuse programs specifically intended for lesbians and gay men, such as those offered by Pride Foundation in Minneapolis, enable a single staff to provide integrated substance abuse and risk-reduction counseling.

Youth. Young people are recognized to be at higher risk of AIDS because of their particularly strong sense of invulnerability, their tendency to experiment with sex and drugs, and the possibility that they have been sheltered from adult sources of information. The long incubation period in HIV-related disease means that they very rarely see apparent infections in their peers, which may contribute to their inaccurate perception of freedom from risk. The especially powerful role of social factors such as support networks and perceived peer norms in teens' lives must be taken into account in planning interventions. Gay or drug using young people may be at elevated risk because of being isolated from mainstream society while not yet integrated into a subculture society. Through agencies such as IPLGY, educators can attempt to overcome the "self fulfilling negativism" of such isolated youth by integrating them into supportive, nonsexual social networks and providing positive models of healthy, loving relationships.[39] The provision of supportive nonthreatening socializing opportunities may in itself help build social skills, norms, and networks that reduce the prevalence of risk behaviors.

With youth, educators have a unique opportunity to prevent risk behaviors before they are formed or fully entrenched.[39] Young people's risk is only increased by withholding complete prevention information from them. Those who would prohibit discussion of protective behaviors other than abstinence need to acknowledge that many youths will become, or are already, sexually active. As a society we can either deny this reality or, more responsibly, educate for responsible sexuality as completely as possible. Hoping that young people will abstain until meeting another virgin with whom they will remain mutually monogamous for life may not be realistic in most instances. The need for explicit education for teens is brought into clear focus by a survey of behavioral changes in Massachusetts teens in response to AIDS; 35% of the teens stated they were protecting themselves by "being more selective in partner choice." An even more ambiguous response, "being careful," was reported by 25% of the teens. Only 10% said they were using condoms, while another 10% reported that they now abstain from sex altogether.[63] To encourage health-protective behavior in young people, frank sex and AIDS education programs are needed both in the schools and on the streets. Anything less than complete and explicit education wastes precious time and money in the fight against the epidemic of HIV infection.

Clarity, Simplicity, and Specificity of Messages

As public concern about the HIV epidemic continues to rise, individuals are increasingly likely to feel inundated with AIDS information from the media and other sources. While media attention has markedly helped increase the general awareness of AIDS in various populations, there has not necessarily been a comparable increase in the quality of specific knowledge. One reason for this has been the failure to speak frankly, clearly, and specifically about risk behaviors and preventive techniques. In addition, early conceptualizations of risk groups and inaccurate assumptions about their characteristics facilitated the denial of personal risk among certain individuals.

For example, early prevention messages which encouraged gay men to limit their risk by reducing number of partners, avoiding anonymous contacts, and avoiding the exchange of body fluids may have been counterproductive if men assumed the three recommendations to be of equal importance. Evidence that this may have been the case is provided by a 1985 study of the behavior of gay men in New York over 1 year.[54] It was found that total elimination of the three risky behaviors studied (nonmonogamy, out-of-home sexual contact, and unprotected anal-genital/oral-genital contact) was found in only 4% of the sample and, for 40% of the sample, change did not occur in the form of total elimination of any one behavior. A similar persistence of high-risk sexual behavior was observed in the 1984–1985 Chicago MACS study of gay men. It appears from participant reports that this persistence was in part due to confusion about risk factors; 75–80% of the men asserted that limiting their number of partners put them at low risk.[29] When semen, blood, or vaginal secretions are exchanged, it is possible to be infected by even a single partner, regardless of how well known the partner is. Men who assumed otherwise may have been tragically misled by educational messages which failed to single out this most important point. In the interest of providing a simple, accurate, and unambiguous message, future educational efforts should emphasize the danger of semen, blood, or vaginal secretion contact with sexual partners.

Many people have tended to put a great deal of weight on partner choice when estimating their risk. Like teenagers in the Massachusetts survey, many adults consider "being careful in choice of partners" an appropriate preventive measure. Many others are coming to rely on the belief that risky behavior is permissible in any mutually monogamous relationship in which both partners have tested negative. Any educators discussing this alternative must make it totally clear that 100% accuracy of negative test results cannot be guaranteed for anyone with an exposure history. Partners should also be encouraged to discuss monogamy expectations openly and explicitly, as well as alternatives available in the event these expectations are ever compromised by either partner. Both partners must also be free of all blood exposures as well. Even the transmission of infectious agents other than HIV cannot be excluded. For absolute protection, the practice of safer sex cannot depend on partner choice. To be safest, care in the exchange of body fluids should be taken with all partners.[64] This should be any AIDS educator's conclusive statement.

So that there is no doubt about the meaning of "body fluid exchange," specific sexual activities must be addressed in whatever terms are clearest to the target population. At the same time, specific and explicit means for preventing fluid exchange must also be communicated. This is imperative as people are more likely to dismiss or react fatalistically to a health message when not presented with concrete steps to protect themselves.[65] Currently this factor presents difficulties for appealing to the HIV-infected population, since cofactors for AIDS have yet to be clearly identified. Stevens and colleagues found that repeated exposure to the virus is associated with development of AIDS and ARC in HIV-infected individuals.[13] Until more information on strategies to enhance the odds of staying healthy is available, studies such as this should be cited to encourage the continued practice of behaviors limiting fluid exchange for both infected and noninfected individuals.

People tend to change behavior in gradations, not absolutes. Moreover, there remains in the minds of many some confusion regarding what changes are needed to limit risk while still maximizing fulfillment of other desires.[53] Clearer preventive messages should help speed the change process. Unfortunately, our ability to frame simple and clear preventive messages is limited by the disagreement and uncertainty which persist in the medical community regarding the risks of certain sexual practices, such as oral sex and wet kissing. Such disagreement and the conflicting reports which result merely increase public confusion. Many well-informed, at-risk individuals are, in fact, able to cite such reports selectively as justification for their persistence in "possibly risky" activities.[66] A common drive of educators to be in control of all the "answers" often leads them to "clear up" this confusion with black and white statements based on limited information or personal opinion. Alternatively, they may choose to address only that which is known conclusively and steer completely clear of any "gray area." Too many programs therefore confine safer sex discussion to condom use during intercourse. It is crucial for educators to acknowledge overtly what is ambiguous in HIV transmission knowledge; individual audience members need to get used to making decisions based on less than complete answers regarding, for example, oral transmission. Both educators and those they address must, for the time being, accept the ambiguities.

Acknowledging and Dealing with Barriers to Change

The health belief model classification for the determinants of health behavior provides a framework for understanding the complex barriers to behavioral change. These barriers should be explicitly considered in any AIDS education program. An educational intervention telling individuals that they must make significant changes in deeply entrenched behaviors, without acknowledging the real difficulties in bringing about such changes, is overly simplistic and unlikely to succeed. It is not always easy to pinpoint barriers relevant to specific individuals, as they are often not consciously aware of them themselves.

One barrier to change may be confusion regarding facts about AIDS transmission and prevention resulting from conflicting sources of information. Professional AIDS educators cannot assume that their qualifications guarantee that they will be perceived as credible sources of information. Along with providing factual information to address knowledge deficiencies, it is therefore important to assess the degree to which individuals believe the prevention information provided.[67] Individuals with strongly preconceived notions or who depend on unreliable sources of information may require a different style of intervention than of those who are merely ignorant of AIDS facts.

Once knowledge deficiencies have been addressed, motivational barriers become prominent. Many health beliefs, including perception of personal risk, perceived effectiveness of change, belief in the power of science, and social norms, directly impact motivation to change. Interventions that address these factors are described under Examples of Educational Interventions.

It is also important to acknowledge the potential tension, stress, and loss involved in making significant behavioral changes, as individuals may be unable to incorporate changes fully until they have processed associated feelings. Individuals who express the anger or grief they are experiencing because of the AIDS crisis, and who find they are not alone in owning such feelings, may be more ready to move on to take positive steps to respond to the crisis responsibly than those who do not. It should be acknowledged that change comes slowly for many people and that "backsliding" is not uncommon, but that there are always potential health benefits to be derived from continuing to change behavior in the risk-reducing direction. Individuals should be encouraged to seek reinforcement and find ways to reward themselves for their positive changes.

Evaluation Strategies

Although educational programs frequently target knowledge or attitudes, in the final analysis, changes in behaviors that impact health outcomes are the true measure of success in health education. The extent to which reported knowledge and attitudes are predictive of behavior is always a matter of uncertainty. Likewise, self-reported behavior or behavioral intent cannot be guaranteed to represent actual behavior, especially for highly personal or stigmatized behaviors. Further adding to the challenges of evaluation is the fact that program participants are often unavailable for follow-up to assess behavior in health outcomes over time.

Measures of Behavior

Although self-reporting has its limitations, certain steps can be taken to maximize its usefulness in evaluation. Pre- and postintervention reports may be obtained using either retrospective recall or diaries as data collection techniques. Checks on the reliability of responses should be employed by asking for the same information in different ways and asking the same questions on separate occasions.

Because it is crucial to maintain behavior changes indefinitely to reduce risk of HIV infection effectively, it is important to assess temporal and decay aspects of change. Optimally, evaluation is conducted repeatedly over a long enough period to assess whether recidivism is affecting the behavioral gains of the interventions. This can be difficult, especially for one-time interventions that assemble a loosely defined group of participants who may not be available for follow-up. In such cases a mail-back evaluation can be distributed with instructions to return it after a set period of time. Although response rate can be expected to be low, it may be enhanced by offering cash or other incentives.

In highly controlled settings, ordinarily available only to well-funded educational researchers, more aggressive techniques can be employed to obtain measures of behavior other than self-report. Such protocols of course would require informed consent and strict confidentiality provisions. For some of the sexual behaviors related to HIV transmission, it may be possible to obtain certain corroborating information from clinical examination. A positive rectal gonorrhea culture at follow-up in a man denying receptive anal intercourse, for example, could serve to invalidate his self-report. It may also be useful to make a direct assessment of the health-related outcome for purposes of evaluation. Some evaluators of AIDS educational interventions have, for example, used protocols that include periodic HIV antibody testing.

Control Studies

Unfortunately for evaluators, influences on behavior other than the educational intervention are numerous. This creates another difficulty in evaluating a program for its impact on behavior. As no single intervention is likely to result in a complete change in behavior, and the many factors outside of the program which influence decisions can be difficult to assess, an effort to isolate the effects of the program is essential to fully understanding its impact. One frequently used method for evaluating health behavior interventions is to provide the educational intervention in one group while using a well-matched peer group as a control. The two groups are presumed to be subject to similar outside influences on behavior. There are, however, serious ethical considerations in enrolling at-risk participants in an ongoing study without giving them effective AIDS risk-reduction information. Because of the urgency of communicating AIDS prevention information to all at risk, alternatives to the classical "no-intervention" control group may have to be considered. One attractive alternative is to give alternative educational interventions to two or more groups and evaluate their relative effectiveness. Educational researchers at Gay Men's Health Crisis recently evaluated three different types of intervention, involving differing degrees of group interaction, processing of feelings, and practicing of new behaviors.[68]

It should be stated that observable behavior change in all at-risk individuals, while being our most critical objective, should not be the sole criterion upon which educational programs are evaluated. Since ultimate control over behavior rests with the individuals rather than with educators, it may be important to also assess the extent to which a program addresses individuals' rights to knowledge, assists in clarifying their needs, and serves to improve their decision-making skills. In addition to health status goals, an important corollary objective of health education should always be to enable individuals to make their own informed decisions regarding their health, whatever those decisions might be.

EXAMPLES OF EDUCATIONAL INTERVENTIONS

Examples abound of programs that have focused primarily on increased knowledge regarding AIDS and HIV transmission risks. Many of these programs have attempted to dispel misconceptions about the power of medical technology to combat AIDS and to document the effectiveness of risk reduction methods such as the condom. These are elements of the health belief model that may be easily addressed through conventional didactic techniques. More innovative techniques for addressing other elements of the model will now be considered.

Targeting Efficacy and Social Factors through Modeling

To be effective, educators must deal with the emotional needs and underlying social motivations of those they serve.[3,21,23] Video modeling of ways to handle conflict, embarrassment, and stress surrounding the awkward social transactions required in risk reduction was found to be effective in favorably changing attitudes about condom use in an educational program targeting blacks entering a clinic for gonorrhea treatment. The television-quality soap opera style video was characterized by the absence of any authority figure, the free use of slang, and a script tailored to the attitudes and values of the target audience to maximize viewer identification and emotional involvement with the characters.[11] In the experience of Solomon and DeJong, it has been most useful to focus on problems of communication and interpersonal skills in order to build confidence for difficult negotiations involving prophylaxis. When peer models are observed overcoming barriers to condom use, both peer norms and feelings of self-efficacy are swayed in a health-promoting direction.

AIDS educators, too, have used videos to raise awareness of possible risks in social situations and to explore ways to effectively cope in these situations.[68,69] Such videos explore with audiences the influence of factors such as sexual energy, peer pressure, loneliness, stress, and alcohol or drug use on health-related judgment. After watching such "trigger films" or reading a social scenario, the group explores the issues involved and discusses possible solutions. In individual or specialized small group interventions, real-life scenarios contributed by participants can be discussed to personalize the problem-solving approach of this type of intervention.

Sexually explicit videos and printed materials have also been used to model the feasibility and desirability of safer sexual practices. In a study of gay men conducted by Michael Qualard of the Gay Men's Health Crisis, a higher degree of risk-reducing behavior change was reported 2 months after the intervention by men who saw an erotic safer sex video as part of an educational program than by men who took part in a discussion of safer sex and received only written materials.[70] It is possible that the modeling provided by the explicit video enhanced the response efficacy of viewers; that is, they may have developed an enhanced perception of the feasibility of making such changes themselves by seeing desirable models incorporate these changes into their sexual activity. Quadland's findings suggest that there may be educational benefits to advocating or providing incentives for increased depiction of safer sex in sex industry videos and printed materials.

Some programs have attempted to enhance response efficacy by using peers as models. For example, in one program educating a small group of persons with ARC, the lover of a person with ARC was invited to speak about the reality of having a mutually satisfying sex life after diagnosis.[71]

Building Social Skills to Enhance Response Efficacy

Many educators have used small group discussions and role playing to better equip individuals to implement risk-reduction recommendations.[72] Role plays and similar skill-building activities may be particularly important because they provide an opportunity for participants to practice and receive reinforcement for the behaviors they are expected to carry out in real life. Since encouraging a resistant partner to use a condom is recognized to be a very difficult type of social interaction for many people, a common activity in many programs is role playing the negotiation of condom use. In addition to verbal negotiations, small groups in Gay Men's Health Crisis interventions also practice written and nonverbal negotiation skills.[35] Such activities are readily adaptable to negotiation issues beyond the use of a condom, such as defining personally acceptable oral sex behavior or resisting psychoactive substance use during sexual activity.

Gay Men's Health Crisis groups also practice general communication and assertiveness skills. After discussing feelings about safer sex recommendations and barriers to implementing them, participants work together to set goals and develop individual plans of action.[35] Similar activities attempting to build self-efficacy in social situations have been used successfully (decreasing teenage smoking, for example) in social skill-building programs designed to lower teenage susceptibility to various peer pressures.[73,74]

Targeting Perception of Risk with PWA Spokespersons

Marmor and colleagues expressed interest in using peer counselors with AIDS or HIV infection, specifically in the prisoner population, to dispel misconceptions of at-risk individuals and enhance the impact of prevention messages.[61] People with AIDS have also been used in addressing gay and bisexual men during prevention programs.[72] These individuals' personal experience with AIDS may give them special status as opinion leaders and enable them to have an impact as educators. Particularly in low-prevalence areas, the general perception of risk is likely to rise when someone from within the community steps forward to speak as a person with AIDS. Pitfalls of such an approach include the possibility that the PWA spokesperson may express inaccurate information or attitudes that do not represent all persons with AIDS. Alternatively, he or she may be viewed by audience members to be different from themselves, and therefore the bearer of warnings that do not necessarily apply to their own lives.

Norm-Setting through Social Networks and Opinion Leaders

Established social networks and the norm-setting power of their leaders can be effective vehicles for inducing change.[4,11] For this reason, group education among established social networks may be particularly appealing for AIDS interventions. Such sessions allow participants to interact, sharing anxieties, conflicts, and perceptions of barriers to change. Such interaction is conducive to the strengthening of supportive social networks. In addition, individuals are able to learn problem-solving strategies from their peers. Generating lists of creative safer sex practices (through brainstorming or nominal group techniques), for example, provides all in the group with useful ideas for maintaining a satisfying sexual life while helping individuals realize that their peers really are changing their behavior.

Associations between observed behavior changes and specific educational approaches taken by the Houston KS/AIDS Foundation suggest that campaigns stressing the social acceptability and prevalence of safer sex practices may be more effective than those provoking fear and anxiety by concentrating on the risks of dangerous practices.[66] Consistent with psychological theory that positive reinforcement is more effective than aversive conditioning, images of fun and fashion have been found to be better motivators than fear. Humor also can play a key role in relieving tension as individuals develop new attitudes about the legitimacy of recommendations for difficult behavior changes.[75] Resistant individuals will be more likely to adopt safer sex practices if they experience a new consensus—if they come to feel that "everybody's doing it."[66]

In addition, recommended new behaviors are more readily adopted if they appear to be attractive replacements for past behaviors. Educators at the KS/AIDS Foundation made early efforts to "eroticize" safer sex, affirming the gay identity by keeping their messages "sex-positive." A Play Safe/Playmate contest was part of their campaign in 1984. The contest was held to select 12 attractive men from the Houston community to appear in a Safer Sex calendar. The Men's pictures appeared together with personal quotes on the safer sex them (e.g., Chuck: "My friends were skeptical when I chose a healthier life style; now they ask me how to. . . ."). In this way, peer opinion leaders served as role models supportive of healthy change.[75] Because of their effectiveness it is crucial that such "sex-positive" approaches to education be continued, in spite of political opposition. The moral objectives of some should be clearly separated from public health objectives of all to deal with this epidemic as efficiently as possible.

Many individuals remain isolated from peer support and information networks and may be unaware of changes in peers' behavior.[66] Other individuals, although not necessarily isolated, may experience little or no support for change. Some heterosexuals, for example, may have experienced little change in peer norms. AIDS educators should mobilize opinion leaders in such communities to spread the message that change is taking place, in order to begin addressing this key determinant of health behavior. Peer education programs in IV drug-user, inner-city, and university communities are among those which are beginning to mobilize key opinion leaders.

Social Marketing

Kirby[23] stated that linking educational programs to readily available services (e.g., school-based clinics dispensing contraception) would further increase their effectiveness. Kotler and Zaltman have used the term "social marketing" to describe such a technique for the promotion of social goals.[76] It is distinguished from health education by its promotion of specific products (e.g., condoms), as opposed to ideas (e.g., disease prevention). An advantage of this approach is that it lends itself easily to successful strategies of commercial marketing, including creative, stimulating, and humorous advertising. In developing their gonorrhea education video, Solomon and DeJong identified the marketing strategy of equating condom use with desirable concepts (status, pleasure, peace of mind); viewers' changed attitudes would seem to demonstrate the success of this approach. Incentives such as subsidies, free distribution, and a wider variety of points of purchase have also been used to encourage condom use in response to the AIDS crisis.

Skill Building to Influence Cognitive Cues

Structured activities designed to enhance coping behaviors can be used in educational/support groups for persons with ARC/AIDS, positive-testers, or "worried well" individuals. Barnes instructed those in a persons with ARC support group in the techniques of cognitive restructuring, whereby "negative self-statements" are consciously suppressed and replaced by "coping statements."[71] Exercises encouraged participants to generate common negative thoughts, and possible coping thoughts to replace them, in response to various situations (e.g., "A friend mentions AIDS in a conversation," or "you see a sexually attractive man and would like to catch his eye").

Many educators have also attempted to educate individuals in relaxation techniques (such as progressive deep muscle relaxation) in order to relieve stress and tension. Mental distress, whether due to AIDS anxiety or other stressors, may weaken the body's defenses and/or present a barrier to positive behavior change. Those who are prone to relieve tension through high-risk behavior may benefit from learning alternative techniques for relaxation.

Interventions to Reinforce and Maintain Positive Changes

In addition to motivating those who have not yet adopted safer sex practices, educational programs must concern themselves with reinforcing and maintaining positive changes in those who have.[66] Once initial sacrifices have been made and new habits developed, many individuals may find it relatively easy to maintain safer behaviors. Many others, however, may be prone to recidivism, for reasons that may include the introduction of new life stresses, changes in primary relationships, changes in perception of risk, or changes in psychoactive substance use patterns.

Educators at Gay Men's Health Crisis are planning programs specifically targeting those who have participated in previous programs. A four-session program on dating and intimacy is designed to reinforce prior behavior changes by building additional skills and support systems in the dating context (in which safer sex practices must actually be applied).[35] Participants will consider such topics as the role of dating in their lives, their goals in romantic relationships, and the impact of their self-image on dating behaviors. Educators will evaluate the effects of the reinforcement program by comparing reported attitudes and behaviors of participants to those of individuals who receive no reinforcing sessions.

CONCLUSIONS

The complex picture emerging from studies of risk-reducing behavior change indicates that much is yet to be learned about effective intervention. Meanwhile, prevalence of HIV infection continues to increase, raising the toll in human suffering and lives lost and increasing the likelihood over time that any one individual will encounter an infected partner. In spite of this, studies of gay men show that many continue to engage in risky behaviors, with some actually increasing their risk over time,[54] and many heterosexuals have yet to make any changes at all because of failure to recognize personal risk. As broadly based efforts to promote risk reduction continue and expand, thoughtful setting of objectives and targeting of specific audiences will remain vital determinants of effectiveness. Thus far many studies have documented changes in knowledge, attitudes, and even behavior in specific populations. The emphasis must now shift to exploring more rigorously the determinants of changes in behaviors posing risk of HIV infection.[64] Such knowledge is required for the continued improvement of educational interventions.

Rigorous evaluation of present programs to discern their true impact on behavior and health outcomes is also required if interventions are to improve. There is a particular need for more research and evaluation of creative nondidactic educational programs. For example, further evaluation of techniques for teaching social skills to adults may reveal important differences between their responses and those of children exposed to such interventions. It is unfortunate that the work of many creative AIDS educators is not reported in scholarly journals. Better avenues for networking and sharing successful intervention and evaluation strategies need to be explored, as the potential value of learning from the experience of fellow educators is great. Finally, in all future efforts, attention should always be paid to the ways in which programs address the core determinants of health behavior, both in program implementation and evaluation. If possible, the long-term behavioral and health-related outcomes of AIDS education efforts should be evaluated, in order that we may develop and refine programs that effectively enable individuals to adopt and maintain risk-reducing behavior.

REFERENCES

1. Becker M (ed): *The Health Belief Model.* Thorofare, New Jersey, Slack, 1974.
2. Maimon L, Becker M: The health belief model: Origins and Correlates in physiological theory. *Health Ed Monog* 2:236–263, 1974.
3. Emmons C, Joseph J, Kessler R, et al: Psychosocial predictors of reported behavior change in homosexual men at risk for AIDS. *Health Ed Q* 13:331–345, 1986.
4. Joseph J, Montgomery S, Emmons C, et al: Magnitude and determinants of behavior risk reduction: Longitudinal analysis of a cohort at risk for AIDS. *Psychol Health* 1:73–96, 1987.
5. McKusick L, Wiley J, Coates T, et al: Reported changes in the sexual behavior of men at risk for AIDS, San Francisco, 1982–84—the AIDS Behavioral Research Project. *Publ Health Rep* 100:622–629, 1985.
6. Fujita B, Wagner N, Pion R: Contraceptive use among single college students: A preliminary report. *Am J Obstet Gynecol* 109:787–793, 1971.
7. Chilman C: Adolescent Sexuality in a Changing American Society: Social and Psychological Perspectives. DHEW Publication HIH 79-1426, 1979.
8. Weinstein N: Reducing unrealistic optimism about illness susceptibility. *Health Psychol* 2:11–20, 1983.
9. Aral S, Cates W, Jenkins W: Herpes: Does knowledge lead to action? *Am J Publ Health* 75:69–71, 1985.
10. Green L, Krueter M, Deeds S, et al: *Health Education Planning: A Diagnostic Approach.* Palo Alto, California, Mayfield, 1980.
11. Solomon M, DeJong W: Recent sexually transmitted disease prevention efforts and their implications for AIDS health education. *Health Ed Q* 13:301–316, 1986.
12. Ostrow DG: Medical and psychological implications of HTLV-III antibody testing, in Ostrow DG (ed): *Biobehavioral Control of AIDS.* New York, Irvington Publishers, 1987, pp 19–27.
13. Stevens C, Taylor P, Zang E, et al: HTLV-III infection in a cohort of homosexual men in New York City. *JAMA* 255:2167–2172, 1986.
14. DesJarlais D, Friedman SR, Marmor M, et al: Development of AIDS, HIV seroconversion, and potential cofactors for T4 cell loss in a cohort of intravenous drug users. *AIDS* 1:105–111, 1987.
15. McKusick L, Coates T, Horstman W: Response from McKusick et al. (Letter.) *Am J Publ Health* 75:1449, 1985.
16. Osborn J: AIDS, social sciences, and health education: Personal perspective. *Health Ed Q* 13:287–299, 1986.
17. Ostrow DG, Altman N, Baker A, et al: Chronic hepatitis B in gay men: Prospective risk and prevention studies, in *Proceedings of the International Society for STD Research,* 1983, p 67.

18. Foreit K, Foreit J: Correlates of contraceptive behavior among unmarried U.S. college students. *Stud Family Planning* 9:169–174, 1978.
19. Hazuda H, Stern M, Gaskill SP, et al: Ethnic differences in health knowledge and behaviors related to the prevention and treatment of coronary heart disease. The San Antonio Heart Study. *Am J Epidemiol* 117:717–728, 1983.
20. Kessler R, Neighbors H: A new perspective on the relationships among race, social class, and psychological distress. *J Health Soc Behav* 27:107–115, 1986.
21. Duryea E, Okwumabua J: An exploratory study of the health decision-making variables of New York and Montana ninth-graders. *Adolescence* 20:899–908, 1985.
22. Rogers EM: *Diffusion of Innovations,* ed 3. New York, The Free Press, 1982.
23. Kirby D: Sexuality education: A more realistic view of its effects. *J School Health* 55:421–424, 1985.
24. Joseph J, Kessler R, Wortman C, et al: Coping and change: A summary of major psychosocial findings, in *Proceedings of the Annual American Psychiatric Association Meeting, Chicago,* 1987, p 10.
25. Waters J, Newmeyer J: AIDS risk-factors among IV drug users: Needle use and sexual practices, in *Program and Abstracts 114th Annual Meeting of the American Public Health Association, Las Vegas,* 1986.
26. Ostrow DG, Joseph J, Monjan A, et al: Psychosocial aspects of AIDS risk. *Psychopharmacol Bull* 22:678–683, 1986.
27. Stall R, McCusick L, Wiley J, et al: Alcohol and drug use during sexual activity and compliance with safe sex guidelines for AIDS: The AIDS Behavioral Research Project. *Health Ed Q* 13:359–371, 1986.
28. Ostrow DG, VanRaden M, Kingsley L, et al: Drug use and sexual behavioral change in a cohort of homosexual men, in *Proceedings of the Third International Conference on AIDS, Washington, DC,* 1987, p 157.
29. Ostrow DG, Kaslow K, Fox R, et al: Sexual and drug use behavioral change in men at risk of AIDS, in *Program and Abstracts of the 114th Annual Meeting of the American Public Health Association, Las Vegas,* 1986, p 96.
30. Harvey S, Beckman L: Alcohol consumption, female sexual behavior and contraceptive use. *J Stud Alcohol* 47:327–332, 1986.
31. McClelland D, Davis W, Kalin R, et al: *The Drinking Man.* New York, The Free Press, 1972.
32. Ostrow DG: Barriers to the acknowledgment of the role of drugs and alcohol in the AIDS epidemic and the treatment of drug and alcohol problems in persons with AIDS and HIV infection, in *The Joint Meeting of the American Society on Alcoholism and Other Drug Dependencies and the Research Society on Alcoholism,* April 1986.
33. Wilson T, Lawson D: Expectancies, alcohol, and sexual arousal in male social drinkers. *J Abnorm Psychol* 85:587–594, 1976.
34. Zucker R, Battistich V, Langer G: Sexual behavior, sex-role adaptation and drinking in young women. *J Stud Alcohol* 42:457–465, 1981.
35. Mantell JE, Kochems LM, Divittis AT, et al: Prevention of human immunodeficiency virus (HIV): AIDS risk reduction interventions with high risk groups, in *Annual Meeting of the American Public Health Association, New Orleans,* 1987.
36. Valdiserri RO, Lyter DW, Kingsley LA, et al: The effect of group education about AIDS risk reduction on improving attitudes. *NY State J Med* 87:272–278, 1987.
37. Smith, DW: Barriers to risk reduction in a southern community, in Ostrow DG (ed): *Biobehavioral Control of AIDS.* New York, Irvington Publishers, 1987, pp 121–123.
38. Shilts R: *And the Band Played On.* New York, St. Martin's Press, 1987.
39. Martin AD, Hetrick ES: Designing an AIDS risk reduction program for gay teenagers: Problems and proposed solutions, in Ostrow DG (ed): *Biobehavioral Control of AIDS.* New York, Irvington Publishers, 1987, pp 137–152.
40. Gross J: The deadly spectre of AIDS brings added turmoil for gay teenagers. New York Times, October 21, 1987.
41. Ostrow DG: Homosexuality and sexually transmitted diseases, in Holmes KK, Weisner P, et al (eds): *Sexually Transmitted Diseases.* New York, McGraw-Hill, 1984, pp 213–234.
42. Cleary P, Rogers T, Singer E, et al: Health education about AIDS among seropositive blood donors. *Health Ed Q* 13:317–329, 1986.
43. Echenberg DF: Education and contact notification for AIDS prevention. *NY State J Med* 87:296–297, 1987.

44. Price JH, Desmond S, Kukulka G: High school students' perceptions and misperceptions of AIDS. *J School Health* 55:107–109, 1985.
45. Wertz DC, Sorenson JR, Liebling L, et al: Knowledge and attitudes of AIDS health care providers before and after education programs. *Publ Health Rep* 102:248–254, 1987.
46. Osborn J: AIDS, social sciences, and health education: A personal perspective. *Health Ed Q* 13:287–299, 1987.
47. DesJarlais DC, Friedman SR, Hopkins W: Risk reduction of the acquired immunodeficiency syndrome among intravenous drug users. *Ann Intern Med* 103:755–750, 1985.
48. Nelkin D: AIDS and the social sciences: A review of useful knowledge and research needs. *Rev Infect Dis* 9:980–986, 1987.
49. Sherr L, Palmer C, Golmeir D, Green J: AIDS information. (Letter.) *Lancet* 2:1040, 1986.
50. Roloff ME, Miller GR: *Persuasion: New Directions in Theory and Research.* Beverly Hills, Sage Publications, 1980.
51. Bostrom RN: *Persuasion.* Englewood Cliffs, New Jersey, Prentice-Hall, 1983.
52. Hastings GB, Leather DS, Scott AC: AIDS publicity: Some experience from Scotland. *Br Med J* 294:48–49, 1987.
53. Bolling DR, Voeller B: AIDS and heterosexual anal intercourse. (Letter.) *JAMA* 258:474, 1987.
54. Martin JL: AIDS risk reduction recommendations and sexual behavior patterns among gay men: A multifactorial categorical approach to assessing change. *Health Ed Q* 13:347–358, 1986.
55. Ostrow DG, Brennen J, Stryker J: AIDS and the Black community: A review of the issues and related literature. *MABRC Newsl* 1:1–13, 1987.
56. Rogers MF, Williams WW: AIDS in Blacks and Hispanics: Implications for prevention. *Issues Sci Technol* 3:89–94, 1987.
57. Mays V, Cochran S: Acquired immunodeficiency syndrome and black Americans: Special psychosocial issues. *Publ Health Rep* 102:224–231, 1987.
58. Zelnik M, Kantner J, Ford K: *Sex and Pregnancy in Adolescence.* Beverly Hills, Sage Publications, 1981.
59. Friedman SR, Sotheran JL, Abdul-Quader AA, et. al: The AIDS epidemic among Blacks and Hispanics. *Millbank Q* AIDS 65(2):455–499, 1987.
60. Williams LS: AIDS risk reduction: A community health education intervention for minority high risk group members. *Health Ed Q* 13:407–421, 1986.
61. Marmor M, DesJarlais D, Friedman S, et al: The epidemic of AIDS and suggestions for its control in drug abusers. *J Substance Abuse Treatm* 1:237–247, 1985.
62. Ralph N: Contraceptive practices among female heroin addicts. *Am J Publ Health* 76:1016–1017, 1986.
63. Strunin L, Hingson R: Acquired immunodeficiency syndrome and adolescents: Knowledge, beliefs, attitudes, and behaviors. *Pediatrics* 79:825–828, 1987.
64. Becker MH, Joseph JG: AIDS and behavioral change to reduce risk: A review. *Am J Publ Health* 78:394–410, 1988.
65. Darrow WW, Siegel K: Preventive health behavior and STD, in Holmes KK, et al (eds): *Sexually Transmitted Disease*, 2nd ed. New York, McGraw-Hill, 1989, pp 85–92.
66. Bye L: Designing an effective AIDS prevention campaign strategy for San Francisco: Results from the first probability sample of an urban gay male community, in Ostrow DG (ed): *Biobehavioral Control of AIDS.* New York, Irvington Publishers, 1987, pp 91–108.
67. McKusick L, Horstman W, Coates T: AIDS and sexual behavior reported by men in San Francisco. *Am J Publ Health* 75:493–496, 1985.
68. Mantell JE, Mastroianni P, Divittis AT, et al: Three educational models for AIDS risk reduction, in *Annual Meeting of the American Public Health Association, New Orleans,* 1987.
69. Tross S, Hirsch DA: Project B.O.S.S. facilitator training manual. Memorial Sloan-Kettering Cancer Center Psychiatric Services, New York, 1987.
70. Kolata G: Erotic films in AIDS study cut risky behavior. New York Times, November 3, 1987.
71. Barnes RA: A short course for gay men diagnosed with ARC, in Ostrow DG (ed): *Biobehavioral Control of AIDS.* New York, Irvington Publishers, 1987, pp 153–165.
72. Palacios-Jimenez L, Shernoff M: *Facilitating Safer Sex.* New York, Gay Men's Health Crisis, 1986.
73. Botvin GJ, Willis TA: Personal and social skills training: cognitive–behavioral approaches to substance abuse prevention. *NIDA Res Monog Ser* 63:8–49, 1985.

74. Pentz MA: Prevention of adolescent substance abuse through social skill development. *NIDA Res Monog Ser* 47:195–232, 1983.
75. Wilson MB: AIDS prevention suggestions of "safe sex" promotional campaigns, in Ostrow DG (ed): *Biobehavioral Control of AIDS*. New York, Irvington Publishers, 1987, pp 119–120.
76. Kolter P, Zaltman G: Social marketing: An approach to planned social change. *J Marketing* 35:3–12, 1971.
77. Ostrow DG, Gayle TC: Psychosocial and ethical issues of AIDS health care programs. *Q Rev Bull* 12:284–293, 1986.

4

AIDS Prevention among Gay and Lesbian Youth

Psychosocial Stress and Health Care Intervention Guidelines

RITCH C. SAVIN-WILLIAMS and RAND E. LENHART

OVERVIEW

A forgotten, largely invisible minority in twentieth-century society is the gay adolescent. This condition is changing fairly rapidly, primarily in urban and collegiate areas, as increasing numbers of youth are claiming a sexual identity other than the heterosexual one traditionally assumed and desired by society and its agents. These gay and lesbian adolescents must, however, confront a hostile audience which disbelieves that one can be homosexual during adolescence. The premise of this chapter is that the psychosocial stresses that result from this denial may have profound medical consequences in the current reality of the AIDS epidemic.

These stresses exist for youths who discover the reality and inevitability of their homosexuality primarily because there are few sources of psychological, social, or legal assistance. Robinson[2] reminded his colleagues:

> Few individuals or organizations have been willing to challenge the myth that homosexuality is a phenomenon of adulthood. Whether due to inadequate professional knowledge, fear of jeopardizing professional positions, or simple lack of interest, personnel in youth-serving agencies and school districts (many of whom are gay themselves) have, for the most part, not been willing to speak out on behalf of gay youth. (p. 14)

Many gay and lesbian organizations have also been reticent to offer assistance to young gay and lesbian adolescents—perhaps because they fear by so doing they would be

Portions of this chapter, especially the first half, were derived from an earlier volume.[1] For further elaborations, see Chapters 1, 3, 7, and 10 of that book.

RITCH C. SAVIN-WILLIAMS • Department of Human Development and Family Studies, Cornell University, Ithaca, New York 14853-4401. RAND E. LENHART • Formerly, Psychological Services, Cornell University, Ithaca, New York 14853–4401.

charged with trying to "recruit" young people or they would drain their limited supply of personnel, time, and funds that are needed for other social and legal efforts.[2]

For adolescents struggling against great odds with little external support, the stigmatization of being known as homosexual can have a number of dire consequences. These include ostracism, violence, and expulsion by peers and families; self-destructive behavior such as substance abuse or suicide attempts; prostitution or dangerous sexual activities; and feelings of isolation, alienation, and confusion. Yet, most lesbian and gay adolescents, even those who face the portrait presented in this chapter, evolve into psychologically and socially healthy lesbian and gay adults—unless their life is prematurely ended by disease. High-risk behavior that has life-threatening health repercussions and experiencing psychosocial stress may be directly connected with each other.

This chapter highlights some of the conditions confronted by adolescents that increase their susceptibility (direct and indirect) to human immunodeficiency virus (HIV) infection or, if previously infected, to acquired immune deficiency syndrome (AIDS) complications. Much of this information is applicable for both lesbian and gay male youths. Because the only current recognized solution to the control of AIDS is to prevent its introduction into the bodily system, it is of paramount concern that health care providers consider the sexual behavior of this population of youth that has heretofore been perceived as either nonexistent or of little concern.

Recent public and medical awareness of the incidence and prevalence of AIDS in adult populations has led to increased concern and research regarding potential cofactors of a disease that handicap health care.[3–5] Similar attention has only recently been targeted toward adolescents, especially the health care needs of lesbian and gay adolescents from both medical and psychosocial perspectives. Its absence has been particularly tragic because some adolescents behave in ways that must be considered dangerous given (1) the current medical understanding and dismal forecast for the future treatment of those infected with HIV, and (2) particular stress theories that emphasize the significance of psychosocial sources of stress in increasing the susceptibility of the human system to external agents. Although relatively few reported AIDS cases have been adolescents between the ages of 13–19 years,[6] teenagers represent a sexually active population that frequently engages in risky behavior and that has recently shown marked increases in other forms of sexually transmitted disease (STD).[7] Taken together, these considerations strongly suggest that adolescents, although presently relatively unaffected, may be particularly vulnerable in the future to much higher incidence rates of AIDS and therefore in need of appropriately designed intervention programs and well-defined health care guidelines. Because the concern is with prevention and control, hence education, it is of paramount importance to consider the unusual challenge posed to health care providers of youths who engage in high-risk sexual behavior.

Primary prevention here refers to intervention measures—medical, psychological, and social—that attempt to reduce or eliminate diseases in high-risk populations and to promote disease-specific and general positive health practices. Devising effective and appropriate preventive programs with respect to the potential proliferation of AIDS among adolescents requires consideration of the nature of disease transmission, the sexual practices of this group, and various risk factors related to being a gay or lesbian youth in an openly antigay society.

Other publications also address the crisis of AIDS for adolescents,[8–14] including suggestions for education and prevention programs.[15–19] A comprehension overview of the major issues is Hein's[13] report to the Carnegie Corporation. She presents a multidisciplinary perspective that includes medical, behavioral, psychological, ethical, legal, and economic aspects. Two concerns relevant for this chapter are briefly discussed: The existence of gay youth and the importance of the interrelationship between psychosocial factors (e.g., peer pressure, denial, feelings of invulnerability) and medical status. The major divergence between many of these contributions and the current chapter is that they tend to be concerned with all adolescents, regardless of sexual orientation. For example, Mantell and Schinke[12] presented an AIDS intervention model with primary emphasis (two-thirds of the chapter) on practice and therapeutic frameworks for AIDS prevention, including hands-on suggestions for programs with adolescents. Brooks-Gunn et al.[11] noted that little is known about AIDS among homosexual adolescents; they recommended increased research activity in this regard. The usual tactic is to omit any reference to gay youth and focus instead on "dangerous" or high-risk (i.e., homosexual) behavior among adolescents.

A rare exception to these studies is the research of Rotheram-Borus and her colleagues[20,21] on runaway and gay youths. Because these youths are uniquely at risk for HIV infection, they have begun a 2-year longitudinal study that includes educational and intervention programs and examines the mediating factors of stressful life events and social support on sex practices. The youths are primarily of minority group status and are quite knowledgeable about AIDS (e.g., means of transmission), but they also engage in many high-risk behaviors with very little protection (e.g., use condoms). The 60 gay male youths in the study appeared uniquely at risk for HIV infection in part because of issues surrounding coming out and sexual identity (Rotheram-Borus, personal communication).

In the current report we explore and expand this last point: We target specifically the plight of gay and lesbian adolescents and some of their unique concerns. Other reports[22,23] have addressed AIDS and gay youth, but only in the most general terms. In keeping with the biobehavioral emphasis of this volume, the conceptual model presented here is broader than therapy, encompassing the initiation of HIV into the gay and lesbian adolescent population, its transmission to others, and preventive and education programs. More specifically, this chapter reviews several of the unique concerns posed by gay and lesbian adolescents for the biobehavioral control of AIDS. The first issue is a consideration of the role of psychosocial stress for the initiation and growth of disease. Second, the unique psychosocial sources of stress for homosexually active youth and for gay and lesbian adolescents are addressed, especially in regard to high-risk behaviors and the possibility of acquiring AIDS. Gay youths are invisible to society at large, to health care professionals, and even among adolescents. Finally, suggestions are made that will, we believe, benefit in (1) controlling the spread of AIDS in the adolescent population, and (2) assisting those who encounter youths who have the virus.

PSYCHOSOCIAL STRESS, ADOLESCENCE, AND AIDS

A paradigm recently applied to better understand issues of health and disease integrates concepts and research from the behavioral and biomedical sciences.[24–26] A complete discussion of this approach is beyond the scope of this manuscript. In general, there are two primary ways in which psychosocial factors may have an impact on the development of disease: (1) psychosocial resilience or protective mechanisms, and (2) vulnerability or risk variables.[25] The potential applicability of the first approach lies in addressing the question: "Why do some youths place themselves in situations of unsafe sexual or drug behavior?" The second question is: "Why do some who come into contact with HIV appear to contract the disease while others withstand its assault?" The focus here is on these two in the hope that the development of protective mechanisms and the reduction of risk factors will become the long-term goal of many health care workers.

Protective mechanisms are generally considered to consist of variables such as personality characteristics (e.g., positive self-esteem), family cohesion (e.g., intimate parent–child relationship), and external support systems (e.g., strong extended family).[27] Rutter[25] noted that these factors—"processes" and "mechanisms" are preferred terms—are of limited preventive utility, "because any one may act as a risk factor in one situation but as a vulnerability factor in another" (p. 317). Thus, one research goal is to discover mechanisms that directly or indirectly protect an individual against "risky situations."

The mediating mechanism most relevant in examining AIDS and gay youth is alteration of exposure experiences, especially high-risk situations such as prostitution, or involvement in risky behaviors, such as unprotected anal intercourse. The former might be reduced by parental supervision of the adolescent's activities and acceptance/support of the adolescent's sexual orientation; the latter, by exposure to safer sex education. In addition, self-efficacy or a positive self-esteem frequently serves as a crucial mediating immunization, achieved through (1) close, interpersonal relationships (especially with parents), (2) successful completion of tasks, and (3) turning points in life (e.g., successful resolution of the coming out process).[1,25]

Research on the second major category of psychosocial variables, vulnerability, has generally followed a typical medical model. Prior research on infectious diseases has demonstrated that "psychosocial factors may increase susceptibility to disease, influence the course of the disease, and contribute to health-promoting or health-damaging behaviors" (p. 1309).[24] Levy and Ziegler[28] suggested that AIDS is an opportunistic disease that is most "successful" in those who are at the time immunocompromised. This state may be the result of recent diseases, malnutrition, drug or alcohol use, poor health care, antibiotics, and psychosocial stress.[28–30] Coates et al.[24] concluded, "Even if sexual activity is primary in exposing persons to AIDS, it is important to identify the variety of factors that may compromise immune function and determine host response" (p. 1310).

One factor that has received considerable interest is stress. According to Mechanic,[31] undue and frequent attention to inner feelings, bodily changes, and thoughts of self may have the effect of increasing their ability to provoke distress and its symptoms. Because youth are especially susceptible to both the impact of pubescence, psychosocial growth, and self-awareness, adolescence is a prime time to investigate these issues. Mechanic[31] reviewed the relevant literature and concluded that individuals who experience acute self-monitoring and self-introspection, similar to Buss's[32] notion of private self-consciousness, also report more instances of various physical and psychological symptom and discomforts (e.g., depression). Beyond a moderate level, with increasing introspection there is a corresponding greater intensity and magnitude of emotional and inner distress.

Coates et al.[24] suggested several causation models between stress and AIDS susceptibility. Stress, especially in sustained quantities, may result in immunosuppression, that in turn is linked to a predisposition to acquiring infectious diseases. Or, stress may further depression, low self-esteem, and withdrawal which may in turn affect the immune system.[30]

Inducers of self-scrutiny may be internal (e.g., disease symptoms) or external (e.g., events that encourage self-comparisons). Mechanic[31] argued that "isolation and self-consciousness appear to be encouraged by discontinuities in ecological settings, in home circumstances, and in peer relationships" (p. 10) that seem to demand self-evaluation. The more significant the external agents, the greater the self-appraisals. For adolescents these significant others are most likely to be parents and peers who have important meaning for one's self-regard and identity development.[1] The constant fear may be of social isolation.

In particular, adolescent peers can be quite harsh on those who dare to be different. Their effect can be of two varieties, breaking one's resilience and exposing one to increased stress. Mechanic[31] noted that the recipients of this scorn are

> more likely to be psychologically and socially isolated, and often lack the confidence to establish appropriate relationships that direct their attention away from themselves and their personal shortcomings. Such perceived shortcomings probably contribute to behavior associated with health risks, such as drinking, drug use, promiscuous sexual activity, fighting, and fast and aggressive driving. . . .
>
> The humiliation of being scorned increases adolescent secretiveness and the unwillingness to share feelings with parents, teachers, and peers. Secretiveness makes it doubly difficult to correct faulty or unconstructive attributions to inner experiences (p. 11).

Relevant for this chapter is the applicability of Mechanic's view to the experiences of lesbian and gay adolescents. As illustrated below in the discussion of homosexual behavior, gay identity, and the coming out process, gay and lesbian adolescents are frequently subjected to social ostracism and scorn from both peers and family members. The resulting increased self-absorption, low self-regard, and inner distress of gay and lesbian adolescents are of both theoretical and empirical importance.

PSYCHOSOCIAL STRESSES FOR LESBIAN AND GAY ADOLESCENTS

Several investigators[33] have reported that lesbian and gay adolescents are more likely than heterosexual youth to manifest aspects of the classic "storm and stress" syndrome. This may be due largely to the struggle to discover a "deviant" sexual identity in the homophobic social environment of one's childhood and youth. Rigg[34] noted:

> As time passes and the realization comes that the homosexual drive is not being dispelled, but is becoming stronger, an identity crisis may occur which may be handled in a variety of ways, and therefore may be associated with varied new symptoms. The most obvious one is depression, which may be manifested by withdrawal, lack of interest in schoolwork, lack of interest in activities which involve associating with peers, irritability and moodiness. Loss of peer relationships naturally produces a sense of isolation, which heightens the fear of abandonment already present and increases depression (p. 827).

In this section, the unique experiences of gay and lesbian adolescents that increase the likelihood of leading a stressful life are reviewed. The struggles of feeling different during childhood and of finding a coherent sense of identity during adolescence may help explain the vulnerability of lesbian and gay youth to HIV exposure and to its consequences.

Homosexual Behavior and Gay Identity

An initial issue is defining what is a gay or lesbian adolescent. This may be difficult because during this age period adolescents are likely to experience cross-orientation sexual contact but are unlikely to define the self as homosexual. An important differentiation for this chapter is to distinguish homosexual behavior from homosexual identity.

Homosexual activity connotes sexual, genital behavior between members of the same sex. Gay and lesbian identity, by contrast, represents a consistent, enduring sense of recognition of one's sexuality in which one repeatedly experiences sexual feelings, thoughts, and/or behaviors with respect to members of the same sex. The two are usually highly correlated with each other, although this may be more of a future than a present reality. These issues are particularly crucial in reference to teenaged populations because many forms of sexual activity with partners varying in age, sex, and other variables are commonplace—regardless of self-professed sexual identity.

Two seemingly opposite facts are important to consider: Some gay and lesbian adolescents are homosexual virgins and some "straight" adolescents have engaged extensively in homosexual behavior. Several studies[1,35–38] of gay and lesbian youths document the fact that some individuals accept the self-label of gay and lesbian before they have had same-sex sexual experiences. For example, of 317 gay and lesbian youths between the ages of 14 and 23 years[1] 5% of the males and 12% of the females were homosexual virgins. Manosevitz[39] reported 22% of his sample was homosexual virgin during the ages of 13–17 years and 4% during the ages of 18–24 years. Dank[40] concluded: "It is theoretically possible for someone to view himself as being homosexual but not engage in homosexual relations just as it is possible for someone to view himself as heterosexual but not engage in heterosexual relations" (p. 117).

First awareness of same-sex arousal begins for some during early adolescence. Homosexual activity may have previously taken place or be delayed until late adolescence or adulthood.[36,37,41–43] Although Kinsey et al.[44] believed that homosexual behavior precedes homosexual feelings, most studies report the reverse.[1,32,35–37,42] For example, in a reanalysis of Kinsey's data,[45] the mean age of first homosexual arousal for males was 13.2 years; first homosexual orgasm averaged 15.0 years of age. Labeling oneself as "homosexual," however, occurred much later, averaging 19–21 years of age in the above studies. The delay in identifying oneself as gay or lesbian is usually attributed to societal homophobia and discrimination and their effects on developing adolescents.[46]

By contrast, clearly not all adolescents who engage in homosexual behavior are gay or lesbian. Homosexual arousal or behavior is fairly common, especially during adolescence. Malyon[47] speculated that about 9 of 10 reports by youth of same-sex erotic interest are made by those predominantly heterosexual in orientation. Ross-Reynolds[48] concluded: "The majority of adolescents who engage in homosexual behavior do not continue this practice into adulthood. Conversely, as many as 31% of gay adults engaged in no homosexual behavior until they were out of high school" (p. 70).

There is, however, ample evidence that lesbian and gay adolescents are more likely than other youths to engage in both prepubertal and pubertal homosexual behavior. Compared with heterosexuals, Manosevitz[39] noted that gays engaged in earlier and more frequent sexual behaviors of all types but this difference disappeared by adolescence. Early encounters were primarily with same-sexed partners with a shift to both heterosexual and homosexual behavior during adolescence and early adulthood. During childhood (5–9 years), more than 40% of homosexual males had same-sex sexual activity, and this proportion steadily increased to nearly 60% during preadolescence (10–12 years), to 70% during adolescence (13–17 years), to more than 95% during early adulthood (18–24 years). The heterosexuals' percentages for homosexual behavior during the same age period were considerably lower: 5%, 25%, 15%, and 5%. Clearly, there is a direct relationship between adult homosexuality and pubertal sexual contact with members of the same sex.[33,45]

To explain the relatively high frequency of homosexual experiences among teenagers, some[34,49] have argued that sexual experimentation involving an exploration of bodies and reactions with same-sex peers occurs because such experiences are likely to be more familiar and therefore less threatening than similar heterosexual physical contact. Others[50] view these "transient homosexual activities" as the product of typical adolescent crushes, hero-worshipping, and intimate same-sex friendships. Consistently, these authors have referred to teenage homosexual activities as a product of a "normal phase" in adult heterosexual development and "need cause no anxiety that they are the harbingers of lifelong homosexuality" (p. 828).[34] Although soothing to concerned and frightened parents of gay and lesbian youth, these views may be a source of great anxiety for the teenager who is becoming aware of a sexual identity that does not fit these expectations. The experience is not one of a temporary "phase" but of a comprehensive and stable sexual orientation.

It is crucial that the health provider is aware and knowledgeable of these facts in developing AIDS intervention or prevention programs. First, knowledge of a youth's self-identification as gay or straight may be relatively uninformative in assessing frequency of homosexual behavior. Although adolescents who identify as gay or lesbian are more likely than those who self label as heterosexual to engage in homosexual behavior, such individuals may be homosexual virgins and some self-labeled heterosexual youths may be quite homosexually active. Thus, high-risk behavior is not dependent on self-label. More important than the label for the health care provider assessing AIDS risk is the sexual activity of adolescents.

Second, because many homosexually active youths are also heterosexually active, if an adolescent contacts HIV it is important to inquire as to his or her homosexual and heterosexual contacts. Sexually active teenagers are thus potential contributors to increasing the incidence of AIDS to many populations, including same-age peers—both male and female.

Consequently, this feature of adolescent sexuality mandates that health care providers assess specific sexual practices as opposed to self-selected descriptive labels (e.g., "straight"), as the latter may provide relatively little information regarding possible past or future risk of HIV exposure. Additionally, due to societal discrimination and powerful peer pressure, teenagers may deny a lesbian or gay identity but be willing to discuss the particulars of sexual behaviors with nonjudgmental health care providers and educators.

The delineation of homosexual activity and sexual identity is also important when considering the psychological stresses and consequences of the self-recognition or "coming out" process of youth. We now turn to evidence that supports this conclusion by examining the unique psychological sources of stress for lesbian and gay adolescents.

Feeling Different

Sexual orientation is probably present before the ability to reflect and label sexual feelings and attractions emerges.[51] Thus, relatively few individuals recall precisely when they first became aware of their sexual orientation; it seemed more of a process than an event. In retrospect, however, many gay and lesbian adults report that they first felt "different" at a very early age. They did not know why, but the feeling was extremely pervasive and probably important.[52,53] They recalled that as children and adolescents they were social isolates and outcasts; compared to heterosexuals, they ranked low on social involvement, number of friends, popularity, dating, and participation in same-sex games.[33,54,55] Within the family they became half-members: "afraid and alienated, unable ever to be totally open and spontaneous, to trust or be trusted, to develop a fully socialized sense of self-affirmation . . . stress characterized by secrecy, ignorance, helplessness, and distance" (p. 1).[52] The "secret" must be hidden—from peers, family, and self—as the adolescent learned the wisdom of invisibility and dishonesty.[60]

Troiden[56] quoted a gay male student who noted this sense of apartness during preadolescence: "I never felt as if I fit in. I don't know why for sure. I felt different. I thought it was because I was more sensitive" (p. 363). In several samples, more than 70% felt this sense of being different.[33,56] Reasons given for feeling different included lack of interest in the other sex, little participation in same-gender activities or sports, and gender-nonconforming personality and behavioral traits. These gender atypical behaviors and interests are frequently ridiculed by adolescent peers. Their high prevalence among "pre-gay" children and adolescents has been documented by a number of investigators; some posit gender nonconformity as a causative agent in the development of adult homosexuality.[33,57] Saghir and Robins[55] described its effects on the male child and adolescent: "All of them were called sissy and were teased about it by their schoolmates. It was an unhappy experience that most of them recalled very vividly" (p. 19). The impact on female youth was less severe.

Coleman[58] noted that "on a conscious or pre-conscious level, the child and family members know even then that the child's sexual orientation 'differs' " (p. 32). By incorporating familial and social external values, the child learns that homosexuality is wrong, sick, and, certainly, undesirable.

> A major crisis is created for the individual, the family, and ultimately for society when a child appears about to break with these expectations. Minimally, the child feels different, alienated, and alone. As they grow up, many such children develop low self-esteem. If acknowledged, same-sex feelings would mean rejection and ridicule; consequently, individuals protect themselves from awareness through defenses, such as denial, repression, reaction formation, sublimation, and rationalization. . . The consequences of this concealment can be enormously destructive (p. 33).

These conflicts may be expressed in adolescence in various behavioral arenas, such as acting out in school, rebellion against authority, and dangerous sexual behavior. More common, however, are the more subtle, pervasive expressions that affect self-image.[59]

> Every time a homosexual is denied the validity of his feelings or restrains himself from expressing, he does a small hurt to himself. He turns his energies inward and suppresses his own vitality. The effect may be scarcely noticeable: joy may be a little less keen, happiness slightly subdued; he may simply feel a little run down, a little less tall. Over the years, these tiny denials have a cumulative effect (p. 249).

Some adolescents thus learn that they are among the most despised in society. They are faced with a number of decisions that must be made, but the ability to make the right choices is not yet mature.[60] Should she play it safe and pass as heterosexual, aware of her own deception and of living a lie? Should he compartmentalize his life, separating his sexual self from all other activities and relationships? Should she disclose to others and risk the potential for ostracism, denial, and violence? Theoretical models of the coming out process have been proposed to describe the sequence of feelings and psychosocial stresses that are prototypical for gay and lesbian adolescents.

Coming Out

Psychological and sociological models of the coming out process trace the development from these early feelings of alienation and unease to full scale inner and outer turmoil during adolescence. The realization that being "different" may mean being "gay" appears to occur between the ages of 10 and 18 years.[41,51,56,58,61] The repercussions of this sexual awareness are usually considered to be fairly severe[47]:

> . . . the adolescent who is struggling with homoerotic impulses must contend with a fear of social disapproval along with significant intrapsychic conflict. . . often leading to a fragmentation of identity. Homophobic content becomes internalized and often causes protracted dysphoria and feelings of self-contempt. The juxtaposition of homosexual desire and acculturated self-criticism is inimical to healthy psychological development (pp. 323–324).

The strategies used by adolescents to cope with these sexual feelings include rationalization ("Something I'll outgrow"); relegation to insignificance ("Did it only as a favor for a friend"); compartmentalization of sexual desire ("I mess around with other girls but that does not make me a dyke"); withdrawal from provocative situations to remain celibate or asexual ("I'm saving myself for the right guy"); denial, frequently engaging in heterosexual dating or sexual behavior ("I can't be gay, I've had a girlfriend for years and I like her"); and redirection of energies to other efforts, such as intellectual or work pursuits.[33,38,47,55,60,61,63]

"Passing" as heterosexual is probably the most common adolescent adjustment to the fear of homosexuality.[40,60,63,64] Youth avoid threatening or provocative situations, keep tight control over any mannerisms and dress that might reveal their "true nature," and cultivate a deliberate heterosexual role. Rigg[34] (p. 827) noted, "Refuge may be taken in humor, both telling, and laughing at antihomosexual jokes, or in teasing others suspected of similar tendencies, to point the finger of suspicion in another direction." In such cases, Cass[62] maintained, identity foreclosure is manifested—but the underlying psychological difficulties remain, to emerge later.

Although it may appear to be the safest strategy for the short term, passing may lead to feelings of depression, awkwardness and shame in interpersonal relations, guilt, fear, and anxiety.[64] In research focusing on college students who came to the university psychological services clinic, covert gay men displayed more intrapsychic tensions, social–psychological problems, and social introversion than their overt gay peers.[65] Myrick[66] reached the same conclusion: "Coverts have the most concern over self-esteem, self-acceptance, and status and feel the most social isolation, powerlessness, normlessness, and personal incompetence" (p. 234).

Passing negates personal authenticity and validation of the self as a person of self-worth. Humanistic psychologists[67,68] maintain that healthy personality development requires significant and substantial self-disclosure to others. A person establishes contact with the real self as she or he makes the public self congruent with this real self.[67] To forego this engenders feelings of hypocrisy and not being able to be oneself.[60,63]

Malyon[47] outlined three adaptations that are the most frequent responses to the dilemma of being a homosexual adolescent (from least to most satisfactory): repression of same-sex desires, but eventually the impulses must emerge; suppression of homosexual impulses, which frequently results in a temporary developmental moratorium with a truncated identity formation; and disclosure to self and others, with the potential for ostracism and ridicule. Malyon concluded:

> Self-acknowledged homosexual adolescents, then, are often an alienated and neglected population. The personal, social, and institutional support systems that assist the adolescent heterosexual minor are not available to the homosexual minor. As might be expected, this situation often produces rather morbid psychological consequences. The homosexual adolescent must either try to complete the developmental process in a hostile and psychologically impoverished heterosexual social environment or must decide to seek peer support and social opportunities in the homosexual community (p. 328).

But a move to the gay community may also have negative consequences, such as separation from the family and having to assume adult responsibilities prematurely.[47]

It is frequently difficult to assist adolescents in overcoming these obstacles. They may not be able to disclose their inner turmoil to others because the tasks at hand are so nebulous and so intensely personal that they experience "identity confusion."[61] Adolescents may feel that they belong neither to society nor to the self; they may take the self-pitying position, "Why me?!" The adolescent's task is a formidable one: to recognize that frequently articulated guidelines for future behavior, ideals, and expectations are meant to ensure a heterosexual identity. They are not available or relevant for them.[52] The decision to come out to self and others may feel like a continual existential crisis.[69] This process of slowly surrendering to a gay/lesbian identity entails weighing the costs to one's own psychic self and one's relations to others, especially to family and friends.[52,58,63]

Few, however, have addressed the question of when is the healthiest time to come out to oneself and to others. Harry and DeVall[70] reported that it was not the behavioral event of coming out that was related to high self-esteem but the phenomenological event of defining oneself as gay at a young age. Such individuals appeared to avoid the negative repercussions of being known as gay in junior and senior high school settings without facing negative psychological consequences such as denial, repression, suppression, and rationalization. They took their time, disclosing their sexual identity to "safe" persons who gave them the necessary social and psychological support.[58] They learned crisis competence[46] and developed an internal sense of self-respect and ego integrity[47] that prepared them to face the cruelty of a homophobic peer society.

The Effects of the Social Environment

Societal defects block healthy development for many gay and lesbian youths because[42]

> coming out takes place in an antihomosexual environment where institutional and social support systems are absent. What coming out ultimately symbolizes is the individuals' response to social stigmatization in a struggle to redefine him/herself against a background of antihomosexual prejudice and discrimination. Only with reconstruction of social conditions and attitudes will individuals experience, with pride and dignity, an integration of their feelings, behavior, and identity into a unified and positive self-concept (p. 58).

As the socio-historical time frames change, so too may the experiences of the adolescent coming to terms with same-sex feelings, attractions, and behaviors.

But social attitudes toward gays remain negative. Surveying 278 high school students, Price[71] found a high degree of antihomosexual attitudes when the issue was personal, potentially affecting the youths directly. For example, the youths strongly endorsed the following views: As a parent I would be upset if my child was homosexual, the thought of homosexuality makes me sick, I would not have a close friend who was homosexual, and I do not want to live close to a homosexual. On the other hand, they were relatively neutral on whether homosexuals should be allowed to hold important jobs, are criminals and should be locked up, and should be recognized as like everyone else. Male adolescents held more negative attitudes than female youths. These findings were, for the most part, replications of earlier studies of adolescent attitudes toward homosexuality.[72,73] Rofes[74] was not optimistic about the current plight of gay adolescents in today's society:

> While some of us imagine a drastically changing world for gay teens, this appears to be more an activist's fantasy than reality. Gay teens still feel isolated in their homes, neighborhoods, and schools. It's a rare gay teenager who finds support in his or her high school—either from another gay student or an openly gay teacher (p. 15).

Conclusions

It is important for health care providers, clinicians, and educators to better understand and appreciate the conditions for lesbian and gay adolescents growing up in today's environment. We have highlighted the day-to-day pains and crises that lesbian or gay adolescents may encounter, from both those they love and those they may not. Most cope and survive to become healthy, life-fulfilling adults. Some, however, are not so fortunate: "It should therefore surprise no one that breakdown, depression and attempted suicide are often the end product of pressures that become unendurable" (p. 172).[52] Our ignorance of these issues of coming out has had and will have grave consequences for some adolescents. Feeling different and alienated, having to integrate and develop one's sense of identity in a hostile environment, constantly fearing exposure of one's inner most secret, and experiencing ridicule from peers for being effeminate or masculine may enhance one's susceptibility to AIDS.

These psychosocial factors may increase an adolescent's vulnerability to HIV in several ways. First, they may serve as an impetus for dangerous sexual activity, thus increasing the risk of contacting the virus. Second, because of social rejection and feelings of alienation gay or lesbian adolescents may attempt to escape from the resulting intense self-introspection through alcohol and drugs, thus compromising one's immunological system to fight a possible HIV infection. A third link between psychosocial factors and AIDS acquisition is less clearly documented. At a 1985 symposium on AIDS at the American Psychological Association meetings, preliminary reports were given that indicated that those who develop AIDS are more highly dependent on social approval and have not yet come to terms with their gay identity. Other papers noted that stress increased the likelihood of acquiring AIDS because it helped to create the somatic conditions that handicapped the immune system from fighting diseases. Finally, the stress of the coming out process frequently evokes multiple forms of denial, that may include a delay in seeking treatment. Early treatment may be an affective intervention or prevention process (p. 1310),[24] especially given recent advances in drug therapies that prolong both the quality and quantity of life.

These psychosocial factors are worth investigating in any biobehavioral model of prevention and control, perhaps especially so for adolescents because of the critical nature of their life course time. The conclusion of Coates et al.[24] is most apt:

> Thus, psychosocial factors, including personality variables and transient states, partially influence susceptibility to environmental stressors. Genetic and environmental factors would also influence susceptibility to stress. Thus, we propose that it is the interaction of genetic, environmental, and psychosocial factors that may, at various times, protect the organism, predispose the organism to disease onset, or influence the course of disease once contracted. The implications are that each of these factors needs to be included in research designs, or at least that findings in one area need to be interpreted in light of indications in the others (p. 1311).

The cumulative effects of the coming out process are crucial in assisting health care providers to better understand the behavioral and cognitive processes that contribute to the increased risk among gay and lesbian adolescents of HIV infection. One response to the longstanding daily pains is to "burst out" of all inhibitions in sprees of reckless, dangerous sexual activity. For some, seeking transient sexual encounters with relatively unknown partners assuages isolation, rejection, and pain. Unlike heterosexual adolescents who have social sanctions and opportunities to evolve healthy sexual/intimate relations, many lesbian and gay adolescents have had to repress and suppress their true sexual identity.[52,54,60] Outlets may take place in parks, theaters, or public restrooms with anonymous others. Feeling freed from "the overpowering tensions of hiding" some adolescents may seek frequent casual sexual contacts under these conditions.[60] With each episode adolescents increase the likelihood of exposure to HIV.

One extreme manifestation of this "I'll catch up for lost time" or "I don't care what happens to me" attitude is street prostitution. Gay male and lesbian adolescents may become prostitutes as a means of self-support or as a sexual outlet, with often dire consequences for increasing one's chances of contact with HIV.[7,75–79] Many of these adolescents began as homeless or runaway youth in large urban centers, escaping from family and peer group ostracism, and have limited options in their new environment for surviving.[78–81] One youth in Roesler and Deisher's[37] study of 60 gay youths in Seattle had more than 3000 self-reported sexual encounters; the group averaged 20 years of age and 50 sexual partners. These behaviors clearly carry in today's world a high lethal probability. The difficulty in communicating the urgency of the situation is compounded by an egocentric attitude common among many adolescents: "I'm young and healthy, it won't happen to me" or "I am not gay so I won't get AIDS."

Individuals experiencing extreme psychological stress may be relatively impaired in their ability to engage in health-promoting and self-protecting behaviors and, perhaps more importantly, may behave in ways that place their overall health at serious risk. Consequently, it is crucial for any intervention program to focus not only on preventing specific health-damaging behaviors, but also to promote good health practices and fortify positive psychological health.

Although the determinants of "dangerous and reckless sex" are certainly complex, a healthier attitude on the part of society toward homosexual behavior and a gay/lesbian identity would encourage youths to evolve their sexuality as a natural process with appropriate experimentation, acceptance, and positive feelings. Then, the frequency of these behaviors would be reduced and the spread of AIDS would be contained among gay, lesbian, and homosexually behaving adolescents.

STRESS REDUCTION THROUGH HEALTH CARE

One strategy to reduce the amount of stress that lesbian and gay adolescents must inevitably feel is to provide supportive services. Health care providers can assist in alleviating adolescents' psychological distress and in facilitating the process by which adolescents are less likely to engage in high-risk sexual behavior and more likely to seek and then continue medical care.[24] In the following sections of this chapter, guidelines for health care providers and educators are reviewed for those times when they encounter lesbian and gay adolescent clients.

Health Care Industry Denial of Adolescent Homosexuality

In the provision of services and treatment to specific populations, systems and institutions of education and health care often embody, reflect, and advocate the attitudes and beliefs of the larger culture. Nowhere has this been more evident than in the relationship between the health care industry and gay and lesbian adolescents. Despite the fact that striking changes have occurred during the past decade in the visibility of the gay population and most recently of gay youth,[60,82] it is instructive to note that many archaic, antihomosexual attitudes, theories, and treatment approaches remain as part of the belief system of a considerable number of professionals. These views have been most pronounced in psychiatry and less so in psychology, medicine, nursing, and the social sciences.[83] Almost exclusively, however, the focus has been on adult sexual behavior and orientation, with only occasional reference to adolescents. Nevertheless, these theoretical frameworks necessarily influenced the education and training of health care personnel, and consequently forms of health care and intervention strategies employed during contact with gay and lesbian adolescents.

Relying on psychodynamic theories of development, health care providers have frequently viewed homosexually oriented individuals, by definition, as immature in psychological development and homosexuality as symptomatic of deep-seated emotional illness.[84] The health care professional's role was viewed as a referral source so that "treatment" for the "condition" could be initiated by a psychiatrist. These contentions and proclamations were frequently based on theoretical notions and clinical descriptions of distraught patients who presented themselves to mental health professionals for some form of cure.

By comparison, adolescents who were troubled or uncertain as to their sexual behavior and orientation often escaped such condemnation; the psychodynamics of their sexuality accepted an "allowable" homosexuality which would be gradually replaced by heterosexuality.[85] In clinical psychology a "normal" homosexual stage in early adolescence was viewed by some as comparable to sleep disturbances or enuresis: Teenagers were expected to outgrow these developmental problems. Normal boys and girls only engage in homosexual behavior for physical release; such experiences were more readily available in our sex-repressive society. Homosexual behavior may even be necessary for some heterosexual youths because it fosters same-sex bonding and support. Typically, this so-called normal homosexual stage was presumed to last into early to middle adolescence, followed by a move to heterosexuality. To some, such as Glasser,[49] homosexual adolescents did not exist because it was only after the immaturity and experimentation of adolescence were completed that one could determine sexual orientation. If adults attempted to interfere, then homosexual attachments could become intense and exclusive. More overt homosexual activity would develop with a concomitant absence of motivation to "advance" to sexual activity with the other sex. Throughout these writings, it is emphasized that adolescents *must* make the choice to "progress" to heterosexuality.

In the medical literature Schwanberg[83] noted that in the decade before AIDS awareness (1974–1983) the psychological health of gay men and lesbians was generally ignored by health care providers. Many lesbians and gays reported problems with the doctor–patient relationship because of the naivete and homophobia of the medical profession and their fear that the quality of health care would decrease if they revealed their sexual orientation.[86] This situation is particularly problematic for pediatricians who are responsible for the care of young "pre-gay" or gay children and adolescents.[34,87]

In 1969 the journal *Pediatrics* first recognized the importance of adolescent homosexuality for scientific and humanistic reasons, but it was still considered to be a "developmental deviance."[88] Fourteen years later the American Academy of Pediatrics' Committee on Adolescence[10] had a quite different perspective. They asserted that homosexuality is established before adolescence; homosexual behavior is common in the development of conventional heterosexuality; homosexual behavior may occur given particular environmental contexts (incarceration, single-sex boarding schools, military barracks); and problems with homosexuality are usually the consequence of social conditions rather than of mental illness. It was now argued that pediatricians needed to maintain a positive attitude toward homosexuality:

> The pediatrician must be entirely non-judgmental in posing sexual questions if he or she is to be at all effective in encouraging the teenager to share his or her concerns, experiences, and beliefs. Only with adequate information of this kind can there be proper medical assessment of the potential consequences of homosexual practice or fears. If the history includes open-ended questions about homosexual beliefs, practices, and experiences, then the pediatrician may elicit items that require either further investigation and evaluation, or possibly referral (pp. 249–250).

If unable to be nonjudgmental, the pediatrician should refer the patient to someone who can be. The physician's responsibility is

> [to] provide health care for homosexual adolescents and guidance for those young people struggling with problems of sexual expression. The pediatrician can play a role in the evaluation and care of those adolescents who are concerned about their expression of sexual preference by offering reassurance to those in discomfort because of early adolescent homosexual experience; willingness to help or refer for help those in difficulty with family, peers, or institutions; and by being familiar with community resources for teenaged homosexuals and their parents if referral for social and emotional stress is required (p. 250).

Some gays and lesbians use psychological services to help them cope with discrimination and homophobic attitudes, and to assist them in developing a positive, fulfilling gay/lesbian lifestyle. Indeed, some mental health professionals refuse to "treat" those who wish to change their sexual orientation.

All too frequently, however, these services are available only to adults and not to adolescents. This deficiency is due primarily to the invisibility of lesbian and gay adolescents in society at large, and to the attitudes and beliefs of health care providers. These occurrences contribute to a sense of alienation and stress for individual adolescents that is frequently noted by various theoretical models and, occasionally, by empirical evidence. As a result, those concerned with the education and health of adolescents frequently deny that youth are at risk for health related problems and thus in need of intervention programs. The urgency of a more open and informed health care community is clear in light of the prevalence of AIDS and the growing realization that some youth may be especially susceptible.[34,87]

Strategies for Health Care Professionals

To receive appropriate, informed, and nonjudgmental medical care it is crucial that a positive relationship is developed between adolescents and health care professionals. In light of the reported incidence of homosexual activity among adolescents, it is highly likely that most pediatricians, nurses, psychologists, and other health care professionals have cared for teenagers who are gay/lesbian or at least who have had same-sex contact. In some cases, health care providers maintain an objective treatment stance toward their clients regardless of sexual orientation or sexual experiences. Other health care providers, however, may be less than objective and harbor traditional antihomosexual biases in interactions with clients who are self-identified as lesbian or gay. In these instances, adolescents may expect to receive less than optimal professional services (e.g., refused certain examinations), to be subjected to outright discrimination (e.g., refused particular services), or to undergo outdated and/or inappropriate care (e.g., automatic referral to a psychiatrist for treatment).

A more pervasive but less obvious form of inadequate professional care may be the result of a heterosexist bias. It may be assumed that all adolescents are heterosexual in orientation and only engage in heterosexual behaviors. The potential danger of making such an assumption is multifaceted. For example, adolescents may assume they are not in danger as a result of their sexual activities because they were not discussed by their physician; important medical examinations peculiar to homosexually active teenagers may not be included or inappropriately performed (e.g., cultures taken from wrong body areas); and youths may perceive the attitudes and actions of the health care professional as one more attack on their sexual identity. As a consequence, adolescents may continue to hide their true self, failing to share important and appropriate information the next time they seek assistance from health care providers. Exposure to HIV may be undiagnosed with the additional danger of an increased probability of contaminating others. Needless to say, health care personnel must be aware of the unique problems of lesbian and gay youth, must eliminate all forms of heterosexist bias and misinformation when conducting a sexual history, and must strive for a nonjudgmental, objective attitude in interactions with adolescents if adequate, sensitive care is to be provided.

There are, we believe, appropriate guidelines to be followed by health care providers during their professional interactions with adolescent clients, regardless of actual or supposed sexual orientation. These are reviewed in the sections that follow.

Use Nonjudgmental Language

Assessments of sexual history and current sexual practices should be in terms free of judgmental language, such as "You aren't gay are you?" or that reflect a heterosexist bias, such as "Did you protect yourself from pregnancy in your sexual contact?" One of the most important features of communicating an objective, caring attitude is using language devoid of common misconceptions, preconceived assumptions, and discriminatory stereotypes. Questions should invite openness and acceptance regarding all forms of sexual behavior and sexual orientation—"Have you ever had sex? Was it with a boy (man) or girl (woman)?"—and should allow adolescents to speak freely and honestly about any and all sexual behavior. A brief rationale for asking such questions can be provided: "In order to provide you with the best care, I need to ask some specific questions about some sexual experiences. I make no assumptions about who you are, who your partners have been, and what sexual activities you might have had." Such questions may be preceded by a brief description of sexual behavior common during adolescence and by an explanation that these queries are asked of all youths.

Take the Opportunity to Educate

In their interactions with adolescent clients, health care personnel may also serve as valuable educational resources regarding homosexuality and homosexual behavior, thus correcting public stereotypes while also insuring strict confidentiality. Health care specialists should supply factual, nonjudgmental information with respect to issues of sexual orientation, such as noting the importance of differentiating sexual behavior and orientation. A continuum[43] model of sexuality without clear separation of heterosexuality and homosexuality but with a range inclusive of many varieties of sexual impulses, feelings, attractions, and behaviors can be discussed. Where one places oneself on this continuum, especially for adolescents, may vary with time, circumstance, and experience. It should also be emphasized that homosexual behavior *per se* need not be prohibited (and, indeed, is likely to occur regardless of what is said), but that adolescents must reduce potentially high risk behaviors and sexual practices without adequate protection.

Appreciate the Sexuality of Adolescents

Awareness of the varied sexual lives of teenagers is a great asset in providing relevant health care and preventive measures related to AIDS. Regardless of reported orientation, adolescents tend to engage in a variety of sexual practices with members of both sexes, thereby making it critical to assess specific sexual behaviors and experiences rather than reported sexual identity. In medical examinations, a set of evaluation questions that invite openness and communicate that unbiased, informed, and sensitive care is to be expected should be developed. A reasonable rationale for assessment questions and for the importance of avoiding the dangers of making assumptions about others' sexuality should be provided.

Learn about Homosexual Activity and Homosexuality

Health care workers should apprise themselves of the special medical risks and appropriate tests and cultures that need to be considered when learning that patients have experienced or might engage in homosexual activities. One should be abreast of current knowledge concerning AIDS, especially in regard to its nature, transmission, risk behaviors, and preventive and educational programs. Sensitivity to various social, psychological, and behavioral problems that stem from sexual orientation confusion or a recognition of gay/lesbian identity is to be encouraged. Because health care providers may be selected as the first person with whom these issues are explored, open discussion and appropriate medical information should be provided.

Serve as a Referral Source

An important part of the evaluation process is a sensitivity to emotional and psychological distress that may emanate from coping with what adolescents might perceive to be a deviant sexuality. Referrals should be made to supportive, caring, and nonjudgmental mental health professionals who are willing to assist youth in the process of exploring sexual feelings, thoughts, fantasies, and life-styles in an environment that does not promote a particular orientation or that is unfettered by expectations of certain developmental outcomes. If warranted, referrals to various community homophile organizations might be made.

Provide Professional Leadership in Righting Wrongs

Given that the helping professions in our society have assumed an increasing responsibility in proclaiming moral evaluations in regard to appropriate sexual behaviors, such personnel should support and follow their professional organizations' resolutions that affirm the rights of gay and lesbian people. It is incumbent upon the professional to assume the responsibility of assuring patients that first-rate, nonjudgmental mental health and medical care will be rendered regardless of sexual orientation and to assist their teenaged clients in accepting their sexual orientation. In their positions as health care providers, these professionals can begin to eliminate many of the societal stigmas regarding gay and lesbian individuals. Because gay and lesbian adolescents may greatly benefit from knowledge of and contact with gay-identified health professionals who lead positive, self-affirming, and fulfilling gay/lesbian lifestyles, health care workers who are "out" may provide a critical leadership function. Others may provide leadership by ensuring that education and training experiences that foster the development of accurately informed attitudes and beliefs in accordance with current professional standards are made available to all trainees during professional education. Continuing education programs are strongly advised as well. Finally, because community agencies affiliated with health care need to develop resource materials regarding professional referral sources, health care leaders who are particularly interested and willing to become involved in and improve the physical and psychological health care of lesbian and gay teenagers are needed.

Summary

Regardless of specific profession or sexual orientation, health care personnel can serve as (1) educators, providing both heterosexual and gay and lesbian teenagers with accurate, unbiased information regarding homosexual behavior and gay lifestyles; (2) sources of referral for individuals experiencing physical, psychological, or behavioral difficulties; and (3) agents of change, correcting stereotyped and misinformed attitudes and supporting a positive, accepting viewpoint of homosexuality.

Strategies for Health Educators

Homosexuality and homosexual behavior should be included as a significant portion of school health education material because (1) a substantial number of students have same-sex sexual feelings, engage in homosexual activities, and/or are gay-oriented; (2) many youths have misconceptions and accept inaccurate information about homosexuality; and (3) homosexuality necessarily raises certain fundamental moral issues for some individuals (e.g., should one act on one's homosexual feelings?).[89] These factors emphasize the unique position of health educators to contribute significantly to the education of students with respect to these issues. Many of the guidelines noted with health care providers are also appropriate here. There are, in addition, several other strategies for health educators.

Educational Source

As instructor, health educators can assist students in developing an objective, knowledgeable, and positive stance toward various sexual life-styles by providing accurate and descriptive accounts of adolescent sexuality, homosexual behavior, and sexual orientation development. This form of intervention not only supplies support and guidance for lesbian and gay adolescents but it also encourages peers to develop and maintain a more enlightened, informed attitude system and corrects cultural stereotypes, misinformation, and discriminatory attitudes. Critical issues include noting the continuum of human sexuality; differentiating sexual behavior and sexual identity; clarifying the origins and nature of homosexual behavior and gay identity; discussing the "normality" or "naturalness" issue; and emphasizing that all students, regardless of sexual orientation, should have the possibility to live a satisfying fulfilling life. With respect to the last of these, exposure to a variety of gay and lesbian members in the community may be quite powerful in providing positive role models who assist in the process of dispelling stereotypes.[50]

Referral Source

Similar to health care providers, health educators should be knowledgeable as to community referral sources for adolescents who are experiencing personal problems with sexual behavior, identity, family members, behavioral consequences, and so forth. Appropriate guidance and continuing support should be provided. To do otherwise might contribute to the development or persistence of a number of the psychosocial and stress-related problems described earlier.

Agent of Change

Health educators assume the role of an agent of change in society de facto as a result of their position in education. This responsibility needs to be recognized and accepted. Coincidentally, these professionals are products of the same society in which they are trying to bring about change; they may hold the same biased viewpoints, demonstrate homophobic attitudes, and be susceptible to peer and societal pressure. Yet, they hold a very unique position in terms of encouraging and initiating attitude change, and therefore they must ask themselves if they are willing to accept and appreciate the social impact of their position. Auxiliary supervision and/or training and educational experiences may help in fulfilling these expectations.

Summary

Chng[50] suggested specific strategies for health educators to accomplish these goals. First, educators can serve as role models in communicating appropriate societal attitudes to the young and by correcting misinformation. This goal can be achieved in all interactions, both in and out of the school, and in various subtle and deliberate ways. Second, role playing, the technique of assuming the posture, attitudes, and feelings of another, may encourage empathy and insight into the emotional and personal lives of lesbian and gay students. Finally, adolescents can expand their experiences and notions of gay men and lesbians and their life-styles through exposure to gay and lesbian members of the community. The support and cooperation from a broad spectrum of school personnel, administrators, and social agencies may be highly significant in achieving these ends. It is unfortunate that relatively few data exist that impinge on the issue of efficacy of such intervention programs.

One critical area that is amenable to change is the representation of homosexuality and gay life-styles in publications of health science and sex education. Given that these sources are readily available to both educators and students and are frequently used to supplement classroom discussions, the importance of the manner in which homosexuality is treated becomes evident. Newton[90] reviewed coverage of homosexuality in 35 publicly available textbooks, trade books, and pamphlets. Only 10 referred to homosexuality, with one giving it significant attention. An edited volume of 464 pages by Coates et al.[91] on adolescent health includes three sentences referring to homosexuality. Generally, discussions of homosexuality contained numerous hidden biases and factual errors. For example, most investigators appeared to hold the "liberal" belief that homosexual behavior can be tolerated during adolescence, as long as it does not continue beyond middle adolescence. The professionals who authored these publications contributed not only to the invisibility of homosexuality but frequently reiterated and supported common stereotypes and misinformation. Reading materials for health education classes should conform to two important standards: an accurate and objective reporting of the most recently available factual information regarding homosexual activity and gay life-styles and an absence of moralistic and judgmental proclamations.

Creating a more accepting climate for homosexuality in the high school setting may be extremely difficult. Greenberg's[92] study showed little impact on students' faith in people, their acceptance of differences of others, or their masculinity and femininity as the result of a unit on homosexuality that entailed 15 40-min/day sessions for 3 weeks. Similarly, Calicchia and Governali[93] discovered that when students role-played a homosexual, a more accepting attitude toward homosexuality was not demonstrated. These studies suggested that longstanding attitudes cannot be altered easily, nor are they likely to be strongly influenced by a single educational event. Additional, and perhaps more creative, techniques are needed, and it may be more advantageous to institute such programs before adolescence. It will be important to conduct program evaluation studies in order to indicate which intervention strategies are most effective in producing attitude changes. They will likely only succeed if they have the approval and support for such interventions by parents, other staff members, and school administrative personnel.

NEEDS OF GAY AND LESBIAN ADOLESCENTS

Gonsiorek[94] maintained that gay and lesbian adolescents need social support services as much as they need mental health services. The latter implies that something needs "fixing"; the former, that a hostile psychosocial environment is a primary cause and promoter of both the external plight of lesbian and gay youth and their internalized homophobia. If psychotherapy is elected by youth, then the focus should include pressures society creates for lesbian and gay individuals.[95] Many gay and lesbian adolescents come out not because of an internalized need for "self-actualization" or self-consistency, as implicated in many of the coming out models, but because they are "forced" or "pushed" out by peers or because their previous denial strategies collapsed.[94] Peer support groups might be helpful for many but, with few exceptions, they are unavailable—or adolescents do not know how to find one.[74]

Although support groups and programs have been established in some communities, usually urban, few youths know about or attend them. Exposure to issues of homosexuality commonly revolves around media coverage that tends to focus on the "disease of homosexuals" (AIDS), the fringes of homosexuality (drag queens, leather bars), and homosexual crimes (sexual molestations of children).[95] These are not positive gay images for developing youth. If minority group members hold their group in low esteem then they too tend to have low self-esteem and self-attitudes.[96] McDonald[42] confirmed this for gays: Negative-identified individuals felt guilty and ashamed of being homosexual. The negative views can only be changed if youth are exposed to nonprejudicial, antigay attitudes.[60]

Several writers have outlined what they feel are the kinds of intervention programs lesbian and gay adolescents need. Here we take Martin's[60,79] outline as a starting point.

1. Access to accurate information—especially related to homosexuality as a normal sexual, psychological, and behavioral variation—in public libraries, schools, novels and fiction, and textbooks. Thus, adolescents will be open "to the possibility

of maintaining one's personal, social, ethical, and professional integrity with the homosexual attribute" (p. 63).[60]

2. Greater and more accurate coverage of homosexuality in sex and health education classes that includes invitations to appropriate medical personnel to participate. The curricula should discuss health care activities (e.g., exercise, eating habits, coping with stress, relaxation paradigms); provide accurate and realistic information regarding learning "safer sex" behavioral repertoire, developing conversation skills for gathering information about potential partners, and learning to negotiate specific sexual behaviors; and suggest guidelines for how adolescents can further discuss these issues on a personal basis with private physicians.
3. Availability of positive adult lesbian and gay role models in schools, churches, community organizations, and elsewhere in the natural world of adolescents. This requires gay and lesbian adults who have the courage and strength to be open[60] and who can create a nonsexual and nonjudgmental atmosphere.[78,94]
4. Places where lesbian and gay adolescents have the opportunity to engage in meaningful peer environments and to develop interpersonal skills and psychologically healthy attitudes and behaviors free from anxiety, exposure, and censure.[60,94] These places should provide a nonsexual setting for teenagers to have social contact with other gays and lesbians that promotes positive social interactions and an interpersonal atmosphere that permits the formation of friendships and supportive relationships. Detailed discussions regarding being gay or lesbian in a homophobic society should be conducted with the goal of providing a desensitization experience through disconfirmation of widely-held stereotypes, correcting misinformation, and confronting participants' internalized homophobic attitudes. Specific psychological and behavioral strategies for reducing depression and anxiety, improving self-esteem and feelings of self-worth, and countering internal criticisms should be reviewed and encouraged. Role plays and discussions regarding interactions with nongay friends and peers should be conducted in order to foster a sense of self-confidence and to provide a behavioral repertoire for coping with these situations.
5. The formation of support/education groups, led by informed, supportive, and concerned mental health professionals with a special interest in this area. Particularly beneficial would be gay and lesbian leaders who could become positive role models.
6. Opportunities to address familial relationships on terms that gay and lesbian youths find acceptable.[79,94]

These are not easy agenda items, and yet they are mandatory intervention strategies if lesbian and gay adolescents are to reduce the amount of psychosocial stress that they feel due to spending their formative years in a homophobic society. With such efforts, the incidence of AIDS among adolescents would be kept to a minimum.

CONCLUSIONS

We believe that the best paradigm to reduce the incidence of AIDS among gay, lesbian, or homosexually behaving adolescents is a biobehavioral one. The emphasis in this chapter has been to describe in some detail (1) the sources of stress that gay and lesbian adolescents frequently encounter, (2) the role of psychosocial stress in compromising adolescents to make contact with and then handicap their ability to counter HIV and AIDS, and (3) guidelines for intervention strategies that will reduce the prevalence of (1), hence (2) above.

These conclusions must be considered tentative, largely because the connection between stress and AIDS reduction among adolescents is speculative at this point. Clearly this must be a top research priority—and there is evidence that creative and concerned scientists have undertaken this task.[31]

Because the prevalence of AIDS among adolescents has been, quite fortunately, low, we fear complacency and inattention to the risks that many adolescents are encountering as a result of engaging in many high-risk sexual behaviors. Empirical research should be continued that monitors the sexual practices and the health-promoting and health-damaging behaviors of adolescents that will, we hope, make us less than prophetic concerning a future catastrophe of youthful people with AIDS.

Finally, Coates et al.[24] stressed the need for research that (1) assesses the current attitudes, beliefs, and practices of health care providers toward homosexuality in general and AIDS in particular; (2) distills basic information on the issues discussed in this chapter (e.g., contribution of psychosocial stress to medical status); and (3) explores knowledge and strategies that are needed to develop intervention programs that have potential to help health care providers improve their ability to address the psychosocial and medical needs of their clients. We wholeheartedly concur.

The balance of providing the next generation with a healthy group of lesbian and gay adults rests with our ability to conduct the biobehavioral research and educational programs necessary to prevent and control AIDS among our lesbian and gay adolescents. We cannot afford to fail.

REFERENCES

1. Savin-Williams RC: *Gay and Lesbian Youth: Expressions of Identity*. Washington, DC, Hemisphere, 1990.
2. Robinson G: Few solutions for a young dilemma. *Advocate* pp. 14–16, 1984.
3. Albert TJ, Cline F, Feigen GM, et al: Medical problems of homosexuals. *Med Aspects Hum Sex* 17:58–81, 1983.
4. American Medical Association's Council on Scientific Affairs: Health care needs of a homosexual population. *JAMA* 248:736–739, 1982.
5. Ostrow DG, Sandholzer TA, Felman YM: *Sexually Transmitted Diseases in Homosexual Men: Diagnosis, Treatment, and Research*. New York, Plenum, 1983.
6. Centers for Disease Control, AIDS Activity Division: AIDS Weekly Surveillance Report, July 24, United States, 1989.
7. Sladkin KR: Counseling the sexually active teenager: Reflections from pediatric practice. *Pediatrics* 10:681–684, 1985.
8. DiClemente RJ, Boyer CB, Morales ES: Minorities and AIDS: Knowledge, attitudes, and misconceptions among Black and Latino adolescents. *Am J Public Health* 78:55–57, 1988.
9. Rotheram-Borus MJ, Bradley J: Prevention of HIV infection among adolescents, in Blumenthal S, Eichler A, Weissman, G (eds): *Women and AIDS: Promoting Healthy Behaviors*. Washington, DC, American Psychiatric Press, in press.
10. Bingham CR: AIDS and adolescents: Threat of infection and approaches for prevention. *J Early Adolesc* 9:50–66, 1989.

11. Brooks-Gunn J, Boyer CB, Hein K: Preventing HIV infection and AIDS in children and adolescents: Behavioral research and intervention strategies. *Am Psychol* 43:958–964, 1988.
12. Mantell JE, Schinke SP: The crisis of AIDS for adolescents: The need for preventive risk-reduction interventions, in Roberts AR (ed): *Contemporary Perspectives on Crisis Intervention and Prevention.* New York, Prentice-Hall, in press.
13. Hein K: AIDS in adolescence: Exploring the challenge. *J Adolesc Health Care* 10:10S–35S, 1989.
14. Rotheram-Borus MJ, Koopman C: AIDS and adolescents, in Lerner R, Peterson A, Brooks-Gunn, J (eds): *The Encyclopedia of Adolescence.* New York, Garland, in press.
15. Flora JA, Thoresen CE: Reducing the risk of AIDS in adolescents. *Am Psychol* 43:965–970, 1988.
16. Jaffe LR, Wortman RN: The fear of AIDS. *J Adolesc Health Care* 9:84–86, 1988.
17. Remafedi G: Preventing the sexual transmission of AIDS during adolescence. *J Adolesc Health Care* 9:139–143, 1988.
18. DiClemente RJ, Boyer CB, Mills SJ: Prevention of AIDS among adolescents: Strategies for the development of comprehensive risk-reduction health education program. *Health Educ Res* 2:287–291, 1987.
19. de Neergaard L: Reaching adolescents in school in Denmark about AIDS. *Hygie* 7:32–33, 1988.
20. Rotheram-Borus MJ, Koopman C: Adolescent AIDS awareness for runaway and gay youth: A preliminary report of the Triple A Project. *Multicult Inquiry Res Aids* 3:1–4, 1989.
21. Rotheram-Borus MJ, Selfridge C, Koopman S et al: The relationship of knowledge and attitudes towards AIDS to safe sex practice among runaway and gay adolescents, in *The International Conference on AIDS, Montreal, Canada,* 1989.
22. Owen WF: Medical problems of the homosexual adolescent. *J Adolesc Health Care* 6:278–285, 1985.
23. Zenilman J: Sexually transmitted diseases in homosexual adolescents. *J Adolesc Health Care* 9:129–138, 1988.
24. Coates TJ, Temoshok L, Mandel J: Psychosocial research is essential to understanding and treating AIDS. *Am Psychol* 39:1309–1314, 1984.
25. Rutter M: Psychosocial resilience and protective mechanisms. *Am J Orthopsychiatry* 57:316–331, 1987.
26. Temoshok L: Emotion, adaptation, and disease: A multidimensional theory, in Temoshok L, Van Dyke C, Zegans LS (eds): *Emotions in Health and Illness: Theoretical and Research Foundations.* New York, Grune & Stratton, 1983, pp 207–234.
27. Garmezy N: Stress resistant children: The search for protective factors, in Stevenson J (ed): *Recent Research in Developmental Psychopathology.* Oxford, Pergamon, 1985.
28. Levy JA, Ziegler JL: Acquired immunodeficiency syndrome is an opportunistic infection and Kaposi's sarcoma results from secondary immune stimulation. *Lancet* 1:78–80, 1983.
29. Berkman LF, Syme SL: Social networks, host resistance and mortality: A nine-year follow-up study of Alameda County residents. *Am J Epidemiol* 109:186–204, 1979.
30. Kaplan GA: Psychosocial aspects of chronic illness: Direct and indirect associations with ischemic heart disease mortality, in Kaplan RM, Criqui MH (eds): *Behavioral Epidemiology and Disease Prevention.* New York, Plenum, 1985, pp 237–269.
31. Mechanic D: Adolescent health and illness behavior: Review of the literature and a new hypothesis for the study of stress. *J Hum Stress* 9:4–13, 1983.
32. Buss AH: *Self-Consciousness and Social Anxiety.* San Francisco, WH Freeman, 1980.
33. Bell AP, Weinberg MS, Hammersmith SK: *Sexual Preference: Its Development in Men and Women.* Bloomington, Indiana: Indiana University Press, 1981.
34. Rigg CA: Homosexuality in adolescence. *Pediatr Ann* 11:826–829, 1982.
35. Boxer AM: Betwixt and between: Developmental discontinuities of gay and lesbian youth, in *The Society for Research on Adolescence, Alexandria, Virginia,* 1988.
36. Remafedi G: Male Homosexuality: The adolescent's perspective. *Pediatrics* 79:326–330, 1987.
37. Roesler T, Deisher R: Youthful male homosexuality. *JAMA* 219:1018–1023, 1972.
38. Sanders G: (1980). Homosexualities in the Netherlands. *Alternative Lifestyles* 3:278–311, 1980.
39. Manosevitz M: Early sexual behavior in adult homosexual and heterosexual males. *J Abnorm Psychol* 76:396–402, 1970.
40. Dank BM: Coming out in the gay world. *Psychiatry* 34:180–197, 1971.
41. Koodin H, Morin S, Riddle D, et al: Removing the Stigma. Final Report. Task Force on the Status of Lesbian and Gay Male Psychologists. Washington, DC, American Psychological Association, 1979.

42. McDonald GJ: Individual differences in the coming out process for gay men: Implications for theoretical models. *J Homosex* 8:47–60, 1982.
43. Saghir MT, Robins E, Walbran B: Homosexuality. II. Sexual behavior of the male homosexual. *Arch Gen Psychiatry* 21:219–229, 1969.
44. Kinsey AC, Pomeroy WB, Martin CE: *Sexual Behavior in the Human Male*. Philadelphia, WB Saunders, 1948.
45. Van Wyk PH, Geist CS: Psychosocial development of heterosexual, bisexual, and homosexual behavior. *Arch Sex Behav* 13:505–544, 1984.
46. Kimmel D: Adult development and aging: A gay perspective. *J Social Issues* 34:113–130, 1978.
47. Malyon AK: The homosexual adolescent: Developmental issues and social bias. *Child Welfare* 60:321–330, 1981.
48. Ross-Reynolds G: Issues in counseling the "homosexual" adolescent, in Grimes J (ed): *Psychological Approaches to Problems of Children and Adolescents*. Des Moines, Iowa State Department of Education, 1982, pp. 55–88.
49. Glasser M: Homosexuality in adolescence. *Br J Med Psychol* 50:217–225, 1977.
50. Chng CL: Adolescent homosexual behavior and the health educator. *J School Health* 61:517–520, 1980.
51. Savin-Williams RC: An ethological perspective on homosexuality during adolescence. *J Adolesc Res* 2:283–302, 1987.
52. MacDonald GB: Exploring sexual identity: Gay people and their families. *Sex Educ Coalition News* 5:1, 4, 1983.
53. Robertson R: Young gays, in Hart J, Richardson D (eds): *The Theory and Practice of Homosexuality*. London, Routledge & Kegan Paul, 1981, pp 170–176.
54. Grellert EA: Childhood play behavior of homosexual and heterosexual men. *Psychol Rep* 51:607–610, 1982.
55. Saghir MT, Robins E: *Male and Female Homosexuality*. Baltimore, Williams & Wilkins, 1973.
56. Troiden RR: Becoming homosexual: A model of gay identity acquisition. *Psychiatry* 42:362–373, 1979.
57. Green R: *The "Sissy Boys Syndrome" and the Development of Homosexuality*. New Haven, Yale University Press, 1987.
58. Coleman E: Developmental states of the coming out process. *J Homosex* 7:31–43, 1982.
59. Fisher R: *The Gay Mystique: The Myth and Reality of Male Homosexuality*. New York, Stein & Day, 1972.
60. Martin AD: Learning to hide: The socialization of the gay adolescent. *Adolesc Psychiatry* 10:52–65, 1982.
61. Jay K, Young A: *The Gay Report*. New York: Summit, 1977.
62. Cass V: Homosexual identity formation: A theoretical model. *J Homosex* 4:219–235, 1979.
63. Lee JA: Going public: A study in the sociology of homosexual liberation. *J Homosex* 3:49–78, 1977.
64. Weinberg MS, Williams CJ: *Male Homosexuals: Their Problems and Adaptations*. New York, Penguin, 1974.
65. Braaten LJ, Darling CD: Overt and covert homosexual problems among male college students. *Genet Psychol Monogr* 71:269–310, 1965.
66. Myrick FL: Homosexual types: An empirical investigation. *J Sex Res* 10:226–237, 1984.
67. Jourard SM: *The Transparent Self*, ed 2. New York, Van Nostrand, 1971.
68. Maslow A: *Motivation and Personality*. New York, Harper, 1954.
69. deMonteflores C, Schultz SJ: Coming out: Similarities and differences for lesbians and gay men. *J Social Issues* 34:59–72, 1978.
70. Harry J, DeVall WB: *The Social Organization of Gay Males*. New York: Praeger, 1978.
71. Price JH: High school students' attitudes toward homosexuality. *J School Health* 52:469–474, 1982.
72. Sobel HJ: Adolescent attitudes toward homosexuality in relation to self-concept and body satisfaction. *Adolescence* 11:443–453, 1976.
73. Sorensen R: *Adolescent Sexuality in Contemporary Society*. New York: World Book, 1973.
74. Rofes EE: Youth: New identities, new issue. *Advocate* November 27, 1984.
75. Deisher RW, Eisner V, Sulzsbacher SI: The young male prostitute. *Pediatrics* 43:936–941, 1969.
76. Gandy P, Deisher RW: Young male prostitutes: The physician's role in social rehabilitation. *JAMA* 212:1661–1666, 1970.
77. Harris M: *The Dilly Boys: Male Prostitution in Piccadilly*. London, Croom Helm, 1973.
78. Letourneau D: Juvenile male prostitution, in *Symposium on Gay and Lesbian Adolescents, Minneapolis, Minnesota, May 30–31, 1986*.

79. Martin D: Social and educational programs for gay and lesbian youth, in *Symposium on Gay and Lesbian Adolescents, Minneapolis, Minnesota, May 30–31, 1986.*
80. Burnison M: Runaway youth: Lesbian and gay issues, in *Symposium on Gay and Lesbian Adolescents, Minneapolis, Minnesota, May 30–31, 1986.*
81. Deisher R, Robinson G, Boyer D: The adolescent female and male prostitute. *Pediatr Ann* 11:819–825, 1982.
82. Remafedi G: *Symposium on Gay and Lesbian Adolescents, Minneapolis, Minnesota, May 30–31, 1986.*
83. Schwanberg SL: Changes in labeling homosexuality in health sciences literature: A preliminary investigation. *J Homosex* 12:51–73, 1985.
84. Kriegman G: Homosexuality and the educator. *J School Health* 39:305–311, 1969.
85. Robinson LH: Adolescent homosexual patterns: Psychodynamics and therapy. *Adolesc Psychiatry* 8:422–433, 1980.
86. Golden E: Health care for gay men and lesbians: Problems and prospects, Unpublished manuscript. Ithaca, New York, Cornell University, 1985.
87. Remafedi GJ: Adolescent homosexuality: Issues for pediatricians. *Clin Pediatr* 24:481–485, 1985.
88. Solnit AJ: Bisexuality gone awry: The child is father to the man. *Pediatrics* 43:913–914, 1969.
89. Newton DE, Risch SJ: Homosexuality and education: A review of the issue. *High School J* 68:191–202, 1981.
90. Newton DE: Representations of homosexuality in health science textbooks. *J Homosex* 4:247–254, 1979.
91. Coates TJ, Petersen AC, Perry CL (eds): *Promoting Adolescent Health: A Dialog in Research and Practice.* New York, Academic Press, 1982.
92. Greenberg JS: A study of personality change associated with the conducting of a high school unit on homosexuality. *J School Health* 45:394–398, 1975.
93. Calicchia CA, Governali JF: Attitudes toward homosexuality: Does role-playing have an impact? Health values: Achieving high level wellness. 4:176–182, 1980.
94. Gonsiorek JC: Mental health problems of gay and lesbian youth, in *Symposium on Gay and Lesbian Adolescents, Minneapolis, Minnesota, May 30–31, 1986.*
95. Hart J, Richardson D: *The Theory and Practice of Homosexuality.* Boston, Routledge & Kegan Paul, 1981.
96. Stephan WG, Rosenfield D: Black self-rejection: Another look. *J Educ Psychol* 71:708–716, 1979.

5

Women at High Risk of HIV Infection

Behavioral, Prevention, and Intervention Aspects

DOOLEY WORTH

INTRODUCTION

The need to know how individual women respond to and make decisions about acquired immune deficiency syndrome (AIDS)-related risk-taking behaviors has only recently come to the attention of psychosocial researchers. Before 1986, there was little recognition of HIV infection as a "women's problem."[1] When public awareness of AIDS as a "heterosexual" problem developed, attention was focused on female prostitutes (who were seen as possible vectors of transmission to their male clients, although there was little evidence for such an assumption)[2] and on women as mothers who were also seen as vectors of transmission—to their unborn children.[3]

Because of the focus of policy-makers and researchers on women as vectors of disease transmission, the psychosocial impact of the risk of human immunodeficiency virus (HIV) infection and illness on women was late in being recognized or researched.[4] For some women, including lesbians, this continues to be the case, although there is a higher rate of intravenous drug use among lesbian and bisexual women than among heterosexual women.[5,6]

Women did not come to the attention of researchers due to several factors; one, the social impact of the disease on women was considered insignificant compared to that on gay men although as Carpenter and Danforth have noted[7]:

> The societal impact of HIV in women is disproportionately large, both because of the effects of maternal HIV infection on family dynamics and because obligations to children often interfere with health care of the mother.

Furthermore, the lack of public funding for HIV-related risk reduction programs meant that the majority of such programs were mounted privately, primarily by volunteer

DOOLEY WORTH • Montefiore Medical Center and Department of Epidemiology and Social Medicine, The Women's Center, Bronx New York 10467.

efforts in the gay community, which responded to the lack of public funding by developing their own programs. Although women were welcome in such programs, many women feel constrained (by social and cultural mores) from discussing their sexual behavior or articulating their sexual needs in the presence of men, making it difficult for them to participate.

Finally, as AIDS was initially perceived by health professionals to be a male, or more particularly, a "gay male disease," women were often not diagnosed until they were in the later stages of AIDS. Sometimes they were not diagnosed at all.[8]

Research that has been conducted since 1986 provides evidence that women's response to HIV risk depends on among other things, their cultural and risk-taking orientations and socioeconomic status.[9–11] Knowledge about the impact of HIV on women has gradually emerged from counseling and education-based research programs targeted specifically at women at risk of HIV infection.[12] This chapter explores the responses and identifies the needs of women who have acknowledged their possible risk of HIV infection in several such programs: The Women's Group, The Womens' Center, and the Lower East Side Health Project. The Women's Group program, which was initiated in 1986 by the author in cooperation with Dr. Richard Elion of the Stuyvesant Polyclinic and with Susan Rosenthal and Karen Solomon of the New York City Department of Health AIDS Unit, has served as the primary source for the following observations. For the past 2 years, it has been staffed by Department of Health HIV counselors. Over a 3-year period the program provided counseling and referral services to over a thousand self-identifying at-risk women from around the city. Many of the women were referred by the Health Department's HIV Hotline (which provides phone counseling and referrals). Participants included intravenous drug users (IVDUs), women partners of male intravenous drug users, lesbian IVDUs, and their partners, sex partner of bisexual men, women infected through blood transfusions, and infected women who have had multiple partners. The Womens' Center AIDS research project at Montefiore Medical Center addresses women IVDUs in methadone treatment. The Lower East Side Health Project, which is a research project of Narcotic and Drug Research Inc., addresses women IVDUs and sex partners of IVDUs both in and out of treatment.

RISK ACCEPTANCE: WHAT IS THE CONTEXT?

The author's experience working in all three programs indicates that many women at high risk due to their own or their partner's behavior do not face their risk or seek information before there is a crisis, a confrontation, or a program asks them to be tested. The crisis is often the discovery of a partner's risk, disclosure of risk, a specific encounter occurring which makes it hard for them to deny risk, or diagnosis of the women, their partners, children or a loved one.[13]

Even when there is a recognition of the possibility of risk, women employ different means to distance themselves from addressing their need for risk reduction—falling into the "them, not us" syndrome. By their own admission, many of the women who eventually came to the Women's Group program resisted seeking help until there was a crisis, only initiating behavior change related to prevention at that point, when it was often too late to prevent primary or secondary HIV infection. The women IVDUs participating in the

Women's Center at Montefiore did not speak openly about their own risk of HIV infection until they had been coming to support groups for nine months.[10]

Women delay dealing with the issue of being at risk because they are frightened by the implications of risk acknowledgement, e.g., the need to re-evaluate their sexual relationships and possibly undertake major life-style changes. The discrimination which surrounds HIV testing and seropositivity also plays a role, as women fear the social consequences of being labeled "bad girls" should it be known they are at risk or infected.

HIV ANTIBODY TESTING AND RISK REDUCTION

The question of what the role of HIV antibody testing and counseling in risk-reduction programs targeted at women should be is an important one. Currently, HIV antibody testing is being promoted as a means of identifying infected women, so that they may undergo early medical intervention. There are, however, no assurances that the funding for such intervention is or will be made available, particularly to women most at risk: IVDUs. This has created fears that the identification of women IVDUs might increase the discrimination they already experience when seeking health, and social services, housing and employment because of their drug-related risk taking.

Research does indicate that women may respond differently to the process of HIV antibody testing and counseling than men do.[14] The decision about whether or not to undergo HIV antibody testing is one of the first women face when they accept they are at risk of HIV infection. The majority of women who participated in the Women's Group Program, upon learning they were at risk, wanted to be tested. The exception was women IVDUs, women who had shared needles and were most at risk of HIV infection,[15] and who are most likely to suffer further discrimination should it be known they were infected. Many female drug users are tested as part of AIDS research, drug treatment, or rehabilitation programs. As such, the decision to be tested was often seen as "having been made for them." They respond by delaying or not picking up their test results for weeks, months, or even years. When asked why, the women IVDUs said they feared having to confront dying and the need to change their drug using and, secondarily, their sexual behavior. Some did not think they could go on if they knew for sure they were infected. The sex partners of IVDUs, who usually have to decide themselves whether to go and be tested were more likely to want to know their HIV antibody test results.

Women IVDUs in recovery responded that they feared that finding they were infected would threaten their recently established sobriety. Those who have been treated in residential treatment centers [TCs] or who are participating in drug-free twelve-step programs often denied their risk of HIV infection until someone they shot up with became sick, or died of AIDS. This person is not infrequently a sibling or relative as family members often share needles.[16] When this occurs the veil of denial is stripped away, the women's defenses collapse, and, in the ensuing anxiety, their sobriety is threatened. If their recovery program does not have an AIDS educational plan in place to help both the staff (some of whom are ex-addicts) and clients cope with risk acknowledgment, HIV antibody testing, and infection, denial will go unchallenged as it did in the early days of the epidemic in many 12-step programs.

Women who are in recovery (whether in formal programs or not) but who lack adequate support systems, or whose support systems have been destabilized by AIDS, are in danger of returning to shooting drugs temporarily or permanently when they find out they are infected.[17]

Given the often traumatic, life-changing nature of the experience of undergoing HIV antibody testing for women, suggestions that specific groups or populations of women be "routinely tested" have serious social implications. The experience of the author is that for all women at risk the issue of HIV testing *itself* raises serious questions about risk taking (theirs and their partners), health, relationships (including dependency), sexual decision-making, reproductive choices, illness, death and dying, regardless of the outcome of testing. Once these issues have been raised they have to be addressed and worked through with the help of both professionals and other women attempting to cope with the same issues—a lengthy, time-consuming, and sometimes expensive process.

HIV antibody testing has recently been proposed as the cornerstone of "risk-reduction" programs for women, in spite of the feeling of some public health officials that this is an improper role for HIV antibody testing.[4] The case for a pivotal role for HIV testing in risk-reduction programs is not clear. There is insufficient evidence on whether or not traditional HIV antibody testing (with one pre- and posttest session of counseling) plays a significant role in reducing sexual risk taking, and most of it applies to men.[18] Furthermore, research on the effects of knowledge of serostatus on gay men shows increased psychosocial morbidity.[19]

Research does indicate that risk-taking related to needle use and sharing among both women and men IVDUs has been reduced but this appears to a result of street based outreach and education rather than HIV testing.[20,21] Also, needle cleaning is not "new" behavior among IVDUs, as many have always cleaned their works with water—educators have been able to build on this practice by introducing the idea of using bleach and by promoting cleaning of cookers and other works.[22]

Studies of the impact of HIV antibody testing on gay men indicate that it is *the integration of education into life-style behavior* that has the greatest impact on encouraging the initiation of sexual behavior change.[23] Research conducted with gay men showed that seroponegative men were less likely to alter their risk-taking behavior.[18] Similar results have been observed among women crack addicts in New York City. Crack-using women (who are not necessarily needle users) who test negative tend to believe that if they are not already infected that they will not be, so they continue to use crack and have sex to obtain it.[24] Cancellieri et al.[25] found that notification of HIV antibody test results led to increased crack use among both seropositive and seronegative women in New York City.

Research among methadone patients in New York City shows that needle heroin users who find out they are infected often respond by returning to or increasing their needle use raising questions about the efficacy of using HIV testing as a risk-reduction strategy for women IVDU's in treatment for chemical dependency.[17]

THE IMPACT OF HIV ANTIBODY TEST RESULTS

Although individual women who undergo HIV antibody testing have varying responses, from denial to a decision to do everything to live, there are observable response patterns. The period of waiting for the test results is uniformly one of high anxiety; one where women may increase their drug use or be fearful about their recovery.

Negative Test Results

The majority of women who received a negative test result are greatly relieved. There are, however, a small minority who have had repeated exposure to infection who disbelieve their test results and may go so far as to develop false symptoms of the disease.[13] Women who respond this way tend to be members of a discordant couple (one where their partner is infected and there is continued exposure to infection) or women IVDUs (who have shared needles with others who are infected and/or have infected or symptomatic partners).

Women in discordant couples who test antibody negative but whose partners are infected are faced with a unique set of problems, as it is someone else's behavior that puts them at risk, behavior that is embedded in complex relationships based on different types of dependency (e.g., legal, sexual, economic, emotional). Some of the women in discordant couples who test antibody negative express the feeling that "it would be easier to be seropositive," this would allow them to avoid the guilt they feel if they want to leave the relationship because of their fear of being infected by their partner, their fear of not being able to have children with their partner (having to reformulate relationship goals, having to choose between their desire for children and continuing their relationship), their fear of their partner's death, their fear of surviving alone, their fear of becoming a single parent, and their fear they will not be able to handle the burdens imposed by a care-taking role.

Heterosexual women in discordant couples who are infected by their partners, or are at risk of infection often have serious problems in accepting their risk. Because they have been inculcated throughout their lives with the idea of "romantic love," they have a hard time accepting that the man they "love" could infect them. Furthermore, they are subjected to sociocultural and familial pressures that promote the role of motherhood for women. How does a heterosexual woman whose partner is infected explain to her and her partner's family why they are not having children (when they previously expressed their plans to) without explaining that her partner is infected, and how he got infected?

The difficulty of coping with these pressures is reflected in the type of risk reduction noted in one women's program, Project AWARE in San Francisco. The project research shows that there is a lack of development of safe-sex techniques among discordant couples, one fourth abstained from sex altogether, another 33% made no changes in their sexual practices, while 30–40% did indicate some use of safer sex techniques.[26] The same research data indicates that women are more likely to change partners or the type of sex they have (reducing anal sex) than to negotiate for the use of condoms with their partners.[2]

Lesbian women in discordant couples face other emotional dilemmas, such as fears that the donor of sperm that they used for artificial insemination or that the father of their child may have been infected, possibly infecting the mother and or child.[27]

Positive Test Results

The fears of seropositive women in discordant couples are usually focused on whether their partners will leave them to be sick and die alone. Blachman and others suggest this is not an unrealistic fear for heterosexual women, that infected or symptomatic women are more likely to be abandoned by their male partners than the reverse.[28]

Studies have, however, shown that effective counseling for discordant couples can help them by providing support for them to cope with their fears and to cope with the difficult decisions they face.[29] Counseling for discordant couples, like that for other relationships, has to be long term, as in most cases it can take months of steady counseling just to help women change the perception that they are "going to die," to make them aware that the outcome of the disease is slowly changing as medical intervention improves, that they have to concentrate on making decisions about how they will *live* rather than focusing on dying.[30]

The perception of a positive test result being a "death sentence" still exists and triggers an emotional crisis in women who test HIV antibody positive. Women with partners and children tend to isolate themselves, pulling back from important relationships with their children and partners out of fear of infecting them or having to explain they may "desert" them through death.[13]

Single seropositive women also isolate themselves, they often stop dating because they believe it is unethical to be involved with someone and not tell them they are infected. They live with the fear that if they disclose their status to potential partners they will never again have the possibility of an intimate relationship, a devastating possibility for a woman in her 20s or 30s. As there are currently relatively few infected women, it is unlikely that a man will decide to start a new relationship with a woman who is known to be infected. As one young infected woman expressed it, "Why would any man want to start a relationship with me, when there are so many women out there who are not infected?" They also believe that the fact that they are being advised not to have children makes them undesirable partners for many men and rather than be rejected they socially isolate themselves.[13,24,31]

Seropositive women often experience feeling a total loss of control over their lives and their bodies, an experience which results in feelings of loneliness, helplessness, hopelessness, frustration, and *anger*. Anger manifests itself as both serious bouts of depression and/or acting out. Some women direct their anger at men. They feel they are asked to be responsible for men, to take care of men, in many cases the men who have introduced them to drugs, the men who continue to put them at risk through unprotected sex, the men who may have "betrayed" them by having sex with other men without their knowledge. Anger may also be directed at societal norms that designate women "risk managers." The anger that women feel extends to male health care providers with whom they find it difficult if not impossible to discuss sexual questions related to AIDS, and who treat them in a way that makes them feel like victims, afraid to ask for or demand what they really need, be it information, referrals, care, or compassion. Unfortunately, this type of behavior is not limited to male health care providers as some female providers also treat women in a manner that increases their sense of victimization and anger.

Anger is not always externalized, as it is socially or culturally unacceptable in many situations for women to verbalize their anger with men. Instead of verbalizing their feelings of anger, seropositive women may berate themselves for having engaged in behavior that led to their becoming infected, or for having stayed in relationships that were destructive to their self-esteem, relationships based on lies, or abusive behavior. When anger is turned inward a woman's self-esteem suffers increasing her risk as lowered self-esteem leads to women feeling they do not have the right to ask for sexual protection against infection, to fear rejection if they insist on it. A diminishment in self-esteem also results in some women resuming or increasing drug use.[17]

Underlying and increasing women's anger is *fear*—fear of abandonment, or death, and of dying. This fear, hard to face, harder yet to talk about, encompasses their anticipation of their own death, the death of a significant other or child, of having to choose to "live" or "die" with AIDS, of having to gain control of a potentially fatal situation, of dying alone, living through the loss of loved ones.

Not all women who are seropositive respond by acting out or becoming depressed or withdrawn. Individual women, including women who are active IVDUs, are galvanized by the experience to "live their lives to the fullest," seizing control of their health and attempting to alter their risk-taking behavior.[32] This response is noted across "risk groups." Among women IVDUs, for instance, those who have "bottomed out" sometimes use the information that they are infected to change their lives while those who are not at the "end of their run" may see being infected as just one more problem.[31] In some instances, spirituality provides the basis to support women who are changing their lifestyles. The effect of spiritual beliefs and social support, on survival needs to be explored as one component of research on what determines how individual women respond to or make choices about living with HIV infection or related illnesses.[33]

DISCLOSURE OF POSITIVE HIV ANTIBODY RESULTS

Once a seropositive test result is confirmed or a diagnosis made, women are faced with deciding who in their personal lives they can or should tell they are infected. Disclosure in many cases is not just a matter of being infected or ill; it involves telling a partner or family member of their own or a partner's drug use or sexual preference which may previously have been hidden to avoid conflict. It may mean having to address cultural pressures to marry and have children, explaining to family members why there will be not children, why social roles cannot be fulfilled as expected.

Women also have to decide about disclosure outside their family. When they seek medical and social services, they have to be aware of the possible implications of disclosure of test results to medical and other service personnel (e.g., loss of private health insurance, and being denied an abortion).[34,45] Women need help in deciding if, how to, when to, and whom to disclose their HIV status to. The fear of rejection and abandonment which accompanies and informs disclosure is reality based, some partners and families are driven by fears that reside in the larger community and do not react well or embrace the infected woman. For women who define themselves by the man they are with, disclosure strikes at the core of their emotional and social stability for it means facing the loss of their partners but also the status that being with him confers on them socially, emotionally and economically.

While disclosure of serostatus can be limited (to support groups members or a counselor for instance), the decision-making process about it is crucial, it is part of women accepting and acknowledging the changes that HIV infection and illness are bringing about in their and their partner's lives. Without such acknowledgement it is harder for women to cope with the complex, often ambiguous issues that they are faced with. The climate of fear which surrounds AIDS, and by association HIV infection, often makes such disclosure extremely difficult. What may be perceived in the interest of promoting public health (disclosure) may not be in the emotional, social, or economic interest of individual women.

POST-TEST DECISION MAKING

For infected women and those with infected partners sexual choices after testing may become life and death choices. The need to change deep-rooted sexual behaviors, to say "no" to risky sex or use condoms, to refrain from certain types of sex, all have to be negotiated. Partners have to be engaged in these negotiations. For many women, this is either a new experience or one that lies outside of culturally dictated behavior.[35] In cultures in which it is not the norm to discuss sex or intimacy, in which women who do attempt to control their sexuality are perceived as deviating from the cultural ideal, or in which women are brought up to believe that the locus of sexual decision making power lies outside themselves, it is extremely difficult for an individual woman to take it upon herself to initiate safe sex negotiations, to realize that she is going to have to participate in "making the rules" from now on.[10,36]

A shortage of available men (an established fact in many inner-city minority neighborhoods with high rates of unemployment and drug-related crime) may also act as an impediment to a woman introducing the subject of safer sex practices or risk of HIV infection as there is more pressure to be "accommodating" in the face of competition and "man sharing."[10]

Economic factors, such as engaging in prostitution to support a habit, or forming a relationship with an older man, one who supports the woman's habit in exchange for sexual favors (and who the woman may or may not live with or dependence on a running buddy,[37] also come into play and are affected by HIV infection. Many women are faced with what they perceive to be a decision between economic or emotional survival that depends on keeping a male partner, placing economic support or intimacy in opposition to protecting themselves against HIV infection).[10,38]

RESPONSES TO THE NEED FOR SEX-RELATED RISK REDUCTION

Before women can address their need to engage in safer sex practices they need to process the loss of old concepts of themselves, linked to sex preference, sexual practices, their potential for childbearing, and sexual risk-taking. Changes in perceptions of sexuality are exacerbated when infected women have feelings of victimization and anger. A sense of victimization is strongest in sex partners of bisexual men (where gender identity is threatened) who claim not to have known about their partner's risk-taking behavior. It also exists for women IVDUs, many of whom have been victims of incest or rape, and in women who have become infected through blood transfusions.[39] One of the most visible signs of victimatization is low self-esteem. The developing of self-esteem is crucial for women at risk, or who are infected and can be addressed by helping the women to become aware that they have the ability and resources to assume control over their situation (by showing them that they can control small things in their lives first).[40] Women who have been victimized (sexually, physically) have to be given the opportunity to express their feelings, their anger, and the uncertainty such feelings create about their ability to control their sexuality, their sexual desirability, childbearing, and physical survival, and they need to do it with other women in the same or similar circumstances.

Women who have been victimized by men often do not trust other women, they may even see them as threatening. Yet it is women who have had similar experiences and who understand their feelings who most often form the basis of new social and emotional support systems that are necessary for the women to cope with having been abused and its effect on them engaging in risk reduction.

Long-term ongoing changes in sexual behavior, such as the introduction and continued use of condoms, are an adjunct to increased self-esteem, which comes about as women empower each other to take more control over their lives. Only after women have dealt with their feelings about the affect of HIV infection and illness on their and their partners sexuality can they begin to experiment with what is often perceived as "restricted" or "unnatural" sexual behavior. Although there is endless talk about condom use, the most common response of women who find they are at risk of infection is limiting themselves to one partner, changing partners, or having less sex.[26,41] For women IVDUs, limiting themselves to one partner may not offer much protection, as 52% of women IVDUs in NIDA's NADR demonstration projects have male partners who are IVDUs, 89% of whom do not use condoms.[42] Changing partners, or limiting partners, or having less sex allows women to avoid having to confront the need to negotiate to engage in safer sex practices such as the use of condoms, to avoid confronting the power imbalances in their sexual relationships.[7] A small number of women eschew negotiating for sexual protection in favor of increasing unprotected sexual activity with multiple partners. They do this out of anger: "Someone gave it to me, so I am going to pass it on to others."

Sexual abstinence is another response seen in infected women.[43] While it is an appropriate response for an initial period, as it gives the woman time to explore her feelings and to emotionally process what is happening to her, it is a poor long-term solution, particularly for healthy infected women. Healthy women who attempt to remain celibate often engage in risky sex later on if they have not worked out how they feel about changing their sexual behavior or engaging partners in negotiations. Women then "slip" (e.g., engage in unprotected sex) because they are unprepared for sexual encounters.

If a woman's feelings about having to change her sexual behavior are not vented, it is likely that she will respond to overwhelming emotions by building a wall of denial. An inability to respond emotionally to the feelings aroused by knowledge of HIV antibody status is not limited to women. It has also been observed in males IVDUs, who have tremendous difficulty getting in touch with their feelings.[44] Counselors in the Stuyvesant Polyclinic HIV-testing program noted that some male needle users came back repeatedly to be retested because of their fears of abandonment should they tell their partners they were infected.[13] Male IVDUs appear to be more "needy" than women IVDUs for emotional support, if they do not have a partner, or lose a partner because of their serostatus they ordinarily try to find a new one, and as a last resort will choose to be with an infected woman rather than be alone.[24,31]

Infected women, who are socially indoctrinated to respond as caretakers and are more worried about infecting partners, are more likely to stay single should their partner leave them, usually stay in established relationships and are more likely to pursue a new relationship with a seropositive partner.[13]

THE HIV-RELATED NEEDS OF WOMEN

Women respond to risk acknowledgment and HIV antibody testing varyingly depending on how their social, sexual, and economic relationships are related to their risk-taking. The majority of women affected by the disease are victims of sexism, racism, poverty, and have chemical dependency problems. They share many HIV-related needs, needs that for the most part existed prior to AIDS and that have been intensified by AIDS. These needs coincide with, and are different from, those of gay men as women's lives are organized "through many family constellations, ethnic groups and lifestyles."[28]

The context of women's lives, the different constellations they participate in, are changed irrevocably as they confront the impact of HIV on their health, sexual behavior, and reproductive decision-making. The alteration of life-style context both intensifies existing needs of women and creates many new needs.

Women's primary need is to have access to the power to *define their own HIV-related needs* and to be able to participate in making the health and social service systems more responsive to their "perceived" needs. These needs include information, legal, health, mental health, social, and drug treatment services. Women also need support to help them satisfy their sexual and economic needs.

It should be noted that women's sexual decision-making is affected by the fact that they have less economic, social, and political power than men, a fact overlooked by many AIDS educators.[11,45] Because of this, sexual decision-making needs need to be addressed as part of a broader examination of gender socialization across race, class, and culture in the United States.

Information Needs

Women need to know how AIDS is and is not transmitted (including perinatal transmission); how to protect themselves their partners and children against infection (e.g., changing needle-sharing patterns, needle-cleaning practices, becoming drug-free, using condoms); undergoing HIV antibody testing and counseling prior to making decisions about pregnancy, as 78% of women IVDUs are in their childbearing years[46]; how to reconcile their need for contraception with the need for protection against sexually transmitted diseases; how to recognize symptoms of the disease, including how AIDS may present differently in women[8]; the impact of AIDS of reproductive choices; and how to seek the medical, social, and legal services they and their families need.

Legal Needs

The legal needs of HIV-infected women vary across class division and socioeconomic status. Women with fewer economic and social resources (those most at risk) need help in protecting themselves against eviction, loss of jobs, welfare, or health benefits as a result of their own, their partner's or child's HIV infection or illness. Women who are mothers (most women IVDUs and sex partners of IVDUs are) need assistance in planning for the custody of their children, should they and/or their partner become ill. Custody is a complex issue when chemical dependency is involved, as the children may already be in the informal custody of a family member or friend. Women may also need advise on their reproductive rights and how to avoid or resolve problems with the police or parole systems related to their drug use activities.

Health Needs

The health needs of the women most affected by AIDS (primarily poor black and Latino women of childbearing age) are not unfamiliar to health care providers working in inner cities. They currently seek services from a fragmented health care system which increasingly has more restrictive reimbursement rules (which do not allow same day service provision, which limit the number of visits per year or per illness, for example). Few have access to home care services (particularly housekeeping and child care) should they become home bound because of HIV-related illness.

Women affected by HIV infection and illness need programs that can go beyond providing services assisting them in advocating for the type of services they and their children need; low barrier, low-cost health care and health education services, (which explain how their bodies work, particularly their reproductive systems and how drugs affect both). Health care providers are needed who do not discriminate against their clients, and who can explain diagnoses and treatment options in a clear, understandable manner.[47] More specifically, high-quality, culturally and gender-sensitive HIV counseling and testing, access for women to experimental drug protocols, better AIDS-related diagnostic protocols for women, and specialized counseling and contraceptive education are needed for high-risk or infected women.[48,49]

Mental Health Needs

The psychological needs of women who are HIV seropositive or whose partners are vary greatly from those of men. For one thing many women need to know it is alright for them to put their own needs first (they seldom do, particularly when it comes to health care as they have been socialized to assume the role of "care taker" of others). This phenomenon has been noted to be particularly prevalent among women who are sex partners of IVDUs.[50] Women who are mothers need to know that someone cares what happens to *them,* not just their children. This is particularly true of women IVDUs who are severely socially stigmatized and who are often offered services which only address them "as mothers of vulnerable children" reinforcing their perception that they themselves are not worth helping.[3] Women IVDUs need to know they *deserve* access to services that will support them in coping with AIDS and that service providers should treat them with dignity.

More concretely, women at risk of HIV infection need low-barrier, low-cost or free, drop-in, crisis-oriented, ongoing HIV-related counseling that is easily accessible but confidential. Peer-based professionally facilitated group counseling models are being used in many women's risk-reduction programs and appear to be very productive.[51] Such counseling is not only cost effective, it has been shown to be a sound approach to counseling women faced with initiating behavior modification.[32,51] The format of such counseling can be varied to suit the population of women being served: gender-specific groups, family groups, couples groups, groups for women at risk, groups for women who are ill, groups for women who are caretakers.

Psychosocial counseling for women at risk of HIV infection, although it touches on many traditional "women's issues," must address issues which are not traditionally considered a component of women's mental health programs (e.g., bereavement counseling for young adults, sexual behavior modification).

Women who find they are at risk of HIV infection or who are infected need help in learning to face and make decisions about a wide range of issues (e.g., survivor's guilt, anger, depression, suicidal ideation, multiple bereavement processes) common to individuals exposed to HIV.[52] Some of these issues are compounded for women by the effects of social isolation (which in the minority community can be increased by seeking mental health services).[26,28] The primary need of women is to learn new mental health skills that will enable them to cope on an ongoing basis with the ambiguity and personal crises (losses) HIV infection and illness bring into their daily lives.

In addition to the impact of HIV, some women need help in coping with the effects of physical and sexual abuse (past and present) that must be addressed in order for them to approach the larger issues of chemical dependency, and sexual dependency. All women need help in dealing with the impact of HIV infection and illness and/or chemical dependency on their family system dynamics.[53]

In order to implement such services, in many cases mental health providers have to reorient their delivery systems, training individual providers in both AIDS-related psychosocial needs and chemical dependency, re-evaluating the use of standard mental health measures to evaluate the functional state of chemically addicted women, and introducing cross-cultural counseling if it does not exist.[9]

Social Needs

The most pressing social need of women at risk of HIV infection or illness is reduction in the social isolation they experience. Women are much more socially isolated than gay men as most have no identifiable support groups or communities in which they can seek social support. Social isolation is most severe for women sex partner's as there is no "sex partner culture" for either the partners of bisexual men or IVDUs.[26] Women IVDUs have access to more support than sex partners as they are members of one of two subcultures, the drug subculture or the recovery subculture.[24] However, while some social support exists within the subcultures of women IVDUs, their drug needle use stigmatizes and isolates within their larger communities and sometimes in their families.[53,54]

The social isolation women experience can be somewhat mitigated or reduced through self-help groups and counseling but the problem really needs to be addressed at its roots in the community.[55] This need is being addressed by grass roots organizations such as the Association for Drug Abuse Prevention and Treatment (ADAPT) and the Lower East Side Health Project in New York City, the Safety Net Program run by Women, Inc. in Roxbury, Massachusetts, and other community-based programs working to reach, educate and support women at risk.[56,57]

In addition to having their social isolation reduced, women need help in coping with unexpected changes in their social roles (confronting the loss of social validation attached to motherhood, being abandoned by a partner who cannot accept their serostatus, becoming widowed at a very early age). Life-styles changes related to HIV infection or illness, such as having to redefine the organizing principle of their lives should they be chemically dependent also have to be addressed and supported. This includes help in finding and arranging for others to care for children, and re-establishing relationships with children women wish to know them before they die.

Sexual Needs

Too often the sexual needs of women are overlooked or assumed to be similar to those of men. Women who, like gay men, are faced with the need to change their sexual behavior, need to mourn the loss of their old sexual identity. They also need to become aware of and confront sexual decision-making processes, which in many cases they are unaware of, or lack the power to control. For women who are chemically dependent sexual behavior is inexorably linked to their drug use. Drug use therefore has to be addressed in order to bring about the possibility of sexual risk reduction. Women who use drugs often exchange sex for money or drugs. Their decision-making is thus determined more by their need for drugs than by their sexual needs.[58]

Women who support their drug use through prostitution very often do not use barrier protection with their partners, as a means of demarcating "personal" from "business" sex. They need to be encouraged to find other ways of symbolically separating the two, allowing them to protect themselves in both situations.[59]

Infected women who are single (unpartnered) are in a particularly difficult situation when it comes to sexual risk reduction. Those who are recently recovering experience reawakened sexuality and are nervous about having sex "straight" (straight sex may seem boring, lacking the excitement involved in sex for money/drugs exchanges). Already anxious, they then suddenly find themselves confronted with losing the possibility of sexual intimacy for the rest of their lives should they disclose their serostatus. Recovering women may also feel resentment at suggested curbs on their sexuality (imposed or suggested as part of the recovery process), have trouble learning to take responsibility for sexual and fertility decision-making, addressing intimacy issues—the loss of drug-based intimacy, with sexual dysfunction (their own or their partner's), and with the linking of sex with death and its affect on their sexual relationship. Women IVDUs who forgo needle use also need to mourn the loss of sexual pleasure that many gain from needle drug use (in particular needle heroin use).[3,13]

The current portrait of a female sex partner of an IVDU does not do justice to the complexity of relationships that exist, ignoring lesbian partners, for instance. There are women sex partners who are intravenous users themselves, those who are addicts but not intravenous users, and those who do not use drugs at all.

Some research has indicated that the majority of female sex partners of male IVDUs are non-drug users.[60] Although many may be non-needle users, the assertion that most women partners are non-drug users is challenged by more recent data.[61] The sex partners seen in the Department of Health Stuyvesant Program for women at high risk were predominantly either needle drug users themselves (many in treatment or recovery programs), or non-needle drug users (many also in treatment or recovery). The totally non-drug-using partner was rare.

Women who are sex partners of IVDUs are at high risk of HIV infection. More than 70% of female heterosexual transmission cases are classified as sex partners of IVDUs (71–85% black and Latina women).[62] Although female sex partners have been characterized as having low self-esteem, feeling powerless, being socially isolated, and having a history of sexual or physical abuse,[63] little is known about their sexual risk taking.[4] There are, for instance, few reliable statistics on how many lesbian partners have been infected by their needle drug-using partners.[6]

Women sex partners who are non-needle users but who are coping with their own recovery process tend to focus on their partners, constantly worrying about whether or not they are staying clean. Often their own risk of infection or need for protection slips into the background of their concerns or is down played.[50]

Non-drug-using partners of needle users are confronted with other issues. Some do not know about their partners use and therefore do not realize they are at risk or have a need to protect themselves. Other women "know" about their partners' needle use but choose not to acknowledge it because they do not want to face the issues that acknowledge raises.[39] When they do acknowledge risk, however, they are more likely to be concerned about their own risk of infection than women IVDUs.

Acknowledgment exposes women to tremendous ambivalence as they face distinct complex psychosocial and sexual problems. Their partners often feel contaminated and doomed, and begin to distance themselves emotionally and physically. The women themselves have ambivalent feelings about having sexual relations with someone they feel could "contaminate" or kill them. This creates a distance in the relationship which exacerbates the stress being experience by both partners and often leads to a lack of intimacy and increased feelings of isolation for both partners[13].

Non-using partners need to learn how to express their real feelings and fears related to their sexuality, their partner's drug use and possible death, their own risk, and their current or potential care-taking role. They have to learn to negotiate with their partners, to create or maintain "romance" with restrictions on sexuality, to mourn the loss of old concepts of sex, self, and physical intimacy, and to deal with uncertainty and fear and their effect on their and their partner's sexuality and their own economic security. While some leave their relationships (especially if the male continues to use needles), many decide to stay to help their partners "see it through."[13,24,31]

Women who are the casual or new sexual partners of recovering IVDUs are even less likely to acknowledge their or their partner's risk of infection. They seem to believe that because "it took place in the past," it does not place them at risk today. This belief is prevalent among non-IVDU women in recovery programs and places them at increased risk. It is common knowledge that some of the older men in 12-step programs, for instance (many of whom are former heroin needle users), attempt to strike up relationships with younger non-needle-using women who are new to recovery—in New York City, commonly referred to as "thirteen stepping" or "pigeon-fucking."

One similarity found in female sex partners is that they tend to put the needs of their partners before their own; for example, "he really needs sex [the way he wants it]; after all he has been sick and he doesn't have much to look forward to. . . ."[13]

Economic Needs

The economic needs of women at risk of HIV infection vary across class and socioeconomic variables. The needs that most concern policy-makers and service providers are those of the majority of women who become ill—poor minority women who use needles or whose partners do. For women who are dependent on men to support their drug habit, alternatives such as becoming drug free or finding other legal means of support have to be explored. As women needle users can usually make much more engaging in illegal activities than they can in legal activities (lacking education and job-related skills), and there is a severe shortage of treatment options for women, this is a formidable challenge.

Another seemingly "intractable" problem is that many women who are HIV seropositive or ill are precariously housed or are already homeless. This problem if it is not addressed prior to a woman's becoming ill can result in her becoming homeless with the onset of the disease and hospitalization.[64] Furthermore, many women lack adequate income and health insurance to cover the cost of medical, mental health, and other HIV-related services. Many chemically dependent women who are eligible for such services lack access to them because of their inability to negotiate the system to obtain the necessary certification (e.g., for Medicaid, welfare benefits).

Chemical Dependency-Related Needs

Female IVDUs comprise the majority of diagnosed AIDS cases and the largest group of HIV-infected women. It is commonly believed they are introduced to the use of needles by men they are involved with sexually.[4] While this may have been true 5 or 10 years ago, today other patterns obtain. Ethnographic work being conducted by the author at The Women's Center Program at Montefiore Medical Center with IV heroin/cocaine using women indicates that it is not uncommon for women to introduce other women to needle use.[58]

What is clear is that female IVDUs are frequently the partners of other IVDUs (male or female). Those who use and share needles with their partners face the most serious obstacles in initiating behavior changes related to HIV risk reduction. Attempts by women to withdraw from injectable drugs is perceived to threaten their primary social, psychological, and economic relationships. As most women who have been studied by the author in various settings have partners who continue to use drugs and needles regularly, it is very difficult for them to stay "clean" (e.g., not use needles) or to engage their partners in condom use.[61] Although women in treatment cyclically go through drug detoxification programs, they are seldom able to stay "clean" for long after leaving them as their partners continue to "use." Drug use also effects sexual risk reduction as sex is often implicitly or explicitly exchanged for drugs, and the effect of the drugs distorts or can cause delays in decision-making to practice "safer sex."[9,58]

Ultimately, women IVDUs who want to stop using but who are in relationships with partners who continue to use needles are faced with a choice between getting or staying off drugs and continuing their relationship (the same is true for male IVDUs who wish to stop and whose female partners continue to use). Recognizing the connection between their and/or their partner's drug use and their risk of HIV infection is often seen as a betrayal of the relationship on which they are economically, socially, and physically dependent. The sense of betrayal is played out in many ways but is particularly dangerous when women are involved in abusive relationships. It is more comfortable for many chemically dependent needle-using women to ignore their risk than confront such threatening issues.[10]

One of the most consistently documented needs of chemically dependent women is access to affordable, low-barrier, "gender-sensitive" treatment for polydrug addiction.[9] Ideally treatment should be integrated with health care and mental health services to provide a comprehensive, cost-effective approach to service provision.[65] However, most existing treatment is fragmented, hard to gain entry to, and based on models developed to treat males addicted solely to heroin.[9]

Today, women are primarily polydrug users and cocaine not heroin is rapidly becoming the drug of choice and is increasingly linked to HIV infection.[58,66] Treatment programs that are available for women must reflect these realities and the reality that most women seeking treatment have children—that treatment must incorporate child care.[65] Furthermore, as many chemically dependent women have partners who are active needle users, "bridge programs" (programs that can help them leave relationships based on chemical dependency) and family systems approaches are needed, as are programs that encourage couples to enter treatment. In addition, staff members of organizations providing health and social services to women need to be trained in chemical dependency so they can recognize and ultimately understand their clients' behavior.

CONCLUSION

Risk assessment, acceptance, and HIV antibody testing all set in motion processes which can bring about irrevocable changes in the lives of women at high risk of HIV infection. They bring into sharp focus existing needs that have either been ignored or inadequately addressed: the need for accessible, nonjudgmental health care and low-cost, gender-appropriate counseling (to address the issues that threaten the emotional, physical, social, and economic stability of women's lives) in populations of women often denied both.

If high-risk women are to be reached earlier on in the HIV infection and illness continuum and engaged in behavior change related to the prevention or reduction of HIV transmission, society is going to have to acknowledge and address these needs, it is going to have to support women who are at high-risk (because of their or their partner's behaviors), in their exploration of the issues which are raised by the presence of HIV infection in their communities.

Much of what we know about how women are responding to the risk of HIV infection has been learned through support groups and other HIV counseling program models for women: models such as the Women's Group, The Womens' Center, the Lower East Side AIDS Project, Project AWARE, and NIDA's sex partner's AIDS risk-reduction projects, all of which offer women "safe" environments to openly express their fears and feelings about HIV risk and infectivity without encountering discrimination—projects that afford women at risk the opportunity to see how other women faced with the same problems are coping, what types of choices they make, and how they find and foster the social support that they need.[32]

Offering women gender-exclusive group processes is extremely important. As has been noted by many researchers and the counselors in the Department of Health/ Stuyvesant program, women behave very differently when men are present in counseling groups, they are less expressive, talk less, discuss intimate subjects less, and laugh less.[13,24,31] To date women's groups are the core of successful programs that are reaching women at risk and helping them acknowledge their risk and help one another to engage in risk reduction.

ACKNOWLEDGMENTS. The author would like to thank the following individuals for their help and cooperation, Dr. Richard Elion and Susan Rosenthal (New York City Health Department), Karen Solomon (Body Positive/New York), Dr. Gerald Friedland, Dr. Ernest Drucker and Kathleen Eric (Montefiore Medical Center, The Womens Center), Dr. Susan Tross and Dr. Abu Quadar (Lower East Side Health Project, Narcotic and Drug Research, Inc.) and the women who shared their sorrows and strengths, their thoughts and triumphs with each other and the author as they confronted AIDS.

REFERENCES

1. Saint Cyr-Delpe M: Update to the Community Response on Women and AIDS, in *Fifth International AIDS Conference, Montreal, Canada, June 8, 1989.*
2. Cohen J: Overstating the risk of AIDS: Scapegoating prostitutes. *Focus* 4(2):1–2, 1989.
3. Mitchell J: Women, AIDS and public policy. *AIDS Public Policy* 3(2):50–52, 1988.
4. Turner CF, Miller HG, Moses LE (eds): *AIDS, Sexual Behavior and Intravenous Drug Use,* Washington, DC, National Academy Press, 1989, p 281.
5. Dorfman DP, Mays MA: AIDS and lesbians: IV-Drug Use is the Risk, in *Fifth International AIDS Conference on AIDS, Stockholm, Sweden, June 12–16, 1988.*
6. Ribble D, Marte C, Kelly J, et al: HIV infection in lesbians, in *Fifth International AIDS Conference, Montreal, Canada, June 7, 1989.*
7. Carpenter CCJ, Danforth S. Societal impact of HIV infection in women, in *Fifth International AIDS Conference, Montreal, Canada, June 5, 1989.*
8. Ribble D, Marte C, Tiersten A, et al: Differences in Stage of Presenting Symptoms Between Men and Women in a Primary Care AIDS Clinic, in *Fifth International AIDS Conference, Montreal Canada, June 7, 1989.*
9. Mondanaro J: *Chemically Dependent Women: Assessment and Treatment.* Lexington, Massachusetts, DC Heath and Company, 1989.
10. Worth D: Sexual decisionmaking and AIDS: why condom promotion among vulnerable women is likely to fail, *Studies in Family Planning,* The Population Council, New York, November–December, 1989.
11. Worth D: Minority Women and AIDS: Race, Culture and Gender, in Feldman D (ed): *Cultural Aspects of AIDS and the Global Pandemic.* New York, Praeger Publishers, 1990.
12. NIDA Community Research Branch/NOVA Research Company: Sexual Partners Demonstration Data, in *Fifth International AIDS Conference, Montreal, Canada, June 7, 1989.*
13. Worth D: Unpublished ethnographic research data, The Women's AIDS Group Program, Stuyvesant Polyclinic/NYC Department of Health, 1987.
14. Hutterer J, Blass P, Oberaver C, et al: Differences in HIV/AIDS counseling for women and for men, in *Fifth International Conference on AIDS, Montreal, Canada, June 8, 1989.*
15. Des Jarlais DC, Friedman SR: Gender differences in response to HIV infection, in Bridge TP, Mirsky AF, and Goodwin FK, (eds): *Psychological, Neurological and Substance Abuse Aspects of AIDS.* New York, Raven Press, 1988, pp. 159–163.
16. Gerstein DR, Judd LL, Rovner SA: Career dynamics of female heroin addicts. *Am J Drug Alcohol Abuse* 6(1):1–23, 1979.

17. Sorrel S, Springer E: The argument against HIV antibody testing in chemical dependency treatment programs. *J Psychoactive Drugs* 21(4):419–421, 1989.
18. McCusker J, Stoddard AM, Mayer KH, et al: Effects of HIV antibody test knowledge on subsequent sexual behaviors in a cohort of homosexually active men. *Am J Public Health* 78:462–467, 1988.
19. Coates TJ, Morin SF, McKusick L: Behavioral consequences of AIDS antibody testing among gay men. *JAMA* 258:1889, 1987.
20. Des Jarlais DC, Friedman SR: AIDS and the sharing of equipment for illicit drug injection: A review of current data. New York, National Institute on Drug Abuse, New York State Division of Substance Abuse, 1987.
21. Watters JK: Meaning and context: The social facts of intravenous drug use and HIV transmission in the inner city, *J Psychoactive Drugs* 20(2):173–177, 1988.
22. Watters JK: Preventing human immunodeficiency virus contagion among intravenous drug users. The impact of street-based education on risk behavior. in *Third International AIDS Conference, Washington, DC, June, 1987.*
23. Ostrow DG: AIDS prevention through effective education. *Daedalus* 118:229–254, 1989.
24. Santiago D: New York City Department of Health, personal communication, July 1989.
25. Cancellieri FR, Holman S, Sunderland A, et al: Psychiatric and behavioral impact of HIV testing in pregnant drug users. in *Fourth International AIDS Conference, Stockholm, Sweden, June 12–16, 1988.*
26. Wofsy C: Women and the acquired immuno-deficiency syndrome: An interview. *Women Med,* 149:687–690, 1988.
27. Case P, et al: The social context of AIDS risk behavior among intravenous drug-using lesbians in San Francisco, in *Fourth International AIDS Conference, Stockholm, Sweden, June 12–16, 1988.*
28. Blachman M: Seropositive women: Clinical issues and approaches. *Focus* 3:2–3, 1988.
29. Kamenga M, Jing K, Hassig S, et al: Condom use and associated HIV seroconversion following intensive HIV counseling of 122 married couples in Zaire with discordant HIV serology, in *Fifth International AIDS Conference, Montreal, Canada, June 1989.*
30. Cochrane SD, Mays VM: Women and AIDS-related concerns: Roles for psychologists in helping the worried well. *Am Psycholog* 44:529–535, 1989.
31. Mesquita L: New York City Department of Health, personal communication, July 1989.
32. Eric K, Drucker E, Worth D, et al: The womens' center: A model peer support program for high risk IV drug and crack using women in the Bronx, in *Fifth International AIDS Conference, Montreal, Canada, June 8, 1989.*
33. Grant D, Anns M: Counseling AIDS antibody-positive clients: Reactions and treatment. *Am Psychol* 44:72–74, 1988.
34. Taylor K: New York City Commission on Human Rights, AIDS Unit, personal communication, 1989.
35. Worth D, Rodriquez R: Latina women and AIDS. *SIECUS Rep* 15(3):5–7, 1987.
36. Hammond E: Race, sex, AIDS: The construction of "other." *Radical America* 20(6):28–36, 1987.
37. Friedman SR, Des Jarlais DC, Neaigus A, et al: AIDS and the new drug injector. *Nature (Lond)* 339:33–334, 1989.
38. Fillilove M, Weinstein M, Fullilove R, et al: Will you still love me tomorrow? Race/gender issues in the sexual transmission of AIDS, MIRA, San Francisco, submitted for publication, 1989.
39. Weissman G: Community outreach and prevention—A national demonstration project. in *American Public Health Association, Boston, November 1988.*
40. Andriote JM, Medina V: For women at risk, prevention begins with self-esteem. *Natl AIDS Network Monitor* Fall, 1988.
41. Cohen JB, Lyons CA, Lockett GJ, et al: Emerging patterns of drug use, Sexual behavior, HIV infection and STD's in high risk San Francisco areas from 1986–1989, in *Fifth International AIDS Conference, Montreal, Canada, June 8, 1989.*
42. Sowder B, Weissman G, Young P: Working with women at risk in a national AIDS prevention program, in *Fifth International AIDS Conference, Montreal, Canada, June 8, 1989.*
43. Poole LE, Cohen JB, Lyons CA, et al: Behavior change to reduce HIV transmission risk in a prospective study of seropositive women, in *Fifth International Conference on AIDS, Montreal, Canada, June 7, 1989.*
44. Solomon K: New York City Department of Health/Stuyvesant Polyclinic AIDS counseling program, personal communication, 1988.

45. Franke K: Discrimination against HIV positive women by abortion clinics in New York City, in *Fifth International AIDS Conference, Montreal, Canada, June 6, 1989.*
46. Wofsy C: Human immunodeficiency virus in women. *JAMA* 257:2074–2075, 1987.
47. Williams AB: Educational needs assessment for women at risk for HIV through intravenous drug use, in *Fifth International AIDS Conference, Montreal, Canada, June 7, 1989.*
48. Marte C, Ribble D, Keyes C, et al: Need for gynecological protocols in AIDS primary care clinics, in *Fifth International AIDS Conference, Montreal, Canada, June 5, 1989.*
49. Long I, Kirchenbaum D, McCarthy M: Women underrepresented in AIDS clinical trials, in *Fifth International AIDS Conference, Montreal, Canada, June 7, 1989.*
50. Wermuth L, Ham L: Perceptions of AIDS risk among women sex partners of IV drug users in San Francisco, in *Fifth International AIDS Conference, Montreal, Canada, June 8, 1989.*
51. Rossi L, Garcia L, Salame E, et al: Changes in the sexual behavior of HIV infected patients in a group process, in *Fifth International AIDS Conference, Montreal, Canada, June 8, 1989.*
52. Dobko T, Benedik B: The medical and emotional support needs of women with HIV, in *Fifth International AIDS Conference, Montreal, Canada, June 5, 1989.*
53. Walker LA: What Comforts AIDS Families, *The New York Times Magazine,* June 21, 1987, pp 16–64.
54. Grief GL, Porembski E: Significant others of IV drug abusers with AIDS: New challenges for drug treatment programs, *J Substance Abuse Treatm* 4:151–155, 1987.
55. Shaw N: Preventing AIDS among women: The role of community organizing. *Socialist Rev* 100:76–92, 1988.
56. Serrano Y, Goldsmith D: Street outreach strategies for intravenous drug and crack users, their sexual partners, and addicted prostitutes at risk of HIV, in *Fifth International AIDS Conference, Montreal, Canada, June 5, 1989.*
57. Portis K: Women Inc., Roxbury, MA, personal communication, 1989.
58. Worth D, Drucker E, Eric K, et al: An ethnographic study of high risk sexual behavior in women using IV heroin, cocaine and crack in the South Bronx, in *Fifth International AIDS Conference, Montreal, Canada, June 8, 1989.*
59. Cohen J: Condom promotion among prostitutes. University of California at San Francisco, unpublished paper, n.d.
60. Des Jarlais DC, Chamberland ME, Yancovitz SR, et al: Heterosexual partners: A large risk group for AIDS. *Lancet* 2:1346–1347, 1984.
61. Snyder F, Sowder B, Young P: NIDA Outreach Demonstration Projects provide insights into drug use risk patterns. *Network* 1:1–7, 1989.
62. Guinan ME, Hardy A: Epidemiology of AIDS in women in the United States: 1981 through 1986. *JAMA* 257:1987.
63. Arquelles L, Rivero AM, Reback CJ, et al: Female sex partners of IV drug users: A study of socio/psychological characteristics and needs, in *Fifth International AIDS Conference, Montreal, Canada, June 8, 1989.*
64. Drucker E, et al: IV drug users with AIDS in New York City: A study of dependent children, housing and drug addiction treatment. Montefiore Medical Center, unpublished paper, 1989.
65. Worth D: The need for comprehensive holistic treatment for female IVDV's, in *NASADAD AIDS Policy Seminar, Denver, Colorado, April 20–22, 1988.*
66. Chaisson RD, Osmond D, Bacchetti P, et al: Cocaine use and HIV infection in intravenous drug users in San Francisco. *JAMA* 261:561–565, 1989.

6

Prostitution and AIDS

CAROLE A. CAMPBELL

INTRODUCTION

This chapter takes up one relationship between acquired immune deficiency syndrome (AIDS) and prostitution. The role that prostitutes play in the epidemiology of AIDS is discussed. Various approaches taken to control AIDS and other sexually transmitted diseases (STDs) are covered. The approach taken in Nevada, where prostitution is legal in some counties, is described as are current legislation efforts aimed at prostitutes.

Prostitution is one type of sex work belonging to what is referred to as the sex industry.[1] In addition to prostitutes, sex industry workers include exotic dancers, nude models, escorts, porn actresses, and workers in massage parlors. Prostitution can be defined as the exchange of sexual services for money or things of monetary value, such as drugs.[2] In the act of prostitution, women exchange access to their bodies for material gain. Usually, the arrangement is negotiated and money exchanged before the service is provided. The person who provides the service is a prostitute. Prostitutes who make their contacts for sexual services on the street are referred to as streetwalkers. The person who requests and pays for the service is a client. The client is sometimes referred to as a "john." There is another type of exchange sometimes involved in prostitution and that exchange pertains to the relationship between a prostitute and a pimp. Prostitutes sometimes give money to a pimp in exchange for protection and affection. Streetwalkers tend to have pimps more often than other types of prostitutes because of their need for protection on the street.

Social scientific interest in behavioral aspects of prostitution began long before the advent of AIDS. James et al.,[3] Davis,[4] and Winick and Kinsie[5] have examined some of these aspects. Winick[6] looked specifically at the prostitute–client relationship. Milner and Milner[7] examined the prostitute–pimp relationship. The relationship between prostitution and intravenous (IV) drug usage is also one that existed long before the advent of AIDS, and Goldstein[8] examined this relationship. Since both prostitution and IV drug use are illegal, prostitutes who use IV drugs are caught up in two illegal behaviors. The relationship among prostitution, IV drug usage, and AIDS is discussed later in the chapter.

Prostitutes, like gays and IV drug users, suffer stigmatization because of their deviant status in society. All three groups have been further stigmatized because of their implied

CAROLE A. CAMPBELL • Department of Sociology, California State University, Long Beach, California 90840.

involvement in the spread of AIDS. Prostitution is of particular interest to a discussion of behavior and AIDS since prostitutes have been implicated in the spread of AIDS and are considered to be a data source on heterosexual transmission. The role of prostitution in the epidemiology of AIDS is discussed in the next section.

ROLE OF PROSTITUTES IN THE EPIDEMIOLOGY OF AIDS*

Infection with human immunodeficiency virus (HIV), the virus that causes AIDS, has occurred in prostitutes in many parts of the world.[9] Prostitutes can become infected with HIV through either sexual or parenteral transmission.

Seroprevalence surveys for antibody to HIV in women with histories of prostitution have shown varying results since testing began in 1984 (Table 1). In sub-Saharan Africa, where HIV is thought to be transmitted primarily through heterosexual exposure, from one (1%) of 98 prostitutes in Accra, Ghana,[10] to 29 (88%) of 33 prostitutes in Ngoma, Rwanda,[11] have had antibody to HIV. HIV seroprevalence appears to be lower among prostitutes in Africa who use condoms frequently (>50% of sexual exposures),[12] have higher socioeconomic status,[13] and who have not been recruited from STD clinics.[11]

In Europe, where homosexual exposures and IV drug abuse are major risk factors for HIV infection, none of 50 prostitutes tested in London,[14] none of 56 tested in Paris,[15] and none of 399 tested in Nuremberg, West Germany,[16] had antibody to HIV (Table 1), but 10 (71%) of 14 prostitutes who abused IV drugs in Pordenone, Italy,[17] and 14 (78%) of 18 who abused IV drugs in Zurich, Switzerland, [18] were infected. Seventeen (<1%) of nearly 2000 registered prostitutes in six West German cities were anti-HIV positive; one half the infected women abused drugs intravenously.[19] In Athens, Greece, 12 (6%) of 200 registered prostitutes were HIV-antibody positive; none abused drugs intravenously.[20]

Data regarding HIV-antibody seropositivity in men who have had sexual exposures with female prostitutes have shown inconsistent results. Among heterosexual European men who have returned from Africa with AIDS, sexual contact with a prostitute is a common finding.[21] Clumeck et al.,[22] found that 47 (81%) of 58 African males with AIDS reported regular contact with prostitutes as compared to 20 (34%) of 58 controls who were healthy men matched in age, income, and ethnic and geographic origin. Similarly, Van de Perre et al.[11] found the rate of seropositivity was 28% (7 of 25) for African male customers of prostitutes but only 7% (2 of 27) for controls who were healthy blood donors. These two case-control studies suggest that male customers became infected from prostitutes. However, few heterosexual men who report sexual exposures with prostitutes in New York City have turned up in STD clinics with antibody to HIV.[23]

The reliability of risk assessments from prostitute contact in studies that are not controlled is questionable.[24] Such studies rely on interviews of patients diagnosed with AIDS who have been identified from surveillance reports. Data from surveillance reports show that 30% of men with no identified risks have reported contact with prostitutes.[24] However, since the rate of contact with prostitutes in the general population is unknown, the fact that these men have had contact with prostitutes does not necessarily indicate that

*The author wishes to thank William W. Darrow, Research Sociologist at the Centers for Disease Control, for his assistance in the preparation of this part of the manuscript.

TABLE 1. Antibody to Human Immunodeficiency Virus in African and European Prostitutes: 1984–1987

Investigators	Study site	Number positive	Number tested	Percent anti-HIV positive
Africa				
Neequaye et al.[10]	Accra, Ghana	1	98	1
Mann et al.[12]	Kinshasa, Zaire	101	377	27
Kreiss et al.[13]	Nairobi, Kenya			
	High status	8	26	31
	Lower status	42	64	66
Van de Perre et al.[11]	Ngoma, Rwanda	29	33	88
Europe				
Barton et al.[14]	London, England	0	50	0
Brenky-Faudeux et al.[15]	Paris, France	56	0	0
Smith and Smith[16]	Nuremberg, West Germany	0	399	0
Tirelli et al.[17]	Pordenone, Italy			
	No IV-drug use	0	10	0
	IV-drug abuser	10	14	71
Luthy et al.[18]	Zurich, Switzerland			
	No IV-drug use	1	103	1
	IV-drug abuser	14	18	78
Schultz et al.[19]	Six West German cities	17	2000	1
Papaevengelou et al.[20]	Athens, Greece	12	200	6

prostitute contact is associated with HIV infection. A control group of uninfected men would make such an association more conclusive. It could be the case that rather than having infected the men who report prostitute contact, prostitutes were infected by them. It also could be that men are infecting each other through semen deposited in prostitutes. An additional consideration on risk assessments of prostitutes is offered by Potterat et al.,[25] who suggest that the risk could in fact be inflated because of the unwillingness of infected persons to admit to homosexual behavior or IV drug usage. The reliability of military data on risk behavior similarly is questionable because homosexuality and IV drug usage are grounds for dismissal from the military.[26]

CDC Multicenter Study

To assess HIV-antibody prevalence and determine risk factors in female prostitutes in the United States, a multicenter cross-sectional study was conducted in 1986–1987 under the auspices of the Centers for Disease Control (CDC).[27] This study was justified on the basis that HIV seropositivity among prostitutes previously had not been correlated with sexual practices, IV drug use and other possible risk factors. The purpose of the study thus was to estimate the prevalence of antibodies of HIV in various populations of female prostitutes and to identify factors associated with HIV seropositivity. Data were collected in seven geographic areas: Atlanta, Colorado Springs, Las Vegas, Los Angeles, Miami, northern New Jersey (Newark, Jersey City, and Peterson), and San Francisco. Any woman aged 18 years of age or older who had exchanged sexual services for money or drugs at least once since January 1, 1978, was eligible to participate. After giving informed consent, participants were interviewed for sexual, drug, and medical histories; were examined for signs of HIV infection and IV drug use; and were asked to provide a blood specimen to be tested for seromarkers for hepatitis B, antibody to *Treponema pallidum* (syphilis), and antibody to HIV. Participants were given educational information on HIV risk reduction when they received their test results.

Recruiting prostitutes to participate in the study was sometimes difficult because of the illegal nature of both prostitution and IV drug usage. The various sites employed several types of recruitment strategies. Some sites recruited women who had been arrested for prostitution. Other sites recruited through STD clinics, methadone maintenance clinics, alcohol rehabilitation centers and women's shelters. Some sites used various outreach efforts to enroll women. One such effort involved listing personal advertisements for "sexually adventurous women" in newspapers. Several sites used vans to go out into areas where prostitution activity occurred. One site rented a room and conducted interviews in a hotel prostitutes frequented and the Nevada site conducted interviews at a legalized brothel.

Participants were not strictly representative of all prostitutes in the United States or even of the cities included in the study. Similarly, women who were recruited from methadone maintenance clinics were not necessarily representative of prostitutes in those cities. The study was limited in that there was an overrepresentation of streetwalkers who tend to use IV drugs more than other types of prostitutes.[1] Since one of the interests of the study was in women who had exchanged sex for drugs, there was some amount of sample bias. Prostitutes who use IV drugs were overrepresented among the incarcerated study participants since these women are not as likely to be bailed out of jail as quickly as women who do not use IV drugs and thus were more likely to be available for interviews. A certain amount of selectivity operated, since the study included those women who were motivated enough to respond. Some women who use IV drugs may thereby have been excluded.

Although there were some initial problems in gaining access to prostitutes, researchers found that many of the prostitutes were eager to participate. The questionnaire contained a number of questions pertaining to number and types of sexual acts. Generally there were no problems in getting participants to respond to sensitive questions. Some of the questions pertaining to the number of sexual partners presented problems in quantification, however. Several of the women said that they didn't keep count of their customers. Similarly, women who use IV drugs reported that they didn't keep count of the number of times they injected (Sterk C: personal communication, 1988).

There were certain advantages to conducting interviews in natural settings where prostitution took place. Women were able to participate in the study without having to leave their world. Had they been required to leave their environment, many may not have participated in the study because of their mistrust for institutional settings. A certain amount of mistrust of the researchers was felt initially by some prostitutes because of the gender of the researchers, since most of the researchers were female and initially were considered competitors for customers. This conflict was resolved once the prostitutes understood the intentions of the researchers. The researchers were able to observe these women in natural settings and to learn more about the dynamics of prostitution. This was especially true of the brothel where business went on as usual while interviews were conducted.

Dealing with illegal behavior required special care on the part of the researchers. Confidentiality could not be compromised, and the participants could not be jeopardized by the study in any way. Researchers who interviewed incarcerated women were careful to make sure that the women understood that their decision to participate in the study had no bearing on their probation or parole. Follow-up work involving test results and risk-reduction educational materials was sometimes difficult to conduct because prostitutes have considerable mobility.[28] One of the sites, however, found that more than half the women could be located 4–6 weeks after enrollment. Most women arrested for prostitution plead guilt and are fined and released within a 24-hr period. Researchers had to be quick in order to interview these women before they were released. Some of the women are given sentences for periods of up to 15 days, but very few are held for 30 days or more. Thus, they were instructed to go to alternate sites for their test results.

Preliminary results showed that more than one half (54%) of 941 tested for hepatitis B had a seromarker, 27% of 998 tested for syphilis had been infected, and 12% of 1048 tested for antibody to HIV were seropositive (Table 2). Seropositivity for HIV ranged from zero in Las Vegas, where most of the women enrolled were employed in a brothel outside of Clark County, to 55% in northern New Jersey, where the women studied were enrolled through methadone maintenance clinics and outreach vans.

Risk factors for antibody to HIV included many variables associated with IV drug abuse, especially attendance at a "shooting gallery," presence of "needle tracks," and having a history of sharing needles. In multivariate analysis, the most significant variables associated with HIV antibody, after controlling for study site, were months of IV drug abuse, a seromarker for hepatitis B, and being a member of a minority group (black or hispanic). After these variables entered a logistic regression model, only one other variable was significant: infrequent or no use of condoms with sexual partners. Women reported using condoms more often with customers than with boyfriends or husbands. These partners sometimes use IV drugs and may play a role in infection. Since this study did not measure bidirectional transmission, it stimulated considerable interest in inter-

TABLE 2. CDC Collaborative Study of Female Prostitutes in the United States

	Seromarkers					
	Hepatitis B		Syphilis		HIV	
Study site	N = 941	%	N = 998	%	N = 1048	%
Las Vegas	9/35	26	0/31	0	0/37	0
Colorado Springs	19/71	27	0/68	0	1/79	1
Atlanta	30/93	32	11/91	12	1/92	1
Los Angeles	152/217	70	71/208	34	11/224	5
San Francisco	74/157	47	16/171	9	9/173	5
Miami	180/309	58	151/342	44	56/355	16
Newark–Jersey City	51/59	86	21/87	24	48/88	55

viewing and testing the customers of prostitutes. The Colorado Springs and San Francisco sites are presently conducting studies of customers. The Las Vegas site emerged as the only site free of HIV infection. The system of legalized prostitution in Nevada is discussed in the next section.

LEGALIZED PROSTITUTION IN NEVADA

Prostitution is considered to be part of Nevada's frontier heritage and dates back to 1859 when silver was being mined at the legendary Comstock Mine. Since 1971 brothels in Nevada have had formal state approval.[29] Prostitution is legal in 11 of 17 counties in Nevada. It is controlled by state statutes and city and county ordinances. Brothels are considered a local option but state law prohibits them in Clark County where Las Vegas is located. They are also prohibited in Reno and Carson City, the two next largest cities in Nevada. Brothels are located in places with populations of 500–8000 and in rural areas.[30] Although they are prohibited in Las Vegas, Reno, and Carson City, they can be found along the closest borders of adjoining counties of all three cities. Currently there are 37 legal brothels in Nevada.[31] No women are allowed to engage in prostitution in any of the bars or casinos in areas where prostitution is legal. Prices in the brothels tend to be cheaper and independent prostitutes cannot compete with these prices. Brothel prostitution is based on high volume.

There are 350 licensed prostitutes in Nevada.[31] More than one third of them work at the Mustang Ranch in Northern Nevada, the state's largest brothel.[31,32] The brothel in Southern Nevada in which the author conducted interviews employs around 20 women ranging in age from 18 to 38.

Community Response

In Nevada there is general tolerance and even acceptance of prostitution by the public. The main reasons for this approval are control achieved through confining prostitution to certain areas and control over venereal disease achieved through weekly medical inspections.[30,32]

Brothels have considerable community acceptance simply because of their historical legacy in Nevada. Brothels with their madams and prostitutes were part of the Old West as were miners and cowboys. Many towns have had brothels as long as the towns have existed and the brothels are just as much part of the town as the grocery store, gas station, and post office. Brothels have always been there and there seems little reason to change. In fact, communities have often reacted to attacks in defense of their brothels. Brothels are part of a way of life in Nevada, so much that they were tolerated in World War II, when prostitution was outlawed as part of an attempt to prevent the spread of venereal disease among servicemen.

Nevada's brothels tend to be integrated into the community. Brothel personnel are known to contribute to community charities and to support local activities. There is considerable economic involvement in the community by brothels.

There are other ways in which brothels and communities are economically related. The brothels in the northern and west central part of the state tend to be town oriented and to get much business from the local residents. The rural brothels in the south are newer and have some local clientele but cater more to nonresidents. The business the brothels get from locals is reciprocal, however. Many of the brothels, especially the large ones, employ persons other than prostitutes in service jobs as hostesses, cooks, bartenders, and security guards. These persons are usually from nearby communities. Brothels as well as their customers buy supplies including groceries, meals, liquor, and gas in addition to other goods from nearby towns. The prostitutes sometimes have bank accounts and go shopping in adjacent communities. In addition, brothels generate local tax revenue.

Other reasons offered for the public acceptance of prostitution by residents are that it keeps young men in the community from being forced into early marriage and from getting venereal disease. A common rite of passage for young men in rural Nevada is a visit accompanied by they fathers to the brothels. Parents also say that legalized prostitution serves to keep their daughters out of trouble. Brothels located near military bases are felt by parents to distract the military men from the local high school girls.

The special restrictions on where legal brothels can exist are said to serve to keep down the level of illegal prostitution in large cities. This suppression is seen as serving to make gambling more attractive to persons who like to gamble but who find prostitution morally offensive. Gambling is considered by some to be a family activity in which both husband and wife can participate. Illegal prostitution thus is seen as threatening the resort, hotel, and casino business, while legal prostitution is seen as protecting the gambling industry.

The main opposition to prostitution in Nevada has come from fundamentalist church groups. Since the legislature formally codified the local option on brothels except in Clark County, a number of lawmakers have tried to ban all brothels. In 1981 there was a bill to outlaw brothels within 25 miles of a city with a population of more than 60,000.[31] This would have included both Las Vegas and Reno. The bill didn't pass, however. In 1985 there was an attempt to ban brothels statewide but it was killed even before it came to a committee.[29,31] It is known as the shortest-lived bill in Nevada's legislative history. There is again a bill proposed for the 1989 legislature that would ban legalized prostitution in Nevada.

Prostitution in Nevada is opposed by some legislators who feel that it hinders the attraction of new business and industry to the state. Prostitution is said to drive off industry and to prevent diversification of the economy. Nevada is otherwise considered to be attractive because of its advantageous tax structure and inexpensive land and labor. Prostitution is not considered a good atmosphere for potential employees and their families. A similar concern that gaming prevents diversification of the state's economy is often expressed. Prostitution and gaming are two activities seen by some as presenting a bad image for Nevada. The response to opposition to prostitution for the most part has been to let local governments continue to control decisions about permitting prostitution in their communities.

One argument against banning legal prostitution is that it would cause illegal prostitution to increase. The ironic effect of prohibiting prostitution in Las Vegas and Reno is that both cities have problems with illegal prostitution. Those cities are attractive to prostitutes because of the number of male conventioneers and tourists who come to gamble with large amounts of cash. Prostitution is considered an act of loitering for the purposes of prostitution and is a misdemeanor offense. In Las Vegas especially, there are concerns expressed by vice cops about the increase in the number of prostitutes during special events such as professional fights and conventions. During such events, prostitutes from out of town often come to work the bars and streets in Vegas. Vice officers are particularly concerned about this influx because it is highly visible.

Control of STDs

Legalized prostitution in Nevada has a formal state policy that to some extent may account for the low incidence of STDs in prostitutes. Mandatory medical exams of prostitutes, including HIV antibody testing, are required by the Nevada Board of Health. In addition, the brothel itself has policies that enforce condom use and inspections of customers. These practices in part also may account for the low incidence of STDs in prostitutes.

Prostitutes are examined weekly for gonorrhea, herpes, and venereal warts and monthly for syphilis. Since March 1986 the Nevada Board of Health has required prostitutes in county-licensed brothels to be tested for HIV antibody as a condition for employment and monthly thereafter. From November 1985 until that time, testing had been done on a voluntary basis and most of the brothels had complied.

If a woman tests positive for the HIV antibody, a second test is repeated on that same serum sample. If the second test is also positive, the serum is then sent for Western blot. The physician is notified and it is recommended that the woman be removed from the line until the presence of HIV antibody can be confirmed or denied by Western blot. If the confirmatory Western blot is also positive, the woman is denied employment as a prostitute (Reich R: personal communication, 1988). She receives an education program on self-imposed restrictions from the physician or State Health Department. Although she is barred from legal prostitution, she would at that point be free to pursue prostitution illegally. Since mandatory testing has been in effect, no evidence of HIV infection has been found in the licensed prostitutes upon initial testing and none of the women have seroconverted. Before mandatory testing started, one woman who was tested voluntarily was found to be HIV-antibody positive.[29,31] She had worked in a brothel the weekend before the results of her tests were known. Eight other women have been found to be positive in pre-employment tests (Reich R: personal communication, 1988).

The brothel that participated in the CDC study adopted an all-condom policy in October 1985. All sex acts including oral sex are performed with a condom. Condom use is now a formal policy and customers are told of this policy when they call. Other brothels in the state seem to be using condoms on a more regular basis but have not as yet established formally all-condom policies. At this writing, there is a bill in the Nevada legislature that would require condoms to be used at all brothels.

The genitals of customers are inspected for any signs of venereal disease. The women have lamps to aid in seeing any unusual symptoms such as lesions or pus. A newly employed prostitute goes through a training period in which she is supervised by a veteran prostitute when she conducts inspections on customers. She must complete this training successfully before she is allowed to conduct inspections by herself. In the event that a woman sees something questionable, she then calls in another woman for a second opinion. If the second woman agrees that the customer is a risk, he is rejected. If he is accepted, he washes with an antiseptic solution and warm water. He is then instructed to put on a condom.

The Social Organization of the Brothel

The brothel has instituted health and safety precautions that make it an attractive place for prostitutes to work. By providing steady work indoors, the brothel offers a safety and security not always possible out on the street. The women live where they work and they have a room that affords them privacy. They can douche and take other health precautions before and after customers. They work for 3 weeks and are off for 1 week, during which time they leave the brothel and often travel.

The owner is usually around and there are always several employees besides the women present including a hostess, bartender, and cook. Outside there is a security fence where a visitor must ring a bell to be let in by the hostess. At night there is a security guard on duty. In addition, brothels are usually located close to sheriff's substations.

Prostitution at the brothel is a highly organized activity. A customer is greeted at the door by a hostess whereupon she rings the parlor bell to beckon the women. The women then enter in their lineup and introduce themselves by saying "hi" and giving their first name. When the customer makes his selection, the woman he selects then takes him by his hand and shows him to a room. After he passes inspection and pays the money, the prostitute gives the money to the hostess. The amount of money, along with the amount of allowable time is recorded. A timer is set for the specified amount of time. When the alarm goes off, the hostess knocks on the door to inform the couple that their time is up. There are also intercoms in the room. This type of monitoring by the brothel staff serves to insure a woman's safety.

Because of the physical protection provided by the brothel, a woman is in a strong position to reject a customer and to enforce condom use. Additionally she has some discretion over the types of sex acts in which she'll agree to participate. She is not obligated to participate in bondage or sadomasochism and has physical safety assurance from the brothel staff against customers who insist on these types of activities.

In addition to physical security, the brothel provides an emotionally supportive environment for the women. When they do not have customers, they can talk and exchange information. Their weekly medical exams are an established routine and they often go together for their exam appointments. This regular contact with medical personnel allows them to get clarification on any health concerns they may have. The women at the brothel were well informed on HIV. Some in fact were so well informed that they seemed to take the role of surrogate AIDS educators with their customers.

The Impact of AIDS

The decision of the owner of the brothel to adopt and all-condom policy was partly the result of pressure from the prostitutes themselves. The women felt that the risk of contracting AIDS without protection was too great, and they threatened to quit unless the owner agreed to enforce stringently an all-condom policy. The women now feel safer with this policy but still take other precautions as well. Now in addition to examining their customers for venereal disease, they look for needle marks. Whenever possible they casually try to inquire about a customer's IV drug or bisexual practices.

The women reported that some customers are resistant to using condoms, especially for oral sex. One woman said that she persuades a customer to use a condom by showing him that he can feel through it when she puts it on his finger and sucks on it. The owner admitted that he has lost some business because of the all-condom policy. He loses a weekly average of 20 customers who leave and go to seek sex where condoms are not required. But there are also customers who insist on using condoms and even bring their own. About one fourth of the customers call beforehand to ask whether condoms are available. Those individuals seem pleased with the all-condom policy. The owner stated that he may be getting some customers who would have formerly sought sex without using a condom but who now consider it to be too great a risk.

The women are often asked by a customer if he is their first customer. They frequently have a full schedule of customers around the clock. With this schedule, it is difficult to determine who is first. Still a man seems to feel some comfort in feeling that he is "first." The owner also has noticed that men who previously would pick another woman after having been with one seem more reluctant to do this now. There also has been a decline in the number of customers who want to "party," a general term used to describe a number of activities including having sex with more than one woman at a time or having sex with a woman along with a female partner the customer brings. Although the extent to which AIDS has changed the types of sex acts requested by customers is difficult to determine, the owner has found that customers are requesting more manual stimulations. They ask a woman to perform dances or fantasy plays and masturbate while watching her.

There is no record of any prostitutes leaving brothel employment specifically because of AIDS.[29] The brothel owner reported that since the introduction of mandatory testing and the all-condom policy, he has seen an increase over the usual number of women seeking employment. In interviewing prospective employees, he uses techniques similar to those used by the women in interviewing prospective customers. He is especially concerned about IV drug practices. When he interviews a woman, he inquires especially about her goals. He looks for any goal she may have such as buying a car or a house or raising a child. An absence of goals is taken to mean that she is on drugs and he will not hire her. If a woman is discovered to be using drugs, she is fired immediately. The brothel's drug policy could account in part for the negative antibody status of the women.

Although precise figures aren't available, Nevada brothels are estimated to be a $15 million/year business.[31] Informal estimates are that with the advent of AIDS, business initially declined 30–50%.[29] A number of brothels went on the market and some were sold. Recent reports are that business is up again and owners hope that the brothel's negative antibody status will entice new customers and bring back former ones.[29] Owners have used this antibody status as a marketing technique. Sex at the brothel is promoted as safer than sex in a less controlled environment.

PROSTITUTION AND SOCIAL POLICY

The idea that the legalized brothel system could replace street prostitution totally has been questioned by those who feel that some customers prefer meeting women in atmospheres other than a brothel. Las Vegas is an example where visiting men still want the freedom to invite women up to their hotel rooms. So even if legal prostitution were permitted in Las Vegas, it never would replace illegal prostitution completely.[32] The effect of the legalized system in Nevada is to reduce rather than to eliminate illegal prostitution.

For this reason, some advocates of the legalization of prostitution argue for total legalization of all types of prostitution.

Total legislation would allow women to work as free agents rather than for a brothel owner. The system of legalized prostitution in Nevada places several restrictions on the women's behavior. Some of these restrictions are of questionable legal validity and may be viewed as direct infringements on the women's civil rights. The women are permitted to leave the brothel only during certain hours and there are restrictions on where in town they are permitted to go. Solicitation of business outside the brothel is prohibited. The system of legalized prostitution in West Germany has fewer restrictions on prostitutes than the brothel system in Nevada. Prostitutes do not work in brothels and instead are confined to certain zones.

Control of STDs

West German prostitutes are required to get regular health examinations. They are given health cards indicating they are free of venereal disease. The German government provides these health examinations. When a woman tests positive for venereal disease (VD), she is referred to a private physician and her health care is confiscated until she is treated. German health authorities consider legalization the only way to control VD.

While the Nevada and West German position is that legalization is the only way to control VD, those who oppose legalization argue that it would have the opposite effect and would cause VD rates to rise. This has not been shown to be the case either in Nevada or in West Germany.[30,33] Available data from European countries suggest that VD rates increase when prostitution is illegal and decrease when prostitution is legal.[3] Smith and Smith[16] found that the rate of HIV seroprevalence among unlicensed prostitutes in West Germany was 20%, as compared with 1% among licensed prostitutes. Unlicensed prostitutes were found to use IV drugs more and condoms less than licensed prostitutes. The lack of seroprevalence among licensed prostitutes could reflect to some extent the exclusion of prostitutes who use IV drugs from licensing.

Control of HIV Infection

Assessing HIV-related behavioral change in prostitution is sometimes methodologically problematic. Many prostitutes used condoms for prophylaxis before the advent of HIV. A well-known trick in prostitute circles is to get a condom on a customer without his ever knowing. The extent to which prostitutes have increased their use of condoms specifically because of HIV has not been determined in any studies to date. There are reports of pimps supplying condoms to prostitutes in some cities. Oral sex has become an increasingly popular request among customers of prostitutes in New York City (Sterk C: personal communication, 1988). The popularity of oral sex is the apparent result of the relative safety of fellatio. To some extent HIV may serve as its own control and some customers may cease seeking the services of prostitutes. There are a few isolated reports[34,35] of women leaving prostitution because of an HIV-related decline in business.

Arrest rates are not the best indicators of behavioral change in prostitutes. Street prostitutes are more visible and consequently they are arrested more often than other prostitutes.[36] Arrest rates thus may reflect the social class of prostitutes more than the actual prevalence of prostitution. Arrest rates are not even good indicators of rates of street prostitution, however. Higher arrest rates, for instance, may reflect a more punitive stance by law enforcement against prostitution rather than an actual increase in levels of prostitution.

Laws on HIV-related sexual offenses currently are being formulated in many states. Most state and local governments that have taken action thus far have made testing mandatory for women convicted of prostitution. Nevada, Illinois, and Florida have enacted statutes mandating testing.[37] Record of HIV seropositivity is recorded in a prostitute's criminal record. The type of action taken against an infected prostitute who is subsequently arrested for prostitution has varied. Prosecutors in most states have sought misdemeanor charges though felony charges have been suggested in some states. In most states, the charge has been reckless conduct or endangering life rather than attempted murder, however.

Quarantine orders restricting travel and activities of prostitutes also have been implemented. There have been cases of quarantine in California, Nevada, and Florida.[38] In one Florida case, a prostitute with AIDS was confined to her home and ordered to wear an electronic transmitter that would signal police if she travelled more than 200 feet from her home. How this would prevent her from practicing her trade is not at all clear.

Mandatory HIV antibody testing has been opposed by the American Civil Liberties Union (ACLU) on grounds that it is an intrusive violation of privacy and Fourth Amendment search and seizure rights. The ACLU also has challenged mandatory testing on the grounds that prostitution has not been correlated with transmission of disease. It seems legally questionable that an infected woman arrested for prostitution could be charged with attempted murder if she used condoms or if she practiced completely safe sex such as manual stimulation or fantasy-oriented sex. Some cities have made testing voluntary for women arrested for prostitution because of the legal issues surrounding mandatory testing. In Albuquerque, New Mexico, women arrested for prostitution are required to get mandatory counseling on HIV, but testing is voluntary.[39]

Given the current state of epidemiologic knowledge, the utility and legal validity of mandatory antibody testing and quarantine are questionable. When these measures are applied specifically to prostitutes but not to other groups that are equally or even more likely to transmit HIV, they stand being challenged in court on the basis of equal protection.

Various approaches are being taken by prostitute advocacy groups to educate women about the risk of HIV infection. COYOTE (an acronym for Call Off Your Old Tired Ethics), a prostitute's support group in California, has organized Bad Girl Rap Groups that meet monthly to discuss personal problems, police harassment, drug use, and safe sex. The Mary Magdalene Project in Los Angeles, organized to support women who are redirecting their lives away from prostitution, provides educational and vocational assistance. The California Prostitutes Education Project warns prostitutes about the danger of unprotected exposures and provides educational sessions on how to prevent infection. In Atlanta the Department of Public Health has conducted safe-sex parties for prostitutes. State health officials in Atlantic City attempted to extend an education project that used current or former prostitutes to distribute condoms and AIDS information to other prostitutes. Although the project never got funded, one prostitute involved in this outreach effort distributed 150 AIDS brochures containing the caption "For Women Only—Work,

Play, Love Safely." The pamphlet contains a single condom with the message "Because of the work you do, your own health may be in danger." The brochure encourages women to require clients to wear condoms and to refuse their business if they won't. Genesis House of Chicago, as part of Chicago's Comprehensive AIDS Prevention Education Program, uses former prostitutes as education outreach counselors and operates a drop-in counseling service. Genesis House distributes a brochure for prostitutes that instructs them to remind customers that "guys who wear condoms last longer."

Prostitutes who use IV drugs are among the most difficult for outreach efforts to reach. In contrast to the general IV drug-using population, prostitutes who use IV drugs are more mobile. They use this mobility to escape the police. Condom use by these women is much less than by prostitutes who do not use IV drugs. Condom use is largely a reflection of the economic reality of a prostitute's situation: those who use IV drugs are more commonly street prostitutes whose addiction often forces them to buy drugs rather than condoms with what little money they earn. These women find themselves involved in one illegal activity in order to support another. Even though they may fear AIDS, AIDS is just one risk among many for these women caught up in day-to-day street survival. Drug treatment for women is limited based on the real need that exists. Most residential drug treatment centers will not accept women who are pregnant and none will take women with children. There are no drug treatment centers specifically designed to serve addicted women with AIDS.

In those states in which mandatory testing of women arrested for prostitution exists, jail facilities provide diagnosis of HIV infection but they do not provide treatment. Clearly, jails are not the best settings for HIV antibody testing. The police take a role in controlling HIV that should be the proper role of public health. The legal and economic reality is such that jail is often the only place that prostitutes get diagnostic services for HIV, let alone treatment.

CONCLUSION

Punitive efforts to control HIV in prostitutes are in need of careful scrutiny. The sensibility of making more laws is questionable since prostitution is already illegal. A prostitute's criminal record is made worse with a felony charge of HIV seropositivity added, since prostitution itself is a misdemeanor in most states. The effect of mandatory testing in reality is to make the criminal penalties related to prostitution more severe. Should a prostitute who has been arrested try to leave prostitution, her criminal record may impede her employment possibilities. Mandatory testing policies could hinder these possibilities even more. The ironic effect of mandatory testing legislation may make it less possible for an infected woman to leave prostitution because of the more serious criminal record she has acquired by virtue of her HIV status. Nevertheless, we can expect mandatory testing of arrested prostitutes to become more widespread. Such testing will create a need for support services and rehabilitation programs for infected prostitutes.

Mandatory testing of prostitutes actually could make prostitutes even more dependent on pimps. Part of the reason prostitutes have pimps is because their behavior is illegal.[36] Pimps are expected to take care of bail when prostitutes are arrested. In addition, they may be expected to provide a lawyer and give prostitutes financial and moral support if they have to serve a sentence. With a felony charge because of a prostitute's antibody positive status, she may need a pimp even more because of the more severe criminal penalties she's acquired.

In most states, prostitution is illegal both for prostitutes and for their customers. Customers are rarely arrested although they are usually the initiators of the transactions. Testing policies for STDs reflect a similar double standard. Generally customers have escaped requirements for medical inspection, although during World War II, the U.S. Armed Forces did adopt a policy that required that male clients of prostitutes be tested.[40] This policy proved far more effective than the actual testing of prostitutes since symptoms of STDs are more visible in males. Also, even if a prostitute is shown to be free of disease at one time, she could be infected by her next customer. Policy on mandatory HIV testing also serves as an effective commentary on society's double standard. Hardly any states or municipalities require the clients of prostitutes to be tested for antibodies to HIV. One exception here is Newark, New Jersey, where anyone convicted of prostitution-related offenses, including both prostitutes and their clients, must submit to antibody testing.[37] Mandatory testing of prostitutes serves to protect the customer more than the prostitute, since it ensures that she is antibody negative but there is no assurance that he is. In this way, mandatory testing policies actually could serve to discourage safe-sex practices. Control of HIV transmission will require recognition of the customer's role in the act of prostitution. Groups that advocate abolishing prostitution might do well to look at this end of the sexual equation since ending prostitution will require reducing the demand for commercialized sex.

Prostitutes face the same occupational disadvantages that many women in other lower-class service occupations face. Efforts toward prostitutes' rehabilitation have not been shown to be a realistic direction for social policy. Most of these women have few skills and job alternatives outside prostitution. Reformed prostitutes do not qualify as displaced homemakers according to current guidelines. We cannot assume that women infected with AIDS can or will leave prostitution. Most do not have the employment skills or social mobility necessary to do so. Additional responsibilities of pregnancy and children may force them to continue their illegal survival activity. Vocational rehabilitation is rarely available to HIV-infected prostitutes. In view of the existing career options, whether infected prostitutes who use condoms and who want to or have to continue work as a prostitute should be advised to leave prostitution may be a moot point.

Prostitutes have long been threatened by arrests, VD, pregnancy, and psychopathic customers. They have always been vulnerable, and AIDS now is seen by them as just one more risk added to their list of occupational hazards. Proponents of legalization see the AIDS crisis as one more reason to legalize prostitution. Social policy aimed at controlling HIV in prostitutes, however, does not appear to be moving in this direction.

The problem of HIV among prostitutes illustrates the gap that sometimes exists between research and policy: epidemiologic data are not being used to formulate social policy. HIV seroprevalence among prostitutes who do not use IV drugs is actually low or absent.[41] Prostitution itself has not been demonstrated to be an additional risk factor in HIV seropositivity among women addicted to IV drugs[41,42] but prostitution may be a factor in the potential spread from the IV drug population to others. Prostitutes who use IV drugs probably pose more of a risk to IV drug users with whom they share needles than to their customers. The absence of HIV infection in prostitutes involved in legal prostitution in Nevada, West Germany, and the Netherlands has not been used by policy-makers as a case for legalizing prostitution in other areas.

Most policy efforts to control prostitution and HIV have been punitive, even though the extent to which prostitutions are infecting customers has not been clearly demonstrated epidemiologically. Moreover, prostitutes have been given far more attention in terms of their potential role as infectors than for the very real risk of infection which their occupation poses to them. There is a general lack of social service programs available to infected prostitutes, particularly in large cities like New York with high rates of HIV infection. This deficiency may reflect a sexist or sex-negative attitude showing a reluctance to recognize prostitution as a sex industry occupation. Legislation has sought mostly to punish prostitutes for their role in infecting customers but has not dealt with the broader structural problems that infected prostitutes face. Controlling HIV in prostitutes will require addressing these fundamental problems.

APPENDIX: RESOURCES FOR PROSTITUTES

Shelters

Genesis House
911 W. Addison St.
Chicago, IL 60613
(312) 281-3817

Mary Magdalene Project, Inc.
6557 Flotilla Street
Commerce, CA 90040
(213) 725-7230

National Task Force on Prostitution Affiliates

National Task Force on Prostitution
P.O. Box 26354
San Francisco, CA 94126
(415) 957-1292

Georgia HIRE/COYOTE
P.O. Box 7781
Atlanta, GA 30309
(404) 876-1212

Los Angeles COYOTE
Box 580
1626 N. Wilcox
Hollywood, CA 90028
(213) 389-4495

Massachusetts COYOTE
P.O. Box 621
Astor Station
Boston, MA 02123-0621
(617) 445-7670

Minnesota COYOTE
P.O. Box 4277
St. Paul, MN 55104
(612) 645-2230

New York COYOTE
P.O. Box 1331
Old Chelsea Station
New York, NY 10011
(212) 242-6449

Rocky Mountain COYOTE
P.O. Box 4157
Boulder, CO 80306
(303) 440-9042

San Francisco COYOTE
P.O. Box 26354
San Francisco, CA 94126
(415) 957-1292 and (415) 232-7762

REFERENCES

1. Delacoste F, Alexander P (eds): *Sex Work*. Pittsburgh, Cleis Press, 1987.
2. Darrow WW: Prostitution and sexually transmitted diseases, in Holmes KK, Mardh PA, Sparling PF, Wiesner PJ (eds): *Sexually Transmitted Diseases*. New York, McGraw Hill, 1984, p 109.
3. James J, Boyer D, Withers J, et al: *Perspectives on Prostitution*. Seattle, Social Research Associates, 1980.
4. Davis NJ: Prostitution, identity, career and legal economic enterprise, in Henslin JM, Sagarin E (eds): *Studies in the Sociology of Sex*. New York, Schocken Books, 1978, pp 195–222.
5. Winick C, Kinsie PM: *The Lively Commerce*. Chicago, Quadrangle Books, 1971.
6. Winick C: Prostitutes' clients' perceptions of the prostitute and themselves. *Int J Social Psychiatry* 8:289–297, 1961–1962.
7. Milner C, Milner R: *Black Players*. Boston, Little Brown, 1972.
8. Goldstein PJ: *Prostitution and Drugs*. Lexington, DC Heath and Company, 1979.
9. Centers for Disease Control: Antibody to human immunodeficiency virus in female prostitutes. *MMWR* 36:157–61, 1987.
10. Neequaye AR, Neequaye J, Mingle JA, et al: Preponderance of females with AIDS in Ghana. (Letter.) *Lancet* 2:978, 1986.
11. Van de Perre P, Clumeck N, Carael M, et al: Female prostitutes: A risk group for infection with human T-cell lymphotropic virus type III. *Lancet* 2:524–527, 1985.
12. Mann J. Quinn TC, Piot P, et al: Condom use and HIV infection among prostitutes in Zaire. (Letter.) *N Engl J Med* 316:345, 1987.
13. Kreiss JK, Koech D, Plummer FA, et al: AIDS virus infection in Nairobi prostitutes. *N Engl J Med* 314:414–418, 1986.
14. Barton SE, Underhill GS, Gilchrist C, et al: HTLV-III antibody in prostitutes. (Letter.) *Lancet* 2:1424, 1985.
15. Brenky-Faudeux D, Fribourg-Blanc A: HTLV-III antibody in prostitutes. (Letter.) *Lancet* 2:1424, 1985.
16. Smith GL, Smith KF: Lack of HIV infection and condom use in licensed prostitutes. (Letter.) *Lancet* 2:1392, 1986.
17. Tirelli U, Vaccher E, Carbone A, et al: HTLV-III antibody in prostitutes. (Letter.) *Lancet* 2:1424, 1985.
18. Luthy R, Ledergerber B, Tauber M, et al: Prevalence of HIV antibodies among prostitutes in Zurich, Switzerland. *Klin Wochenschr* 65:287–288, 1987.
19. Schultz S, Milberg JA, Kristal AR, et al: Female-to-male transmission of HTLV-III. (Letter.) *JAMA* 255:1703–1704, 1986.
20. Papaevangelou G, Roumeliotou-Karayannis A, Kallinkos G, et al: LAV/HTLV-III infection in female prostitutes. (Letter.) *Lancet* 2:1018, 1985.
21. Vittecoq D, May T, Roue RT, et al: Acquired immunodeficiency syndrome after travelling in Africa. *Lancet* 1:612–615, 1987.
22. Clumeck N, Van de Perre P, Carael M, et al: Heterosexual promiscuity among African patients with AIDS. (Letter.) *N Engl J Med* 313:182, 1985.
23. Rabkin CS, Thomas PA, Jaffe HW, et al: Prevalence of antibody to HTLV-III/LAV in a population attending a sexually transmitted diseases clinic. *Sex Transm Dis* 14:48–51, 1987.
24. Padian NS: Heterosexual transmission of acquired immunodeficiency syndrome. *Rev Infect Dis* 9:947–960, 1987.
25. Potterat JJ, Muth JB, Markewich GS: Serological markers as indicators of sexual orientation in AIDS virus-infected men. (Letter.) *JAMA* 256:712, 1986.
26. Potterat JJ, Phillips L., Muth JB: Lying to military physicians about risk factors for HIV infections. (Letter.) *JAMA* 257:1727, 1987.
27. Darrow WW, Cohen JB, French J, et al: Multicenter study of human immunodeficiency virus antibody in U.S. prostitutes, in *Third International Conference on AIDS, Washington, DC, June 3, 1986*.
28. James J: Mobility as an adaptive strategy. *Urban Anthropol* 4:349–364, 1975.
29. Stein MA: Bordellos of Nevada try to lure patrons, banish AIDS. *Los Angeles Times* June 8, 1987, p 3.
30. Symanski R: Prostitution in Nevada. *Ann Assoc Am Geog* 64:357–377, 1974.
31. Swan G: Nevada's brothels are under attack. San Francisco Chronicle, December 1, 1986 pp 1–6.
32. Reynolds H: *The Economics of Prostitution*. Springfield, Illinois, Charles C Thomas, 1986.
33. Yondorf B: Prostitution as a legal activity: The West German experience. *Policy Anal* 5:418–433, 1979.

34. Leishman K: Heterosexuals and AIDS. *Atlantic Monthly* 259:39–58, 1987.
35. Block A: Life on the streets. *San Francisco Examiner* July 27, 1986, pp 15–20.
36. James J: Prostitution: Arguments for change, in Gordon S, Libby R (eds): *Sexuality Today and Tomorrow*. North Scituate, Massachusetts, Duxbury Press, 1976, pp 110–123.
37. Institute of Medicine: *Confronting AIDS, Update 1988*. Washington, DC, National Academy Press, 1988.
38. Decker JF: Prostitution as a public health issue, in Dalton HL, Burris S, and the Yale AIDS Law Project (eds): *AIDS and the Law*. New Haven, Yale University Press, 1987, pp 81–89.
39. Gabbet P: Prostitute counseling sought. *The Independent,* May 30, 1987, p. 11.
40. Bullough V, Bullough B: *Women and Prostitution*. New York, Prometheus, 1987.
41. Rosenberg M, Weiner J: Prostitutes and AIDS: A health department priority? *Am J Public Health* 78:418–423, 1988.
42. Tirelli U: In reply, HIV antibodies in drug-addicted prostitutes. *JAMA* 257:1047, 1987.

7

Intravenous Drug Use and AIDS

DON C. DES JARLAIS, SAMUEL R. FRIEDMAN, and JOYCELYN SUE WOODS

INTRODUCTION

Intravenous (IV) drug users have been the second largest group of persons to have developed acquired immune deficiency syndrome (AIDS) in the United States and in Western Europe. 10,627 (18%) of the 59,287 adult cases reported in the United States have occurred in heterosexual IV drug users, and another 4325 (7%) in IV drug users who also had male homosexuality as a risk factor.[1] In Europe, 1944 (19.5%) of the 9930 adult cases have occurred in heterosexual IV drug users, and another 259 (3%) in IV drug users who also had male homosexual activity as a risk factor.[2]

The drug use most commonly associated with the transmission of human immunodeficiency virus (HIV) is the IV injection of heroin, although cocaine injection may be an increasing problem, and amphetamine injection also a problem to some extent. "Skin popping" (injection just under the skin) rather than IV injection would also be sufficient for transmission. Because so very few persons who inject drugs confine themselves to skin popping, we will use the term "IV drug use" for convenience. This term is meant to include all of the different drugs that are injected as well as the various injection methods.

Because the great majority of IV drug users are heterosexual, once the virus has become established within a community of IV drug users, they form a primary source for both heterosexual and in utero transmission. In New York City, 87% of cases attributed to heterosexual transmission have an IV drug user as the apparent source of the virus, and 80% of the cases of perinatal transmission AIDS have occurred in children who have an IV drug user as a parent (New York City Department of Health: personal communication, February 11, 1988).

This chapter reviews knowledge of the epidemiology and natural history of AIDS in IV drug users, the behavioral changes made by IV drug users in response to AIDS, and the possible futures of the epidemic among IV drug users. Before covering those topics, however, it will be useful to discuss briefly the "nature" of IV drug use in American, Western European, and developing nation societies.

Intravenous drug use has often been described from a variety of perspectives. Among

DON C. DES JARLAIS • Beth Israel Medical Center, New York, New York 10013; Narcotic and Drug Research, Inc., New York, New York 10013. SAMUEL R. FRIEDMAN and JOYCELYN SUE WOODS • Narcotic and Drug Research, Inc., New York, New York 10013.

the public at large, narcotic addiction has traditionally been viewed as immoral and/or a character weakness, although it was not until early in the twentieth century that national laws were passed against the possession of narcotics.[3] During the late nineteenth century, the "typical" American narcotic addict was a middle-class housewife addicted to the morphine in patent medicines. Only after over the counter narcotic sales were prohibited and an illicit market in narcotics developed did a strong relationship between narcotic addiction, lower socioeconomic status, and criminal activity emerge.[4] Law enforcement activities against drug distributors and drug users, and warnings to nonusers never to start using, have been the primary means advocated by persons subscribing to this moralistic perspective on drug abuse.

The view of narcotic addiction as a psychopathology was largely developed by Kolb.[5] While it is currently accepted that there is no unified "addictive personality," substance abuse is currently a classification within the official Diagnostic and Statistical Manual of the American Psychiatric Association.[6] In addition, some narcotic addicts are seen as using narcotics to self-medicate psychiatric symptoms such as depression.

A biologic abnormality perspective is currently most closely associated with methadone maintenance treatment.[7] The discovery of endogenous opioid peptides (endorphins) that naturally occur in the human brain provided a potential mechanism for such a biologic defect.

A deviant subculture perspective emphasizes linkages between the social organization of drug abuse and the larger society, and the initiation and continuation of membership in a group sharing common values.[8] Within this sociological perspective, drug users are considered to vary greatly in both personality and physiology, with the common behavior arising from membership in the group.

The drug use as immoral behavior perspective does not permit scientific testing, although data can be used in support of this perspective. There is supporting scientific evidence for the biologic, psychological, and sociological perspectives on IV drug use, but there is not yet any unified scientific explanation. The importance of which perspective to use in viewing IV drug use goes beyond interdisciplinary academic disputes or political orientations. The choice of perspective greatly determines beliefs about what forms of AIDS prevention among IV drug users are likely to be most effective.

INTERNATIONAL EPIDEMIOLOGY OF AIDS AMONG IV DRUG USERS

Cases of AIDS

The New York City metropolitan area has by far the greatest concentration of IV drug users who have developed AIDS. There have been 4613 cases of AIDS in IV drug users from New York State and 2154 from New Jersey reported to the Centers for Disease Control (CDC) with an additional 3860 cases throughout the United States (New York State AIDS Surveillance: personal communication, April 15, 1988; State of New Jersey AIDS Surveillance: personal communication, March 31, 1988; Centers for Disease Control through April 11, 1988). (IV drug users who also have male homosexuality as a risk factor are not included in these totals).

In Europe, there have been 1918 cases in heterosexual IV drug users, with no single city having a concentration that is equivalent to New York,[2] (Brunet J-B: personal communication, 1987). The countries with the highest numbers of cases are Italy with 871 cases, Spain with 407 cases, France with 354 cases, and Germany with 143 cases. In Italy and Spain, IV drug users constitute more than one half the total cases of AIDS.

Heterosexual IV drug users have remained at approximately 18% of the United States cases since 1983, with a slight increase recently. European IV drug use cases are rapidly increasing as a percentage of the total number of cases, going from 2% in September 1984, to 12% in Sept. 1986, and to 18% in Sept. 1987 (Brunet JB: personal communication, 1987).

HIV Seroprevalence

There is a long "latency" period between initial exposure to HIV and the development of clinical AIDS, which is estimated to average 7 years or longer. Data on cases of AIDS therefore reflect infections that occurred several years prior to diagnosis. Studies of exposure to HIV among IV drug users provide a better indication of current levels of HIV infection and the development of potential future cases of AIDS. HIV seroprevalence data from several studies are presented in Table 1, showing great variation both within the United States and Western Europe. Because of differences in methods of recruiting subjects, comparisons of exact seropositivity percentages are not justifiable. The different cities have thus been grouped into three categories. (For a listing of seroprevalence studies in the United States, see CDC, MMWR[1]).

One factor explaining some of this geographic variation is simply the time that HIV was first introduced into different areas. Studies of historically collected sera show first HIV seropositive samples among IV drug users in 1978 in New York City,[16] 1979 in Milan,[17] 1982 in Berlin,[18] and 1984 in Copenhagen.[19]

HIV may be introduced into a local group of IV drug users from a person in another risk group, or by travel of IV drug users to or from other areas. In New York City, it is likely that HIV spread from gay males to IV drug users, as four of the first ten cases of

TABLE 1. HIV Seroprevalence Rates among Intravenous Drug Users in Selected Cities

High Seroprevalence (>50%)	
New York City	Cohen et al. (1985)[9]
Northern New Jersey	Weiss et al. (1987)[10]
Italy	Angarano et al. (1985)[11]
Edinburgh	Robertson et al. (1986)[12]
Moderate (15–45%)	
Zurich	Schupbach et al. (1985)[13]
West Berlin	Hunsmann et al. (1985)[14]
Low (≤10%)	
San Francisco	Chaisson et al. (1987)[15]
Washington, D.C.	Ginzburg et al. (1988)[a]
New Orleans	Ginzburg et al. (1988)[a]

[a]Personal communication (1988).

AIDS among IV drug users also had male homosexuality as a risk factor.[20] In Los Angeles both male homosexuality and contact with persons from New York were associated with early instances of seropositivity in IV drug users (Mascola L: personal communication, 1987).

Studies of historically collected sera (collected for reasons other than AIDS research and then analyzed for antibody to HIV) show that once HIV has been introduced among IV drug users in a local area, rapid increases in seropositivity can occur. Typically, seroprevalence will stay at a very low level for several years, low enough that only very large-scale surveys will find any seropositive samples. Then when seroprevalence reaches 10–15%, there will be a rapid rise to 40% or more over the next 3 years. Historically, collected serum samples from Manhattan[16] and Milan illustrate this pattern.[17] In Edinburgh, the rise was even faster, with seroprevalence over 50% within 2 years of the first seropositive sample.[12] These studies of historically collected sera show the spread of HIV among IV drug users prior to any awareness of AIDS, hence prior to any AIDS risk reduction within the group. Given our present knowledge of transmission of HIV and the potential for IV drug users to change their behavior, this type of explosive spread should not be permitted to occur again.

Transmission of HIV among IV drug users occurs primarily through the sharing of drug injection equipment. From the studies of behavioral risk factors for HIV exposure among IV drug users, there appear to be three factors associated with seropositivity among IV drug users within individual cities. The first is the frequency of drug injection since the virus was introduced into the area.[9,21,22] Prior to concerns about AIDS, sharing "works" (drug injection equipment) was a "normal" aspect of injecting drugs. Sharing was associated with initiation into IV drug use, served as a social bonding mechanism among IV drug users, and also occurred for many practical reasons—when the drug user did not have enough money to purchase an unused needle, when fear of arrest kept users from carrying their own works, or when unused works were simply not available at the time the drug user wanted to inject.[23]

The second factor, which may be a critical determinant in the speed of viral spread within a local area, is sharing equipment with large numbers of other IV drug users. Clearly, if IV drug users confined their sharing of drug injection equipment to small friendship groups, there would be very limited transmission of the virus from one group to another, and the spread would be rather slow. In New York City and the northeastern United States, the sharing of drug injection equipment across friendship groups occurs most frequently in "shooting galleries," places where IV drug users often rent previously used works. The use of shooting galleries has also been shown to be associated with HIV exposure among IV drug users in other American studies,[22,24,25] (Chaisson RE: personal communication, 1987). In some areas, the sharing of works across friendship groups may occur more frequently with "house works"—a spare set of injection equipment kept by a drug dealer for his customers to use immediately after purchasing the drug—or through groups of casual acquaintances that form in areas where drugs are sold.

A third factor that has emerged in a number of studies is belonging to an ethnic minority. Several American studies found ethnic differences in seroprevalence rates within a single city even after controlling on all other variables.[15,21,26–28] In none of these studies did white American IV drug users have significantly higher rates than black or hispanic IV drug users. The differences between black and hispanic IV drug users were not consistent across the studies.

The reasons why white American IV drug users would have lower seroprevalence rates are not clear. Genetic factors related to HIV susceptibility cannot yet be rule out, although they would seem unlikely. Unmeasured or poorly measured behavioral differences may account for the differences, the precise wording of questions on risk behavior has not been standardized across studies, and ethnic group membership may be associated with different patterns of responding to the same questions. A single city may not be the proper geographic unit for the analysis—most American cities are highly residentially segregated, and the ethnic differences may simply reflect "local epidemics" within a single city. In one study that used subjects primarily from the Lower East Side of Manhattan,[24] a neighborhood that is relatively integrated with respect to IV drug use, the ethnic differences were not statistically significant after controlling for drug use behavior.

One European study has also found ethnic differences. German IV drug users living in Amsterdam had higher seroprevalence rates than did native Dutch IV drug users.[29] Thus, as in the U.S. studies, belonging to an ethnic minority was associated with higher seroprevalence. There may be some generalized aspect of belonging to a minority group associated with higher seroprevalence rates among IV drug users, or there may be different explanations for the American and Dutch findings.

Although IV drug users show a wide range in the frequency of sexual activity, there appear to be few relationships between sexual activity and HIV exposure among IV drug users. The great majority of HIV seroprevalence studies among IV drug users do not show any relationship between sexual behavior and viral exposure after controlling for drug use behavior. One exception to this general rule is that HIV may be initially introduced into a local group of IV drug users through persons who engage in both male homosexual activity and IV drug use. This appears to be the case in New York City.[24] The second possible exception concerns female prostitutes who inject drugs. One study has found IV drug using female prostitutes to have higher seroprevalence even after controlling for drug use behaviors,[22] but this does not appear to be the general case as this has not been found in other studies.

The findings that HIV exposure is strongly associated with frequency of drug injection and with the anonymous sharing of injection equipment in shooting galleries or with house works suggest that prevention programs aimed at these factors are likely to be successful in at least slowing the spread of HIV among IV drug users. While the reasons for ethnic differences in seroprevalence rates among IV drug users are not known, the findings are sufficiently frequent that they need to be taken into account in designing AIDS prevention programs for IV drug users. Heterosexual activity does not appear to be nearly as important as the sharing of drug injection equipment in transmitting HIV among IV drug users, but prevention programs will clearly need to focus on the potential spread of the virus from IV drug users to sexual partners who do not themselves inject drugs.

NATURAL HISTORY OF HIV INFECTION AMONG IV DRUG USERS

Much less is known about the natural history of HIV infection in IV drug users compared to the factors associated with initial exposure. IV drug users engage in a variety of behaviors that may affect the immune system and thus act as cofactors in HIV infection. These include injection of drugs prior to HIV infection, continued injection of drugs after initial infection, and heavy use of noninjected drugs such as alcohol and marijuana. There is evidence for cofactors that influence the outcomes of HIV infection among IV drug users, but there has been no definitive identification of the mechanisms for these cofactors.

It was recognized early in the AIDS epidemic that IV drug users with AIDS are much less likely to have Kaposi's sarcoma (KS) than homosexual men with AIDS,[30] indicating possible cofactors for KS that may be associated with sexual activity. Nitrite use[31] and cytomegalovirus[32] have been suggested as cofactors that lead to KS in the presence of HIV infection. The difference in KS rates between homosexual/bisexual men and IV drug users with AIDS has remained despite the decline in the percentage of AIDS cases in which KS is the initial manifestation.[33]

The percentage of IV drug users who develop clinical AIDS after infection with HIV is currently unknown, although estimates run to 100%. One follow-up study of IV drug users from Queens, New York covered a 3-year period. Twenty-four seropositives were in the initial sample; follow-up information was obtained for 8, 2 of which had developed AIDS.[34] In our first year of a cohort study of HIV-infected IV drug users in New York City, we found a rate of 4% per year of the subjects developing AIDS.[35] Selwyn et al.,[37] also in New York, found a similar rate.

A critical question is whether or not any potential behavioral cofactors accelerate the rate of progression to AIDS. A finding of such a behavioral cofactor would have important implications for both the counseling and treatment of seropositive IV drug users and understanding of the pathogenesis of HIV infection. General immunologic stimulation has been shown to lead to increased viral production and death of HIV infected T4 cells in vitro.[37] This suggests a hypothesis that immunologic stimulation from non-sterile injection would increase the rate of T4 cell loss and increase immunosuppression among IV drug users exposed to HIV.

Two studies show evidence in support of this hypothesis. In one study, high rates of drug injection were associated with an increased rate of T4 cells loss over a 9-month follow-up period among IV drug users seropositive for HIV. The predictive value of continued drug injection remained statistically significant after controlling for initial T4 cell count, alcohol use, marijuana use, and cigarette use.[38] Almost all subjects whose T4 cell counts remained stable or improved over the follow-up period were those who had stopped injecting or were injecting at low to moderate levels. Subjects who were injecting at high levels showed very large declines in T4 cell counts. In a second study, high rates of nonsterile drug injection were associated with the actual development of AIDS, although the relationship did not remain statistically significant when initial AIDS-related symptoms were entered into the regression analysis.[36] Neither of these can be considered definitive evidence that continued drug injection increases the risk of developing clinical disease after initial exposure to HIV, and they indicate only a moderate effect associated with high levels of continued drug injection. Nevertheless, the consistency between the in vitro laboratory studies and the epidemiologic studies should serve as a basis for counseling seropositive IV drug users that continued injection of illicit drugs may endanger their own health as well as possibly transmitting the virus to others through the sharing of injection equipment.

Epidemic level increases in deaths due to tuberculosis, endocarditis, non-*Pneumocystis* pneumonia and other infections[39,40] have occurred among IV drug users in New York City coincident in time with the AIDS epidemic. From 1982 through 1986, there have been approximately 4300 "excess" deaths among known IV drug users compared to a 1979–1981 baseline of slightly more than 500 deaths per year. Less than half these excess deaths occurred from surveillance definition AIDS, the rest were from infections that are not usually considered "opportunistic." Similar increases in deaths from nonopportunistic infections have not been noted in studies of homosexual/bisexual men, the AIDS risk group for which there is relatively good data on outcomes of HIV infection. There are several "cofactors" that could explain high rates of fatal infections occurring in IV drug users but not among homosexual/bisexual men, including differences in rates of exposure to a variety of pathogens, life-style variables such as high levels of alcohol use and poor nutrition, and large differences in health care. Additional research is needed to determine whether any of these potential cofactors are related to the higher fatality rates among IV drug users infected with HIV compared to homosexual/bisexual men infected with the virus.

In summary, recent studies of the natural history of HIV infection suggest several differences between HIV infection in IV drug users compared to HIV infection in homosexual/bisexual men. The rates of Kaposi's sarcoma are higher among homosexual /bisexual men, while HIV-related deaths from "nonopportunistic" infections appear to be very much higher among IV drug users. Cofactors explaining these differences have not yet been identified. There is laboratory and epidemiologic evidence that continued injection after initial exposure to HIV leads to greater immunosuppression among IV drug users, although this also has not been definitively established. The studies of the natural history of HIV infection among IV drug users suggest that stopping drug injection and maintaining an overall "healthy" lifestyle may improve the prognosis of HIV exposed IV drug users to a limited extent. The findings from current natural history studies also reemphasize the need for preventing initial exposure to HIV.

AIDS RISK REDUCTION AMONG IV DRUG USERS

Before discussing the possible future of the AIDS epidemic among IV drug users, it is important to address the belief that prevention cannot work with IV drug users. There is the stereotype that IV drug users are so controlled by their habits that they have no regard for the health consequences of injecting drugs. Research on IV drug users in New York City and other areas clearly shows that this stereotype does not hold for AIDS. In a study of methadone maintenance patients that we conducted in 1984, we found that more than 90% knew that AIDS was transmitted through the sharing of injection equipment and that 59% reported changes in behavior to reduce their risk of contracting AIDS. The most common reported behavior changes included increasing the use of sterile needles (31%), reducing the number of persons with whom one would share injection equipment (29%), and reducing IV drug use (14%).[41] In a similar study of methadone patients and IV drug users under arrest conducted in 1985, Selwyn and colleagues[36] found that 97% of the subjects knew that AIDS was transmitted through sharing injection equipment and that more than 60% reported behavior change in order to reduce the chances of contracting AIDS.[36]

Confirmation of these self-report behavior changes comes from studies of the illicit market for sterile injection equipment in New York City. This market has increased since the AIDS epidemic began[42] and drug dealers have been including sterile needles along with their drugs as a sales strategy.[43] The demand for sterile injection equipment is now strong enough that it also supports the sale of repackaged "counterfeit" sterile needles and syringes. These changes in the marketing of drug injection equipment indicated an increased concern among IV drug users about using sterile equipment that did not exist in New York City prior to the AIDS epidemic.

It is important to consider that the above risk reduction among IV drug users in New York City occurred prior to any formal AIDS prevention programming. The concern arose from information carried in the mass media and through the oral communication channels within the drug distribution network. Specific AIDS prevention programs should be able to improve upon this naturally occurring risk reduction.

AIDS PREVENTION PROGRAMS FOR IV DRUG USERS

A variety of AIDS prevention programs for IV drug users have been established in the United States, Europe and Australia. For the purposes of classification, most of the prevention programs can be divided into "educational" programs that provide information about the need to change behavior to avoid AIDS, and "means" programs that provide actual means for behavior change.

The most common form of AIDS prevention programming has been mass education campaigns, particularly the use of posters and pamphlets containing the basic information that AIDS is spread through the sharing of drug injection equipment. The pamphlets usually advise that all IV drug users should stop injecting drugs and seek treatment if needed, but if they should continue to inject drugs, then they should not share injection equipment and should decontaminate any equipment that might have been used by someone else.

This basic educational strategy is compatible with all of the various "theories" of the nature of drug abuse, which may be one reason for its popularity. If one views drug abuse as a moral failing of the individual, then it is certainly appropriate to inform the individual of the adverse consequences of his or her actions. To the extent that drug abuse is a moral failing, then the self-interest of the individual should be sufficient to lead to behavior change. The psychological, physiological, and sociological perspectives on drug abuse would emphasize that more than simple information would be needed to lead to large-scale behavior change.

To date there have been no formal evaluations of these information campaigns. A rigorous evaluation would be very difficult, as one would probably need to use individual cities as the unit of analysis, and there would be a high likelihood of confounding from mass media stories about AIDS. Given that such a study would be very difficult and very expensive, and that most theories of drug abuse would predict limited behavior change resulting from such educational programs, it is unlikely that a rigorous evaluation will ever be conducted. It is more likely that these mass educational programs will be continued without formal evaluation.

A more sophisticated educational approach to preventing AIDS among IV drug users is to use ex-addicts or other "street wise" persons to provide face-to-face information about AIDS to current IV drug users. The face-to-face setting provides for extensive information transfer, including clarification through questions. It also provides for modulation of the emotional tone of the message, to provoke enough discomfort about sharing injection equipment to motivate behavior change, but not so much that anxiety prevents behavior change. The ex-addict educators also frequently provide information about how used drug injection equipment can be decontaminated through boiling, or through the use of bleach or alcohol. This prevention strategy also uses elements of the sociological conceptualization of drug abuse in that the ex-addicts may not only be better at communicating with current addicts, but they may also serve as "role models" for successful behavior change.[44]

There has been one formal evaluation of an "ex-addict as educator" AIDS prevention program.[45] The research design involved dividing the city of Baltimore into areas, with random assignment of ex-addict educators to some but not all of the areas. Interviews were later conducted with IV drug users in the different areas. Preliminary findings suggest that the ex-addict educators led to increases in knowledge about AIDS without leading to any statistically significant changes in behavior.

The National Institute on Drug Abuse (NIDA) is funding street outreach education programs in 11 cities throughout the country. These programs will be formally evaluated, and there should be enough variation among them to learn much more about the strengths and weaknesses of this prevention strategy.

In addition to prevention programs that provide education about AIDS, a number also provide means for changing behavior. The specific means may vary, from reducing drug use through providing additional treatment to providing sterile injection equipment so that drug use may be continued without using contaminated equipment. Several states have increased the capacity of their drug abuse treatment systems as specific AIDS prevention measures. Prior to awareness of AIDS among IV drug users in New York, the treatment system was already operating at capacity. There were "waiting lists" of approximately 1000 drug users who had applied for treatment, but were not able to be placed into a treatment program at the time of application. The waiting list period averaged between 2 and 3 months. Since then approximately three thousand new treatment positions have been created, roughly a 10% expansion of the system. The waiting list situation, however, has not changed. The new treatment positions have been filled, and the waiting list remains at about the same number. As more IV drug users in New York have learned about AIDS, the demand for treatment has increased.

The expansion of the New Jersey treatment system originated with an ex-addict education program to teach current IV drug users to sterilize their injection equipment.[46] Reports from the ex-addicts indicated that a substantial number of the drug users they contacted preferred entering treatment as a way of reducing their risk of developing AIDS. (Prior to the AIDS epidemic, federal funding reductions had led New Jersey to institute client fees for entry into treatment, which greatly reduced the effective availability of treatment for low income drug users in the state.) New Jersey then instituted a "voucher" program in which the ex-addict AIDS educator distributed vouchers that could be redeemed for free entry into treatment. More than 80% of the vouchers were redeemed for entry into treatment, and interviews with the drug users entering treatment indicated that, for about half of them, concern about AIDS was a major reason for entering treatment.

Providing treatment for IV drug users should be an effective means for preventing HIV infection among those who actually enter treatment. Various treatment outcome studies (e.g., Simpson et al.[47]) have shown dramatic reductions in drug injection among those who enter treatment and are retained for at least 90 days. There are now at least three studies that show lower HIV seroprevalence rates among IV drug users who entered and remained in methadone treatment.[48–50]

As a strategy for controlling the AIDS epidemic among IV drug users, however, there are several major difficulties with this strategy. First, it will be difficult to expand the treatment system in a short time period. The difficulties involve not only the need for additional funds, but also community opposition to the opening of new treatment programs in many neighborhoods, and a lack of trained staff. Controversy over what types of treatment should be provided—with those believing in psychological causes of drug abuse tending to favor drug-free treatment programs and those believing in physiological causes tending to favor chemotherapy programs—also will impede rapid expansion of the treatment system. Finally, there will be a substantial number of IV drug users for whom treatment is not effective, or who simply do not "want" to stop injecting drugs. This group may be growing due to the great increase in cocaine injection in the United States over the last decade and the difficulties in treating cocaine abuse.

The difficulties with relying on providing treatment as a means for IV drug users to reduce their risk of developing AIDS have led to a number of programs that provide means for "safer" injection as AIDS prevention among IV drug users. These safer injection programs are generally opposed by persons holding the moral weakness theory of drug abuse in that they may be perceived as condoning and/or encouraging drug abuse. They are fully consistent with the sociological perspective on drug abuse, which includes the possibility of creating new social norms and rituals around the injection of drugs so that the chances of viral transmission are greatly reduced if not eliminated. Safer injection programs are partially consistent with the psychopathological and physiological perspectives and have received mixed support from treatment program advocates. Proponents of these views of drug abuse agree that for IV drug users it is the drug effect that is sought and not the sharing of injection equipment. They often express doubts, however, about whether or not active IV drug users are able to change their patterns of using injection equipment, and fear that safer injection programs may undermine the willingness of drug users to enter treatment.

Outside of the United States, the preferred means for safer injection has been to provide legal access to sterile injection equipment. Most European countries permitted over the counter sale of needles and syringes prior to AIDS; in France and several cantons of Switzerland the laws have been changed to provide for the sale of sterile needles and syringes without prescriptions. The only places in Western Europe that currently require prescriptions for the sale of needles and syringes are Sweden and some cantons of Switzerland. Studies in Glasgow[51] and in Paris[52] have shown increased purchases of sterile injection equipment by IV drug users, and in Innsbruck, increased use of over the counter sterile injection equipment appears to have reduced transmission of HIV among IV drug users.[53]

"Syringe exchange" systems in which IV drug users can exchange used injection equipment for new sterile equipment have been established in Holland, the United Kingdom, Sweden, and Australia. These programs not only provide the equipment for safer injection, but also usually provide an opportunity for therapeutic contact between health care workers and IV drug users (including counseling regarding heterosexual transmission), and a means for the safe disposal of potentially contaminated drug injection equipment.

These needle exchange programs have not been studied long enough to know whether or not they will reduce the spread of HIV among drug users. The studies from Amsterdam do indicate that the negative outcomes feared by opponents of needle exchanges have not occurred. There has been no decrease in the numbers of IV drug users seeking treatment and there has been no increase in the total numbers of IV drug users.[54] Recent data from ongoing studies in Amsterdam indicate that more IV drug users in that city have been utilizing the syringe exchange as a result of concerns about AIDS. In a study conducted by van den Hoek and colleagues,[29] the percentage of IV drug users who were regularly using the syringe exchange had increased from 8% to 48%. Contrary to some expectations, the frequency of drug injection in the study group decreased rather than increased. The percentage who were injecting at a rate of once or more per day decreased from 87% to 48%. Early findings from U.K. syringe exchanges indicate that they are associated with reduced sharing of injection equipment and not associated with increasing drug use.[55]

At the time of this writing, only two syringe exchange programs have been established in the United States, one in Tacoma, Washington, and one in New York City. Most of the states with large concentrations of IV drug users have laws that require prescriptions for the sale of needles and syringes. Exchange programs have been considered in a number of areas, but face opposition from those who view drug abuse as a moral failing, as well as some opposition from those who view drug abuse as a psychological or physiological problem.

The form of "safer" injection program that has received the widest acceptance in the United States is the distribution of bleach or alcohol to IV drug users for the purpose of decontaminating drug injection equipment. This has been done on a large scale in San Francisco, and on a smaller scale in New York and other cities. The aim of these programs is not only to provide a means for sterilizing injection equipment, but also to develop new norms and rituals for drug injection. The bleach or alcohol is distributed by ex-addicts or others who are familiar with street life. Referrals to a variety of social services are provided as a way of increasing trust between the outreach workers and current IV drug users. In New York, the bleach has been distributed mainly through shooting galleries, while in San Francisco small bottles of bleach are distributed on the streets.

Preliminary data from San Francisco indicate that a large percentage of IV drug users in the city are reporting the use of bleach to clean their injection equipment. Watters and colleagues[56] found that two thirds of their subjects reported using bleach. These represent large scale increases over the less than 5% of drug users who reported using bleach prior to the bleach distribution program, although it is too early to know whether the program will have an effect on the spread of HIV among drug users in San Francisco, the rate of transmission appears to have decreased.[57] Preliminary evaluations of bleach or alcohol distribution have not yet been conducted in other cities.

SPECIAL ISSUES

In addition to the prevention programs discussed above, there are several special issues for AIDS prevention among IV drug users that deserve additional comments. Self-organized groups of gay men have been credited with producing much of the AIDS risk reduction in that group.[58] The threat of AIDS has also produced a limited organizational response among IV drug users. Where IV drug users' organizations already exist—as in the Dutch *Junkiebonden* (drug users' unions)—they have begun to set up risk-reduction projects.[50] In New York City, former and current IV drug users, in cooperation with health professionals, have formed a group call ADAPT to encourage risk reduction and to provide services for IV drug users with HIV disease.[59] ADAPT is one of the groups distributing bleach in New York. A similar group, the AIDS Drug Information Collective (ADIC) has been established in Sydney, Australia.[59] The difficulties in organizing IV drug users to prevent AIDS are formidable, including different concepts of the nature of drug addiction held by current IV drug users, former IV drug users, and society at large. It remains to be seen whether anything like the scale of the gay organizations engaged in AIDS prevention will ever be achieved among IV drug users.

The use of HIV antibody testing has frequently been advocated as a means for controlling the spread of AIDS. There are at least two functions for antibody testing as an AIDS control measure for IV drug users. First it may serve as a warning signal to a local community that HIV is present among IV drug users and that risk-reduction/prevention programs need to be undertaken immediately. Second, antibody testing may lead seropositives to change their behavior so that they do not spread the virus to their drug injecting or sexual partners, or to future children. The effectiveness of this second strategy is likely to depend upon the posttest counseling and supportive services provided.

Three counseling/antibody test follow-up studies involving IV drug users have been reported.[60–62] In all three studies, the process did lead to a period of increased anxiety and depression which was followed by a great reduction in transmission behavior (both sharing injection equipment and sexual behavior) among seropositives. The number of antibody test follow-up studies is rather small compared to the number of seroprevalence studies that have been conducted, however, so one must use great caution in generalizing from these three studies. It is possible that studies with ambiguous or negative results have been conducted but not yet reported.

Heterosexual transmission from IV drug users to persons who do not inject drugs has been a matter of growing concern. As noted in the Introduction, IV drug users are the primary source of heterosexual transmission of HIV in the United States and Europe. Despite this, there have been few studies of programs to reduce transmission of HIV from IV drug users to their sexual partners. Self-reports for IV drug users in many areas suggest that it is easier to get IV drug users to change their drug injection behavior than to change their sexual behavior (see Des Jarlais et al.,[63] for a review). The reasons for the difficulties in changing sexual behavior are not yet well understood but include a general distaste for the use of condoms, the possibility that condoms will serve as a signal of infidelity within a relationship, and fears that relationships may break up over possible sexual transmission of HIV. Preventing perinatal transmission from drug users to their children also has not been well studied, but from informal reports of clinicians this appears to be a formidable problem. Desires for children, either as a way of leaving the drug life-style or as a legacy if one should die, appear to be relatively strong among IV drug users.

Preventing heterosexual and perinatal transmission from IV drug users requires much more systematic research. The only generalization that can be made is that it is greatly preferable to prevent the initial HIV infection among IV drug users than to try to prevent heterosexual and perinatal transmission later.

The ideal point for preventing AIDS among IV drug users, their sexual partners, and their children would be to prevent persons from beginning to inject illicit drugs. This form of prevention would not only prevent AIDS but would also prevent the other health and social problems associated with IV drug use. Two of the different perspectives on the nature of illicit drug injection lead to opposite predictions about the relationship between simple knowledge of AIDS and beginning to inject drugs. The moral weakness perspective, which usually implies a narcissistic self interest to the exclusion of others' interests, would generally predict a strong deterrent effect on beginning drug injection. Indeed, it is this presumed deterrence that leads to the opposition to "safer" injection programs. The psychopathological perspective, which sees drug use as irrational behavior, would predict relatively little reduction in new IV drug use. (Predictions from the physiologic defect and sociological perspectives would not be straightforward, but would depend upon intervening variables, such as whether the defect is inherited or acquired, and the reaction of the IV drug use subculture to the epidemic.)

There has been very little research on the effect of the AIDS epidemic on recruitment into IV drug use. Preliminary results from one study in New York indicate that basic knowledge of AIDS (that the disease exists, is fatal, and is spread through the sharing of drug injection equipment) has relatively little effect on initiation into illicit drug injection. Adolescent and young adult subjects interviewed in 1985 knew of AIDS and how it is transmitted, but did not see it as a reason for not injecting drugs.[38] If a vaccine or effective treatment are not developed soon, research into why people start to inject drugs, and whether they do it "safely" or with sharing of injection equipment, may become a very important area for prevention studies of AIDS and IV drug use.

EFFECTIVENESS OF CURRENT AIDS PREVENTION EFFORTS AMONG IV DRUG USERS

The various studies of AIDS risk reduction among IV drug users indicate that a large percentage have changed their behavior in order to reduce their risks of developing AIDS. Most subjects in almost all studies reported to date have made some changes to reduce their risk of AIDS. These behavioral changes have been only "risk reduction" and not risk elimination. It is not yet possible to predict the effect on this behavior change on the spread of HIV among IV drug users. The current level of behavior change may only serve to slow down the spread of the virus, without reducing the overall "saturation" level of infection within the IV drug using group.

Cohort studies in New York City indicate a new infection rate of approximately 5% per year among seronegatives[36] (Friedland, G: personal communication, 1988), and the seroprevalence rate among persons entering drug treatment programs in Manhattan has stabilized at approximately 55%.[64] While this is clearly a reduction from the rates of new infection prior to AIDS awareness and risk reduction, it is still much greater than the rate among homosexual/bisexual men,[65] and could still lead to a very high percentage of IV drug users becoming infected with HIV before they finished their drug use careers.

The different perspectives on drug abuse lead to clear preferences in prevention programs for reducing AIDS among IV drug users. The present studies of AIDS prevention and risk reduction among IV drug users, however, are not sufficient to determine a "best" type of prevention program. Beyond the generalization that providing means for behavior change is probably more effective than simply providing "AIDS education," there is no empirical basis for selecting a single type of prevention. If anything, the current data would suggest that a variety of prevention programs will be necessary. The different types of prevention programs—and, it is hoped, new types to be devised quickly—may work with different segments of a heterogeneous group of IV drug users. Furthermore, rather than contradicting each other, as one would assume from the different perspectives on drug abuse, the different prevention programs introduced so far seem to be complementary in actual practice.

REFERENCES

1. *Morbidity & Mortality Weekly Report* 36, 15:3S–15S, Atlanta, Center for Disease Control, 1987.
2. *AIDS Surveillance in Europe, Quarterly Report No 16.* Paris, World Health Organization Collaborating Centre on AIDS, 1987.
3. Musto D: *The American Disease.* New Haven, Yale University Press, 1973.
4. Courtwright DT: *Dark Paradise: Opiate addiction in America before 1940.* Cambridge, Harvard University Press, 1982.
5. Kolb L: *Drug Addiction.* Springfield, Illinois, Charles C Thomas, 1962.
6. Spitzer RL et al: *DSM III Case Book: A Learning Companion to the Diagnostic and Statistical Manual of Mental Disorders,* ed 3. New York, American Psychiatric Association, 1981.
7. Dole VP, Nyswander ME: A medical treatment for diacetylmorphine (heroin) addiction. *JAMA* 193:146–150, 1965.
8. Agar HM: *Ripping and Running: A Formal Ethnography of Urban Heroin Addicts.* New York, Seminar Press, 1973.
9. Cohen HW, Marmor M, Des Jarlais DC, et al: Behavioral risk factors for HTLV-III/LAV seropositivity among intravenous drug abusers, in *The International Conference on Acquired Immunodeficiency Syndrome (AIDS), Atlanta, April 14–17, 1985.*
10. Weiss SH, Ginzberg HM, Saxinger WC, et al: Emerging high rates of human T-cell lymphotropic virus type I (HTLV-I) and HIV infection among U.S. drug abusers (DA), in *The Third International Conference on AIDS, Washington, June 1-5, 1987.*
11. Angarano G, Pastore G, Monno L, et al: Rapid spread of HTLV-III infection among drug addicts in Italy. *Lancet* 2:1302, 1985.
12. Robertson JR, Bucknall ABV, Welsby PD, et al: Epidemic of AIDS related virus (HLTV-III/LAV) infection among intravenous drug users. *Br Med J* 292:527–529, 1986.
13. Schupbach J, Haller O Vogt M, et al: Antibodies to HTLV-III in Swiss patients with AIDS and pre-AIDS and in groups at risk for AIDS. *N Engl J Med* 312:265–270, 1985.
14. Hunsmann G, Schneider J, Bayer H, et al: Seroepidemiology of HTLV-III (LAV) in the Federal Republic of Germany. *Klin Wochenschr* 63:233–235, 1985.
15. Chaisson RE, Moss AR, Onishi R, et al: Human immunodeficiency virus infection in heterosexual intravenous drug users in San Francisco. *Am J Public Health* 77:169–172, 1987.
16. Novick DM, Kreek MJ, Des Jarlais DC: Abstract of clinical research findings: therapeutic and historical aspects, in Harris LJ (ed): *Problems of Drug Dependence 1985,* Research monograph series 67. Rockville, Maryland, National Institute on Drug Abuse, 1986, pp 328–320.
17. Verani P: Seroprevalence among intravenous drug abusers in Italy, in *Workshop on Epidemological Surveys on AIDS: Epidemiology of HIV Infection in Europe Spread among Intravenous Drug Users and the Heterosexual Population, Berlin, November 12–14, 1986.*
18. Rex W: Increase of HIV seroprevalence among IVDA in West Berlin prisons since 1982, in *Workshop on Epidemiological Surveys on AIDS: Epidemiology of HIV Infections in Europe Spread among Intravenous Drug Users and the Heterosexual Population, Berlin, November 12–14, 1986.*
19. Worm AM: Incidence of HIV antibodies in IV drug abusers and prostitutes in Copenhagen, in *Workshop on*

Epidemiological Surveys on AIDS: Epidemiology of HIV Infection in Europe Spread among Intravenous Drug Users and the Heterosexual Population, Berlin, November 12–14, 1986.

20. Des Jarlais DC, Friedman SR, Novick D, et al: HIV-1 infection among intravenous drug users in Manhattan, *JAMA* 261:1008–1012, 1989.
21. Weiss SH, Ginzburg HM, Goedert JJ, et al: *Risk for HTLV-III exposure and AIDS among parenteral drug abusers in New Jersey,* in *The International Conference on the AIDS, Atlanta, April 14–17, 1985.*
22. Schoenbaum EE, Selwyn PA, Klein RS, et al: Prevalence of and risk factors associated with HTLV-III/LAV antibodies among intravenous drug abusers in methadone programs in New York City, in *The Second International Conference on AIDS, Paris, June 23–25, 1986.*
23. Des Jarlais DC, Friedman SR, Strug D: AIDS among intravenous drug users: A socio-cultural perspective, in Feldman D, Johnson T (eds): *The Social Dimensions of AIDS:Methods and Theory.* New York, Praeger, 1986, pp 111–125.
24. Marmor M, Des Jarlais DC, Cohen H, et al: Risk factors for infection with human immunodeficiency virus among intravenous drug abusers in New York City. *AIDS* 1:39–44, 1987.
25. Darrow M: Risk factors among prostitutes, in *Workshop on Epidemiological Surveys on AIDS: Epidemiology of HIV Infection in Europe Spread among Intravenous Drug Users and the Heterosexual Population, Berlin, November 12–14, 1986.*
26. Des Jarlais DC Friedman SR: *Ethnic Differences in HIV Seroprevalence Rates among Intravenous Drug Users.* Rockville, Maryland, National Institute of Drug Abuse, in press.
27. D'Aquila RT, Williams AB, Peterson LR, et al: HIV seroprevalence among Connecticut intravenous drug users in 1986–87: Race/ethnicity as a risk factor for HIV seropositivity, in *The Third International Conference on AIDS, Washington, June 1–5, 1987.*
28. Lange WR, Primm BJ., Tennant FS, et al: The geographic distribution of human immunodeficiency virus (HIV) antibodies in parenteral drug abusers, in *The Third International Conference on AIDS. Washington, June 1–5, 1987.*
29. van den Hoek JAR, Coutinho, RA, van Zadelhoff AW, et al: Prevalence, incidence and risk factors of HIV infection among drug users in Amsterdam, in *The Third International Conference on AIDS, Washington, June 1–5, 1987.*
30. Des Jarlais DC, Marmor M, Thomas P: Kaposi's sarcoma among four different risk groups. (Letter.) *N Engl J Med* 310:1119, 1984.
31. Haverkos HW, Pinsky PF. Drotman DP, et al: Disease manifestations among homosexual men with acquired immunodeficiency syndrome: A possible role of nitrites in Kaposi's sarcoma. *Sex Transm Dis* 12:203–208, 1985.
32. Drew WL, Mills J, Levy J: Cytomegalovirus infection and abnormal T-lymphocyte subset ratios in homosexual men. *Ann Intern Med* 103:61–63, 1985.
33. Des Jarlais DC, Stoneburner R, Thomas P: Declines in proportion of Kaposi's sarcoma among cases of AIDS in multiple risk groups in New York City. (Letter.) *Lancet* ii:1024–1025. 1987.
34. Goedert JJ, Biggar RJ, Weiss SH, et al: Three year incidence of AIDS among HTLV-III infected risk group members: A comparison of five cohorts. *Science* 231:992–995, 1985.
35. Des Jarlais DC, Friedman SR, Marmor M, et al: Development of AIDS, HIV seroconversion, and co-factors for T4 cell loss in a cohort of intravenous drug users. *AIDS* 1:105–111, 1987.
36. Selwyn PA, Schoenbaum EE, Hartel D: Natural history of HIV infection in intravenous drug abusers (IVDAs), in *The Third International Conference on AIDS, Washington, June 1–5, 1987.*
37. Zagury D, Bernard J, Leonard R, et al: Long-term cultures of HTLV-III-infected T-cells: A model of cytopathology of T-cell depletion in AIDS. *Science* 231:850–853, 1986.
38. Des Jarlais DC, Friedman SR, Casriel C, et al: AIDS and preventing initiation into intravenous (IV) drug use. *Psychol Health* 1:179–194, 1987.
39. Des Jarlais DC, Friedman SR, Stoneburner RL: HIV infection and intravenous drug use: critical issues in transmission dynamics, infection outcomes, and prevention. *Rev Infect Dis* 10:151–158, 1988.
40. Stoneburner RL, Des Jarlais DC, Benezra D, et al: A larger spectrum of severe HIV-1-related disease in intravenous drug users in New York City. *Science* 242:916–919, 1988.
41. Friedman SR, Des Jarlais DC, Sotheran JL: AIDS and self-organization among intravenous drug users. *Int J Addict* 22:201–220, 1987.
42. Des Jarlais DC, Friedman SR, Hopkins W: Risk reduction for AIDS among intravenous drug users. *Ann Intern Med* 103:755–759, 1985.

43. Des Jarlais DC, Hopkins W: "Free needles" for intravenous drug users at risk for AIDS: Current developments in New York City. (Letter.) *N Engl J Med* 313:1476, 1985.
44. Friedman SR, Des Jarlais DC Sotheran JL: AIDS health education for intravenous drug users. *J Health Educ Q* 13:383–393, 1986.
45. McAuliffe WE, Doering S, Breer, P, et al: An evaluation of using ex-addict outreach workers to educate intravenous drug users about AIDS prevention, in *The Third International Conference on AIDS, Washington, June 1–5, 1987.*
46. Jackson J, Rotkiewicz L: *A Coupon Program: AIDS Education and Drug Treatment,* in *The Third International Conference on AIDS, Washington, June 1–5, 1987.*
47. Simpson DD, Savage JL, Sells SB: *Data Book on Drug Treatment Outcomes: Follow-up Study of 1969–1972 Admissions to the Drug Abuse Reporting Program (DARP),* report 78-10. Fort Worth, Institute of Behavior Research, Texas Christian University, 1978.
48. Abdul-Quader AS, Friedman SR, Des Jarlais DC, et al: Methadone maintenance and behavior by intravenous drug users that can transmit HIV. *Contemp Drug Probl* 14:425–434, 1987.
49. Hartel D, Selwyn PA, Schoenbaum EE, et al: Methadone maintenance treatment (MMTP) and reduced risk of AIDS and AIDS-specific mortality in intravenous drug users (IVDUs), in *The Fourth International Conference on AIDS, Stockholm, June 12–16, 1988.*
50. Blix O, Gronbladh L: AIDS and IV heroin addicts: The preventive effect of methadone maintenance in Sweden, in *The Fourth International Conference on AIDS, Stockholm, June 12–16, 1988.*
51. Goldberg D, Watson H, Stuart F, et al: Pharmacy supply of needles and syringes—The effect on spread of HIV intravenous drug misusers, in *The Fourth International Conference on AIDS, Stockholm, June 12–16, 1988.*
52. Espinoza P, Bouchard I, Ballian P, et al: Has the open sale of syringes modified the syringe exchanging habits of drug addicts, in *The Fourth International Conference on AIDS, Stockholm, June 12–16, 1988.*
53. Fuchs D, Unterweger B, Hinterhuber H, et al: Successful preventive measures in a community of IV drug addicts, in *The Fourth International Conference on AIDS, Stockholm, June 12–16, 1988.*
54. Buning EC, van Brussel GHA, van Santen G: Amsterdam's drug policy and its implications for controlling needle sharing, in Battjes R, Pickins R (eds): *Needle Sharing among Intravenous Drug Abusers: National and International Perspectives.* Research Monograph Series 80. Rockville, Maryland, National Institute of Drug Abuse, 1988, pp 59–74.
55. Alldritt L, Dolan K, Donoghoe M, et al: HIV and the injecting drug user: clients of syringe exchange schemes in England and Scotland, in *The Fourth International Conference on AIDS, Stockholm, June 12–16, 1988.*
56. Watters JK: Preventing human immunodeficiency virus contagion among intravenous drug users: The impact of street-based education on risk-behavior, in *The Third International Conference on AIDS, Washington, June 1–5, 1987.*
57. Watters JK, Case P, Huang, K, et al: HIV seroepidemiology and behavior change in intravenous drug users: Progress report on the effectiveness of street-based prevention, in *The Fourth International Conference on AIDS, Stockholm, June 12–16, 1988.*
58. Coates T: Change in sexual behavior among gay and bisexual men since the beginning of the AIDS epidemic. United States Congress, Office of Technology Assessment, in press.
59. Friedman SR, Des Jarlais DC, Goldsmith D: An overview of current AIDS prevention efforts aimed at intravenous drug users. *J Drug Issues* 19:93–112, 1989.
60. Casadonte P, Des Jarlais DC, Smith T, et al: Psychological and behavioral impact of learning HTLV-III/LAV antibody test results, in *The Second International Conference on Acquired Immunodeficiency Syndrome, Paris, June 23–25, 1986.*
61. Cox CP, Selwyn PA, Schoenbaum EE, et al: Psychological and behavioral consequences of HTLV-III/LAV antibody testing and notification among intravenous drug abusers in a methadone program in New York City, in *The Second International Conference on AIDS, Paris, June 23–25, 1986.*
62. Marlink RG, Foss B, Swift R, et al: High rate of HTLV-III/LAV exposure in IVDA's from a small-sized city and the failure of specialized methadone maintenance to prevent further drug use, in *The Third International Conference on AIDS, Washington, June 1–5, 1987.*
63. Des Jarlais DC, Friedman SR, Goldsmith D, et al: Heterosexual transmission of HIV from intravenous drug users: Regular partnerships and prostitution, in Voeller B, Gottlieb M, Reinisch J (eds): *AIDS and Sex: An Integrated Biomedical and Biobehavior Approach.* New York, Oxford University Press, in press.

64. Des Jarlais DC, Friedman SR: HIV infection among persons who inject illicit drugs: problems and prospects. *J AIDS* 1:267–273, 1988.
65. Winkelstein W, Samuel M, Padian N, et al: The San Francisco men's health study. III. Reduction in human immunodeficiency virus transmission among homosexual/bisexual men, 1983–86. *Am J Public Health* 77:685–689, 1987.

8

Moving beyond Counseling and Knowledge-Enhancing Interventions

A Plea for Community-Level AIDS Prevention Strategies

LARRY L. BYE

SOME DEFINITIONS

Acquired immune deficiency syndrome (AIDS) prevention campaigns are usually part of a broader education effort designed to accomplish the following objectives:

- Increase general public awareness and knowledge about AIDS, its transmission, and risk reduction strategies.
- Reduce general public fears and correct misinformation about the dangers of casual contagion and ordinary social contact with HIV-infected individuals.
- Create support for constructive action by increasing general public understanding of the severity of the crisis, its complexity, and costs.
- Reduce the rate of HIV transmission/infection by changing the behaviors of at-risk individuals.

Within this effort, prevention campaigns are most concerned with reducing the rate of virus transmission by influencing the behavior of at-risk individuals.* This chapter discusses a distinctive approach to the design of such programs—an approach that emphasizes the mobilization of communities and social networks within at-risk populations.

The most effective communication campaigns make use of multiple communication channels. It is possible to use the following approaches in AIDS prevention campaigns:

*By at-risk individuals, we mean homosexual/bisexual men, intravenous (IV) drug users, and heterosexuals with multiple or high-risk sex partners. This latter population includes heterosexuals that are sexually active with many partners or a partner with high-risk characteristics such as a pre-existing HIV infection, history of IV drug usage, or male bisexuality.

LARRY L. BYE • Communication Technologies, San Francisco, California 94111.

Mass Media Channels

- *Media advertising:* These are paid or public service advertisements placed in print, transit, billboards, and television and radio outlets.
- *Press management:* Most information about AIDS comes from news stories. Finding ways to use news formats to correct misinformation or impart new information is extremely valuable.
- *Use of feature and other non-news media formats:* Columns, feature stories, and electronic talk show formats can often be used to disseminate risk-reduction information and other general educational messages.
- *Pamphlets, videos, and collateral materials:* These are materials developed for distribution via mail, public forums, and health care facilities.

Mass media elements can easily be overemphasized in AIDS prevention campaigns. Unfortunately, mass media are not the most effective channels of communication for effecting behavioral change. When used properly, however mass media messages can raise AIDS awareness and knowledge levels and contribute to the adoption of beliefs leading to behavior change.

Centralized Information and Referral (Hotlines)

While mass media channels are useful for raising general levels of awareness and knowledge, most at-risk individuals have additional information and referral needs. Telephone hotlines provide a fast and anonymous way to meet these needs.

Forums, Workshops, and Classes

Panel discussions, lectures, live theater, or video presentations provide the opportunity for at-risk individuals to participate in public dialogue about AIDS prevention.

Peer-to-Peer Interpersonal Communication

These approaches emphasize interactive communication between individuals, either one-on-one or in small groups. The emphasis is on peer-to-peer communication. Unlike professional counseling interventions discussed below, health care professionals play no direct role in the process.

These interventions can be primarily knowledge enhancing. (The "AIDS Tupperware Parties" organized in some cities are an example of this type of intervention.) Others, such as the Stop AIDS Project, go beyond knowledge enhancement and instead have attitude and behavior change as an explicit goal.

Professional Counseling Programs

Whether one-on-one group interactions are emphasized, these programs seek to change individual risk behaviors through:

- Prevention education and counseling offered in conjunction with antibody testing.
- Interventions based on a therapeutic model that are not tied to antibody testing

programs. These interventions sometimes entail group sessions that meet a number of times. Others emphasize individualized counseling sessions where level of risk is assessed and a plan for behavior change is adopted. Whether group or individualized formats are used, these programs usually seek to impart communication skills (e.g., how to negotiate safer sex), safer sex skills (e.g., how to use a condom properly), or an enhanced sense of personal efficacy.

Substance Abuse Treatment Programs

Substance abuse treatment programs seek to control addictive behavior. They address the needs of two groups of heightened risk of HIV infection: IV drug users, and non-needle users likely to engage in unsafe behaviors when under the influence of alcohol and other drugs.

Other Health Care System Access Points

Using various health care system access points to educate individuals about AIDS prevention is important. This is particularly true in the case of sexually transmitted disease (STD) clinics, family planning and perinatal clinics, and other settings that serve large numbers of high-risk persons. In some localities a major effort has also been made to encourage physicians and other direct care professionals to become more effective AIDS educators with their patients.

WHAT IS IN PLACE AND WHAT IS NOT

Most local prevention campaigns are mass media-based; unfortunately, media elements are not being fully used in most of the efforts. In many areas no use is being made of electronic outlets, despite the pervasive influence of radio and television in American life. AIDS educators are instead relying on print advertising and pamphlets, videos, and collateral materials.*

In localities where broadcast media are involved, public service announcements are aired in unfavorable time slots and rarely contain explicit risk-reduction information. A recent National Association of Broadcasters survey indicates that only 20% of radio and television stations are carrying condom advertising.[1]

Recent CDC efforts to distribute announcements with explicit risk-reduction content were frustrated when stations in major markets refused to run the spots. Announcements with noncontroversial awareness-enhancing themes and announcements designed to recontextualize the epidemic along more positive lines were preferred over those that stressed the importance of safe sex practices. Few stations have developed prime-time programming or coordinated, multifaceted campaigns.†

Testing is now widely available across the United States, and demand continues to

*Generalizations in this section are based on data gathered at the AIDS Risk Reduction Campaign Planning Seminars held in Washington, D.C., Chicago, and San Francisco, in May 1988. The seminars were sponsored by the National AIDS Information & Education Program at the federal Centers for Disease Control.

†One exception is the AIDS Lifeline campaign developed by KPIX, Westinghouse/Group W Television.

increase. Many individuals at highest risk are reluctant to be tested, however, and community-based organizations tend not to urge testing because of concerns about discrimination.

Furthermore, there is still ambiguity about whether testing leads to behavior change.† Available evidence suggests that testing is an important milepost in the process of change for some, but not all, individuals. Many individuals alter their behavior prior to testing. Some persist in unsafe sex after learning their sero status. The success of several San Francisco programs suggests that significant behavior change can take place in the absence of widespread testing among at-risk individuals.

Many communities have effective test-linked counseling programs; very few have counseling programs that are not tied to antibody testing. Where these free-standing programs do exist, they serve small numbers of at-risk individuals because therapeutically oriented interventions inherently have limited appeal. Many individuals will not enroll in counseling programs that require attendance at multiple sessions over time.

A major difficulty with all counseling-style interventions is that they view change solely in individualistic terms. They fail to address the critical social nature of risk behaviors and miss the opportunities that flow from viewing AIDS prevention as sociocultural change.

Substance abuse programs often lack the funds and expertise to be effective in AIDS prevention. In addition, there is a critical lack of treatment slots in these programs nationwide. It has been difficult to get physicians to face up to their potential as AIDS educators. Despite data indicating that physicians are a preferred sources of prevention information, they are frequently uninformed about AIDS, or uncomfortable discussing sex and drug-using behaviors with patients. We have been somewhat more successful in marshalling other segments of the health care system for AIDS prevention. Most STD clinics, family planning facilities, and perinatal programs are disseminating information about AIDS prevention.

Few communities have implemented comprehensive campaigns that integrate all of the approaches outlined above. Most have adopted strategies that are primarily knowledge enhancing. Telephone hotlines and events are being used extensively and effectively. Some of the print advertising and pamphlets, videos, and collateral materials are also very effective. The problem is that these approaches are of limited effectiveness in accomplishing behavior change. They may lead to increases in knowledge about AIDS. Knowledge alone, however, does not lead to behavioral change. Despite its efficacy in accomplishing attitude and behavior change, there has been almost no reliance on peer-to-peer communication. Greater emphasis needs to be placed on these approaches, as suggested below.

THE NEED TO VIEW AIDS PREVENTION AS SOCIAL CHANGE

The literature in health education/disease prevention, as well as our experience with AIDS, suggests that community-based AIDS prevention campaigns are most effective in bringing about rapid, large-scale risk behavior change.

*This is the author's assessment based on data presented at the *Fourth International Conference on AIDS, Stockholm, June 1988.*

This is true because there is a critical social dimension to AIDS risk behaviors. Individuals identify within a variety of groups: friends, family, profession, or ethnic groups, for example. What they perceive to be socially acceptable within these groups has an impact on their attitudes and behavior. As perceptions about norms change, behavior often changes as well.

One example of this process is the smoking cessation effort. Due to education programs, anti-smoking legislation and a general increase in public awareness about the dangers of smoking, many individuals have come to perceive smoking as socially unacceptable. This change in perceived group norms has undoubtedly been a factor both in motivating many smokers to stop and in helping many maintain their non-smoking behavior.

Thus, social change, including changes in perceived peer norms, has played a key role in changing the behavior of many individuals. The same is true with AIDS. In areas where dramatic changes in AIDS risk behaviors have taken place, those changes have been accompanied by equally dramatic changes in community norms, values, and institutions.

GAY MALE BEHAVIORAL CHANGE IN SAN FRANCISCO

A number of studies document the significant nature of behavioral change among gay-identifying men in San Francisco.[2–5] One even suggests that the number of new, first-time HIV infections among gay males has been reduced to near zero as of 1987. This unprecedented change in behavior has been accompanied by major changes in gay community norms, values, and institutions—changes in local prevention campaign planners consciously sought to engender.

Gay male cultural norms during the 1970s placed great emphasis on experimentation with sex and drugs.[6] Qualitative research conducted in 1984 suggested that many San Francisco gay men equated their homosexuality with large numbers of sexual partners, anonymous encounters at bath houses, and frequent use of recreational drugs.*

The gay revolution that began at Stonewall in 1969 coincided with other changes taking place in American society—changes encouraging greater freedom of sexual expression and experimentation with drugs. Sexual liberation and drug use attracted many gay men of the baby-boom generation who flocked to San Francisco and other cities in the 1970s.

Bars and sex clubs became institutions of great importance in these settings. As one respondent in the 1984 focus group interview said*

> It was a familiar routine. I used to go to the baths every Friday and Saturday night. I'd usually get high and go and spend some of the happiest times of my life . . . meeting other men and having a great time. And then there would be great parties—all the time great parties. I used to really have the thought that I'd arrived in some kind of magical promised land. It was irresistible!

*Communication Technologies: Focus group research conducted in 1984 with respondents from San Francisco Bay Area gay male communities. The results are summarized in unpublished reports prepared for the San Francisco AIDS Foundation.

Another respondent explained,*

> After years of not knowing who I was nor feeling good about myself I finally had the experience of being out . . . open . . . honest and celebrating my gayness.

Most members of the gay community remained oblivious to the consequences of this life-style. By the late 1970s, however, some gay activists and health care workers were becoming alarmed about the epidemics of STD and substance abuse engulfing the community. Even before AIDS, there was a sense that something was wrong.

By the early 1980s, many rank and file members of the community had come to the same conclusion. Changes were beginning to take place. According to 1984 survey data, many gay men reported fewer numbers of sexual partners and less interest in impersonal sex as well as alcohol and drug use.[7] Some linked the changes to the rising specter of AIDS, while others attributed them to difficult factors.

Designers of prevention programs discerned a desire for self-examination and change emerging within the gay male community, and tried to tie prevention messages to these broader changes. The campaign stressed that the community faces a serious threat from the AIDS epidemic, one more serious than previous political threats posed by conservative anti gay politicians. Thousands of men were already infected and capable of infecting others. The probability of infection in any unsafe sexual encounter was extremely high.

Credible messengers assured the community that AIDS was caused by a virus and that behavioral-change guidelines could be trusted. AIDS was easily preventable, they said. But prevention required major changes in behavior, in community norms, perhaps in the very nature of the way men viewed their gay identity.

The good news was that positive changes were taking place. More and more men were voluntarily abstaining from high-risk behaviors. The community had faced great challenges before and overcome them; it could and would do so again.

The campaign emphasized full-scale community mobilization in order to halt virus transmission. Gay publications were the focus of a major advertising and press relations effort. Community activists forged a partnership with a local network-affiliated television station. As a result, the station began to run prime-time programs with explicit risk reduction information content as part of a coordinated, multifaceted on-air campaign.

Mass media interventions were assigned a secondary role, however. So too were testing/counseling programs. The centerpiece of the campaign was the effort to promote interpersonal communication about the epidemic, its impact and meaning. Bartenders were organized and urged to engage their customers in discussion about AIDS prevention. Gay physicians and psychotherapists were enrolled as health educators. The Stop AIDS Project used hundreds of volunteers to reach 25,000 gay men in face-to-face sidewalk conversations about AIDS prevention. Seven thousand attended evening-long, peer-facilitated Stop AIDS Meetings in homes throughout the city.

Rather than aggressive advocacy of change, the campaign invited community members to realistically confront the AIDS problem and respond in whatever ways they could. Men who could make the commitment to completely halt virus-transmitting behavior were

*Communication Technologies: Focus group research conducted in 1984 with respondents from San Francisco Bay Area gay male communities. The results are summarized in unpublished reports prepared for the San Francisco AIDS Foundation.

urged to do so. Those that could not make this commitment were encouraged to participate in some other way. Everyone was asked to make some contribution to the fight against virus transmission with the community.

The pace of change accelerated. Studies began to document declining incidence of AIDS risk behaviors. STD rates fell. Dozens of gay Alcoholics Anonymous and Narcotics Anonymous groups sprang forth in San Francisco. Sobriety groups rather than political clubs began to be the largest contingents in the city's annual Gay Freedom Day Parade. Attendance at sex clubs declined and many closed because of declining patronage.

As this San Francisco example suggests, it is useful to view AIDS prevention campaigns as social change efforts. Testing/counseling programs are only part of what is needed to combat HIV infection. If we rely only on individual-level interventions, we are going to have to resign ourselves to a slower rate of change within at-risk populations. On the other hand, if we view the process as a social one, we may be able to influence the attitudes and behaviors of more individuals more quickly.

CHANGE IS A DIFFUSION PROCESS

How does the process of social/cultural change work? Everett Rogers and other students of social diffusion describe it in terms of "the communication of innovative ideas of practices through certain channels over time among members of a social system."[8,9] The innovations to be diffused in AIDS prevention are new lower-risk sex and drug-using behaviors or abstinence from established high-risk behaviors.

According to Rogers and other theorists, mass media channels of communication are more effective in increasing knowledge of innovations, while interpersonal channels are more effective in changing attitudes and behavior. In AIDS prevention, the task is to access informal peer networks among communities of individuals who are at risk of infection.

Rogers states: "Most individuals evaluate an innovation, not on the basis of scientific research by experts but on the basis of subjective evaluations of near peers who have already adopted the innovation. These peers serve as models whose behavior is imitated by others in the social system. Thus imitation and social modeling are essential elements in the diffusion process."

IDENTIFYING SOCIAL SYSTEMS

What social systems exist with regard to AIDS related communication? Six groups are particularly important targets for HIV disease prevention: gay-identifying men, IV drug users, sex industry workers, youth (teenagers and young adults), sex partners of needle users, and sexually active adults generally. Closeted homosexual/bisexual men are included in the last group, because they do not identify themselves as gay men.

Gay-identifying men constitute a natural community. Some IV drug users may also have sufficient shared experience to be mobilized on a community basis. The same is true of many individuals who exchange sex for money.

It may also be possible to use community-mobilizing strategies with teenagers and young adults. Age is strongly correlated with AIDS risk. Most studies confirm that young people are more sexually active than older people.[10] Thus, they constitute an important audience for risk-reduction programs.

Some high schools, colleges, and universities have been the focus for student-designed and led campaigns, although much work remains to be done in this area. It may also be possible to reach teenagers and older young adults through campaigns focused off campus.

Partners of IV drug users do not constitute a single social system. We know that they tend to be urban females of lower socioeconomic status. Many are members of racial/ethnic minority groups. It may be possible to target women who share these characteristics—women who believe that their male partners may be using needles. One possible geographical focus for this work is public housing projects or low-income neighborhoods in the center city.

The final group, sexually active adults, is more difficult to mobilize because of the complexity of group identification patterns. Two generalizations can be made, however. First, men who have sex with men but who do not identify as gay are probably best reached through campaigns aimed at the general audience of sexually active adults, rather than through gay-identified campaigns. Second, race/ethnicity and social class are the two critical variables which define the mix of subgroups within the sexually active adult population.

Men who have sex with other men but who do not identify as gay are a difficult group to reach. In attempting to do so, it is important to stress the behaviors that place one at risk of HIV infection without labeling them as homosexual, bisexual, or heterosexual. Labeling only feeds AIDS denial among those men, who do not perceive themselves or their behavior as gay or bisexual.

Blacks, Latinos, and other minorities have been hard hit by the epidemic. As a result there is a strong basis for community-based appeals within these populations. It is important, however, to recognize that social class operates as a cross-cutting variable. For example, a campaign based among lower class blacks in any city will not be successful in mobilizing upscale black professionals. Two separate campaigns will be needed. Each should target singles under the age of 45, since data suggest that they are most sexually active.[10]

Designers of local prevention campaigns need to map these groups carefully in their local jurisdiction. What is the geographical distribution of these groups? How big are they? What demographic characteristics do they have? What meaning do the epidemic and specific risk behaviors have within each of the communities targeted for mobilization? What are group norms? How can the saliency of AIDS be increased in communities where numerous other threats to health and well being exist?

When these questions are answered, an effective mobilization strategy can be formulated. In researching these questions, it is important to involve individuals indigenous to the communities being targeted.

INTERPERSONAL COMMUNICATION ENHANCES DIFFUSION

If diffusion theorists are right in asserting that interpersonal communication is the best way to accomplish behavior change, it follows that AIDS prevention campaigns may be able to accelerate the process of change by providing opportunities for large numbers of at-risk individuals to communicate with one another about AIDS prevention.

One way of configuring the communication is through the use of small groups. Lewin and other pioneering social psychologists in the 1940s perfected the technique of using peer-facilitated small group discussions to effect attitude and behavior change.[11]

In an effort to change the meat-consuming behavior of American women during the years of World War II rationing, Lewin experimented with small group discussions as well as lectures and individualized instruction. He found that small group discussions were the most effective method for changing attitudes and behavior. These discussions were most powerful when individuals were asked to make public declarations of commitment about behavior change to their peers. In other words, the discussions did more than impart information. They provided an opportunity for participants to clarify and express their behavioral intention to their peers.

Small group processes have been used in almost every conceivable setting over the past few decades to accomplish attitude and behavior change. They have been used in psychiatric hospitals, prisons, the military, in drug treatment programs, and many other contexts.

Can Lewin's small group discussion/decision model be used to increase the rate of peer communication about AIDS prevention? The answer may be yes. If significant numbers of at-risk individuals can be motivated to make a commitment to AIDS risk reduction and to communicate this intention to others, it may be possible to accelerate the process of change.

Most members of an at-risk community may not need to participate directly in small group discussions (or any other intervention) in order to be influenced by them. Diffusion theorists argue that once an innovation is accepted by about 15–20% of a population, it cannot be stopped. At a certain point, the process become self-generating. This is true because when opinion leaders adopt innovations they influence the opinions of others in their peer network. These newly influenced individuals then diffuse the innovations through their networks, and so on.

Thus, it may be possible to accelerate community-level norm change through the direct participation of a relatively small number of members of the community. Moreover, it may be possible to bring this about with group sessions that meet only at one or very few points in time.

The Stop AIDS Project has developed a powerful, one-time, evening-long, peer-led session that leads participants to an awareness of beliefs acting as barriers to behavior change. Group leaders (and some of the attendees) function as role models for the others to imitate.

A relatively small portion of the meeting is devoted to dissemination of information about risk reduction guidelines. Increasingly, at-risk individuals are knowledgeable about how to reduce infection. More emphasis is placed on building trust in behavioral change guidelines, encouraging individuals to label high-risk behavior as problematic, and instilling a heightened sense of personal efficacy. Help seeking is also stressed and perceptions about group norms are carefully scrutinized. In short, all of the attitudinal variables in leading AIDS behavior change models are addressed.[12]

Each attendee is asked to declare some kind of personal commitment to the assembled group. For some participants, a commitment is made to reduce or eliminate high-risk behavior. Others pledge to consider making changes or to seek testing, counseling or other assistance. For many, a commitment is made to participate in AIDS prevention activities.

THE IMPORTANCE OF VOLUNTARISM

The San Francisco campaign has stressed participation and involvement. Because of the opportunities it provides for further peer-to-peer communication, designers assumed that participation in AIDS prevention work would strengthen and reinforce a commitment to behavior change. They encouraged at-risk individuals to contribute time to prevention efforts. Considerable emphasis has been placed on community building in the midst of the AIDS crisis.

The campaign has been structured to provide numerous opportunities for involvement. Through techniques borrowed from the field of community organizing, large numbers of individuals have been mobilized for grass-roots outreach activities such as sidewalk discussions, telephone contact, door-to-door canvassing, and public speaking. The purpose of these activities has not only been to promote attendance at Stop AIDS Meetings but to promote ongoing discussion about AIDS prevention generally. This one-on-one communication is an important supplement to that taking place in small group formats.

Outside of San Francisco, or among other risk group populations, different outreach strategies will need to be used. Greater reliance on the telephone may be necessary, for example. However, the more face-to-face contact is used in outreach work, the more powerful will be the impact of peer-to-peer communication.

EVALUATING COMMUNITY MOBILIZING STRATEGIES

As has been pointed out, numerous studies point to the decline in unsafe sexual behaviors among gay-identifying men in San Francisco and to the decline in the number of new HIV infections among this group. Although data analysis is preliminary, campaign effectiveness research suggests that there is high awareness and recall of messages and that acceptance of campaign messages is associated with behavior change.[7,13,14] With regard to attendance at Stop AIDS Meetings, preliminary data from Orange County, California, suggest that significant knowledge, attitude and behavior changes result from participation in the sessions.[15] Orange County is one of the settings outside San Francisco where the Stop AIDS Project has been successfully replicated. It is important to remember, however, that Stop AIDS Projects involve considerable one-on-one communication outside of the meetings, and the impact of this activity has not yet been evaluated.

Methodologies used in the evaluation of individual-level behavioral change interventions may not be appropriate for the evaluation of community level strategies that emphasize sociocultural change. The evaluation task here is complex and difficult. Additional research is needed and should examine the relationship between interventions, informal peer-to-peer communication, changing individual perceptions of norms, and risk behavior modification.

It may never be possible to evaluate the efficacy of alternative prevention strategies rigorously. To do so would require carefully designed experiments, which are not possible given the need to make the best possible interventions accessible to the maximum number of individuals at risk of HIV infection, and the state of flux that exists generally in the area of AIDS prevention program design and evaluation.

APPENDIX: Stop AIDS Projects in the United States

Project name	Contact	Phone number
Stop AIDS Chicago	John Copeland	(312) 871-3300
Stop AIDS East Bay	Tige Foley	(415) 420-8181
Stop AIDS Honolulu	Bob Callery	(808) 924-AIDS
Stop AIDS Long Beach	Mike Barry	(213) 987-0643
Stop AIDS Los Angeles	Jeff Campbell	(213) 659-4778
Stop AIDS New York	Serela Poster	(212) 645-0519
Stop AIDS Orange County	Tim Miller	(714) 534-0961
Stop AIDS Sacramento	Tim Warford	(916) 442-5801

REFERENCES

1. National Association of Broadcasters: Special Report from Research and Planning, Broadcasters Public Service Activities, April 1988.
2. Centers for Disease Control: Self-reported change in sexual behaviors among homosexual and bisexual men from the San Francisco City Clinic cohort. *MMWR* 36:187–189, 1987.
3. McKusick L, et al: Reported Changes in the Sexual Behavior of Men at Risk For AIDS, San Francisco, 1982–84—the AIDS Behavioral Research Project. *Public Health Rep* 100:622–629, 1985.
4. Winkelstein W, Samuel M, Padian NS, et al: The San Francisco Men's Health Study. III. Reduction in Human Immunodeficiency Virus Transmission Among Homosexual/Bisexual Men, 1982–86. *Am J Public Health* 76:685–689, 1987.
5. San Francisco Department of Public Health: Rectal gonorrhea in San Francisco, October 1984–September 1986. *Epidemiol Bull* Vol. 2, 1986.
6. Fitzgerald F: *Cities on the Hill.* New York, Simon & Schuster, 1983
7. Communication Technologies: Designing an Effective AIDS Prevention Campaign Strategy for San Francisco: Results from the First Probability Sample of an Urban Gay Male Community. Unpublished report prepared for the San Francisco AIDS Foundation, December 1984.
8. Rogers, M: *Communication Strategies for Family Planning.* New York: The Free Press, 1983.
9. Bandura A: *Social Learning Theory.* Englewood Cliffs, New Jersey, Prentice-Hall, 1977.
10. Communication Technologies: Planning for the AIDS Epidemic in California: A Population-Based Assessment of Knowledge, Attitudes and Behaviors. Report prepared for the State of California Department of Health Services, Office of AIDS, 1988.
11. Lewin K; Group decision and social change, in Mccaby EE, Newcomb TM, Hartley EL (eds): *Readings in Social Psychology.* New York, Holt, Reinhart and Winston, 1958.
12. Morin SF: Behavior change and prevention of sexual transmission of HIV, in *The Fourth International Conference on AIDS, Stockholm, June 14, 1988.*
13. Communication Technologies: Designing an Effective AIDS Prevention Campaign Strategy for San Francisco: Results from the Second Probability Sample of an Urban Gay Male Community. Report prepared for the San Francisco AIDS Foundation, San Francisco, California, 1985.
14. Communication Technologies: Designing an Effective AIDS Prevention Campaign Strategy for San Francisco: Results from the Third Probability Sample of an Urban Gay Male Community. Report prepared for the San Francisco AIDS Foundation, San Francisco, California, 1986.
15. Miller TE, Booraem C, Flowers JV, et al: Changes in Knowledge, Attitudes and Behavior as a Result of a Community AIDS Outreach Educational Program. Unpublished manuscript prepared for the AIDS Response Program, Garden Grove, California, 1988.

III

Neuropsychiatric Aspects of AIDS

9

Overview:

The Management of the HIV-Positive Patient with Neuropsychiatric Impairment

DAVID G. OSTROW, J. HAMPTON ATKINSON III, and IGOR GRANT

INTRODUCTION: THE CLASSIFICATION OF HIV-RELATED DISEASE

The assessment and management of neuropsychiatric (NP*) disturbances in the patient with acquired immunodeficiency syndrome (AIDS) must begin with an understanding of the criteria by which AIDS and other manifestations of human immunodeficiency virus (HIV) infection are diagnosed. Table 1 shows the criteria used by the Centers for Disease Control (CDC) for the classic definition of AIDS, which in large part, is a diagnosis of exclusion.[1] The core features include a defect in cell mediated immunity with presence of an opportunistic disease, the most common being *Pneumocystis carinii* pneumonia (PCP) and/or neoplasia in the form of Kaposi's sarcoma (KS). With discovery of the agent responsible for the immune deficiency of AIDS, HIV,[2–4] the original concept of an AIDS patient being without a known cause of immune deficiency becomes irrelevant. This means that the occurrence of certain disease processes in the presence of a positive HIV antibody test are taken as diagnostic of AIDS.[5] Included in this list of conditions qualifying as AIDS are two recently added conditions: severe weight loss (the "wasting syndrome") and severe neurological illness (the so-called "AIDS dementia complex" or ADC). It must be kept in mind that none of these diseases is a direct measure of the underlying HIV infectious disease process. The underlying peripheral disease process is a progressive depletion of cellular immune function caused by the destruction of the T-helper lymphocyte population in the course of viral replication,[6–8] whereas the basic

*The term *neuropsychiatric* and the abbreviation NP are used throughout this chapter to indicate both the effects of HIV on the CNS and the psychological/behavioral responses and efforts to cope with HIV infection, disease progression, treatment, and social stigma.

DAVID G. OSTROW • Midwest AIDS Biobehavioral Research Center, Institute for Social Research, and Department of Psychiatry, University of Michigan Medical School, Ann Arbor, Michigan 48109. J. HAMPTON ATKINSON III and IGOR GRANT • Psychiatry Service, San Diego Veterans Administration Medical Center, San Diego, California 92161; Department of Psychiatry, University of California, San Diego School of Medicine, La Jolla, California 92093.

TABLE 1. CDC Surveillance Definition of AIDS (Revised August, 1986)

1. A disease, at least moderately predictive of a defect in cell-mediated immunity, occurring in a person with no known cause for diminished resistance to that disease. Such diseases include Kaposi's sarcoma (KS), *Pneumocystis carinii* pneumonia (PCP), and other serious opportunistic infections.[a]
2. Diagnoses are considered to fill the case definition only if based on sufficiently reliable methods (generally histology or culture).
3. In adults with HIV seropositivity, additional diseases include disseminated histoplasmosis (not confined to lungs or lymph nodes), diagnosed by culture, histology, or antigen detection; isosporiasis, causing chronic diarrhea (over 1 month), diagnosed by histology or stool microscopy; bronchial or pulmonary candidiasis, diagnosed by microscopy or characteristic white plaques of bronchial mucosa, not by culture alone; non-Hodgkin's lymphoma of high-grade pathologic type (diffuse, undifferentiated) and of B-cell or unknown phenotype, diagnosed by biopsy; histologically confirmed KS in patients 60 years or older.
4. Lymphoretricular malignancies diagnosed more than 3 months after any of the above diagnoses will no longer be excluded as AIDS cases.

[a]These infections include specified syndromes involving specific anatomical sites due to one or more of the following agents: candidiasis, cryptococcosis, cytomegalovirus, nocardiosis, strongyloidosis, toxoplasmosis, or atypical myobacteriosis (species other than *Tuberculosis* or *Lepra*); esophagitis due to candidiasis, cytomegalovirus, or herpes simplex virus; progressive multifocal leukoencephalopathy; chronic enterocolitis (more than 4 weeks) due to cryptosporidiosis; or unusually extensive mucocutaneous herpes simplex of more than 5 weeks duration.

etiopathogenic process underlying ADC is, as yet, unknown. Most conditions listed as diagnostic for AIDS probably represent phenomena secondary to the underlying process of immune deficiency.

It would be preferable if we could drop the term AIDS and instead begin to think of a spectrum of diseases secondary to HIV infection (Table 2). The current nomenclature for HIV spectrum disease has four levels, arranged in a theoretical hierarchy of advancing illness.[9] The first category or stage would be that of acute infection or the seroconversion syndrome. This is being recognized as taking place in the first few weeks after exposure. The seroconversion syndrome may resemble acute mononucleosis, or more often a flu or cold occurring around the time of the first appearance of HIV antibodies.[10] Presumably it indicates multiplication of virus within lymphatic tissues and the body's responses, ranging from transitory swollen lymph glands in most cases to an aseptic meningitis picture in a small proportion. The HIV seroconversion illness is generally self-limiting with the newly infected person usually not aware that they have been infected. Nevertheless, as we describe below, there is evidence that early symptomatic infection of the CNS or at least of the leptomeninges may be relatively common.[11]

Category II of the CDC HIV classification hierarchy, chronic asymptomatic infection, is the stage of infection most HIV seropositive individuals are in at any particular time. Category II implies that there are no significant clinical findings as a result of the infection. During this stage, the immune system has not yet been seriously damaged by HIV infection. It has been found that it usually takes at least 1 or 2 years from the time of infection until the immune system actually begins to show the effects of HIV replication and there may be great variation in the length of time an individual stays in category II before progressing to category III or IV.[12]

One of the problems of this classification system is that category III is defined as generalized lymphadenopathy, but it turns out that many of the people who are "asymptomatic" (i.e., category II) during this period appear to have some degree of lymph gland

TABLE 2. Modified CDC Classification of HIV Infection

Group I: Initial infection

Patients in this group may be designated as symptomatic seroconversion or asymptomatic seroconversion.

Symptomatic infections may include a mononucleosislike syndrome, aseptic meningitis, rash, musculoskeletal complaints, and hematologic abnormalities, as well as other clinical and laboratory findings.

Asymptomatic infection may occur with or without hematologic abnormalities.

Group II: Chronic asymptomatic infection

Patients in this group may be designated as having a normal laboratory evaluation, specified laboratory abnormalities, or laboratory evaluation pending or incomplete.

Laboratory abnormalities associated with HIV infection include anemia, leukopenia, lymphopenia, decreased T-helper lymphocyte count, thrombocytopenia, hypergammaglobulinemia, and cutaneous anergy.

Group III: Persistent generalized lymphadenopathy

Patients in this group may be designated on the basis of laboratory evaluation in the same manner as those in group II.

Group IV: Other diseases

Medical evaluation must exclude the presence of other intercurrent illnesses that could explain the symptoms.

Subgroup IVA: Constitutional disease

Patients in this group may be designated as having fever for more than 1 month, involuntary weight loss greater than 10% of baseline body weight, diarrhea lasting more than 1 month, or any combination of these.

Subgroup IVB: Neurologic disease

Category 1: CNS disorders: Includes dementia, acute atypical meningitis (occurring after initial infections), and myelopathy.

Category 2: Peripheral nervous system disorders: Includes painful sensory neuropathy, and inflammatory demyelinating polyneuropathy.

Subgroup IVC: Secondary infectious diseases

Category 1: Patients in this group may be designated as having one or more of the following: *Pneumocystis carinii* pneumonia, chronic cryptosporidiosis, toxoplasmosis, extraintestinal strongyloidiasis, isosporiasis, candidiasis (esophageal, bronchial, or pulmonary), cryptococcosis, disseminated histoplasmosis, mycobacterial infection with *M. avium* complex or *M. kansasii*, disseminated cytomegalovirus infection, chronic mucocutaneous or disseminted herpes simplex virus infection, and progressive multifocal leukoencephalopathy.

Category 2: Patients in this group may be designated as having one or more of the following: oral hairy leukoplakia, multidermatomal herpes zoster, recurrent *Salmonella bacteremia,* nocardiosis, tuberculosis, or oral candidiasis (thrush).

Subgroup IVD: Secondary Cancers

Patients in this group may be designated as having one or more of the following: Kaposi's sarcoma, non-Hodgkin's lymphoma (small, noncleaved lymphoma or immunoblastic sarcoma), or primary lymphoma of the brain.

Subgroup IVE: Other Conditions

This group includes patients with clinical findings or diseases, not classifiable above, which may be attributed to HIV infection and/or which may be indicative of a defect in cell-mediated immunity.

Patients in this group may be designated on the basis of the types of clinical findings or diseases diagnosed, e.g., chronic lymphoid interstitial pneumonitis.

enlargement that is often missed on routine physical examination because of the size or unusual location of swollen lymph glands. The prognosis does not seem to differ between category II or category III, and HIV-infected persons can reside in either stage for anywhere from several months to many years (mean of 9–10 years) before progressing to category IV.[13]

Category IV includes all of what used to be considered AIDS or ARC. The immune system is now damaged enough that the person is beginning to have clinical signs of the secondary processes that can arise in the immunodeficient person. It is those who enter category IV that develop life-threatening complications, including infections and neoplastic diseases. It should be noted that category IVB of this classification system describes neurologic disease caused directly by HIV infection of the nervous system. The CDC has not defined HIV-related neurologic disease more precisely than that, as it is still an area of evolving nomenclature.[14] It may be that some HIV-related psychiatric illnesses should be included under an expanded category IVB of HIV-related neuropsychiatric disorders. The exact frequency and significance of neuropsychiatric disease in the early stages of HIV infection is currently an area of intense scientific research and debate.

A PSYCHOSOCIAL PERSPECTIVE OF HIV SPECTRUM DISEASE

It is important to recognize that once infection with HIV occurs, the tremendous threat of eventually developing category IV illness is very substantial indeed. It used to be said that the chances of an HIV-positive person's developing clinical disease was 10–20%; then these figures were raised to 30–40%. Now we are finding that approximately 6 of every 100 persons being followed who had been infected for 2 years or longer are converting each year to one of the class IV diagnoses.[15] The long-term outlook shows no signs of improving. Those cohorts of seropositive men who have been followed for the longest periods of time (7–8 years) are approaching rates of transition to class IV illness in the range of 40–60% of their members.

Given that tremendous threat, it is not surprising that people who have been told that they have an infection with HIV can suffer virtually any form of stress-related psychopathology. Anxiety disorders are especially prevalent and range from "worried well" or AIDS anxiety to complete immobilization with panic (see Chapter 10, this volume). Mood disorders can include major depression, suicide, and affective psychoses.[16] Psychiatric symptoms related to HIV need not be limited to those who are actually infected. Persons at risk (chiefly gay and bisexual men) who are seronegative might, nevertheless, experience chronic tension, fearfulness, and somatic symptoms because of worry that their behavior might lead them to become infected; some worry that they are infected when they are not. Even among the "general public" one sees people presenting with anxiety and hypochondriacal complaints based on unrealistic beliefs about exposure to HIV. Such psychological responses to beliefs about AIDS need to be kept in mind so that we do not fall into the trap of thinking that all serious HIV-related psychiatric illness results from brain infection by the virus.

The importance of beliefs about AIDS in determining psychological symptoms was illustrated by the results of a large prospective study conducted by Ostrow and colleagues.[17] The investigators examined a cohort of approximately 5000 men in Chicago, Baltimore, Los Angeles, and Pittsburgh, about one half of whom turned out, in retrospect, to be infected by HIV when they entered the study in 1984. About one fourth of the men knew, even in 1984, that they had had sexual contact at one time in the past with someone who had eventually developed AIDS. At that time in Chicago there were only about 300 AIDS cases, but because many men had contacts with individuals from cities with large numbers of person with AIDS, the fear of AIDS in the cohort was extreme. The cohort was assessed regularly using a psychological symptom self-report scale, the Center for Epidemiological Studies—Depression (CES-D) instrument.[17] At baseline assessment it was found that the strongest predictor of depressive symptoms was the number of self-reported possible HIV-related physical symptoms (Table 3). This association was independent of whether the men were infected or not.[18] Since at the time that the initial data were collected HIV was not yet known to be the etiologic agent of AIDS, and no antibody test

TABLE 3. Factors Associated with CES-D and Subscale Elevations by Multiple Logistic Regression Models[a]

Factor	*N*	Depression	Enervation	Negative affect	Interpersonal	Total
Total symptoms						
0–1	4059	1.00	1.00	1.00	1.00	1.00
2–3	531	2.46	3.19	2.01	1.61	2.72
4+	183	4.74	8.17	2.82	2.45	5.46
No one to talk to	182	3.62	2.74	4.00	2.38	3.46
Noticed glands, by HIV						
HIV−						
No	2783	1.00	1.00	1.00	—	1.00
Yes	118	3.02	1.44	2.48		3.33
HIV+						
No	1482	.92	1.02	.96		.95
Yes	301	1.41	1.62	1.22		1.28
Age						
45+	390	1.00	1.00	—	1.00	1.00
25–34	3849	1.32	1.24		1.69	1.28
<25	534	1.75	2.00		2.63	1.77
Education						
Graduate	1641	—	1.00	1.00	1.00	1.00
College	2513		1.29	1.25	1.41	1.23
High school	619		1.27	1.96	1.64	1.68
Had anonymous partners	2681	1.27	1.20	1.21	1.37	—
Had sex with AIDS partner	925	1.38	—	—	—	1.30
Did *not* use cocaine	2990	—	—	1.28	—	—

[a]Only factors with p value of < 0.01 are included in each model; factors not included are indicated by a dash.

existed, this study demonstrates that it is fear of developing the illness independent of knowing whether one has been exposed to HIV or not that drove much of the depressive symptomatology seen in gay men at high risk of AIDS.

Most interesting from an intervention perspective was that the reported number of individuals that participants felt were available to talk to about major life problems (social support network adequacy) was inversely related to CES-D depression symptom scores. Those who said "no one," had the highest depression scores relative to the number of somatic symptoms reported. These results illustrate something that most mental health workers know: the value of an adequate social support network in helping persons deal with chronic sources of stress and distress. It may also be a scientific validation of something that the community AIDS service providers, especially Shanti, have appreciated for a long time: that it is crucial to provide to people with HIV spectrum disease a "buddy" to help them through the problems of dealing with the medical system, social security system, and regular everyday life problems. That approach has been the mainstay of community-based AIDS support measures for several years, and it has demonstrated efficacy in reducing the amount of social role impairment experienced by persons with AIDS.[19]

The clear implication for mental health workers is that listening to patients, not rejecting them and not showing them fear, is very important in preventing additional psychological distress. A useful approach is to start out by asking, "What can I do for you?" Most patients have already been seen by several internists, infectious disease experts, and immunologists, and some have often been to research centers where they have been tested and questioned at length. What many patients want to express is, "I want you to listen to me and not be afraid of me." They may be isolated from the friends and families, and might have found the medical experience to be very isolating, as well. Such patients crave understanding and acceptance of themselves as persons rather than as research subjects or challenging "cases."

Given the very complex medical, psychological, and social support aspects of treating patients with HIV-related illness, a concept of an AIDS or HIV illness care team has been put forward.[20] This is a very useful concept for the inpatient or coordinated outpatient care settings, where most HIV-infected patients sooner or later are seen (Table 4). Every team may not have all these members, but we find that it is very important to have at least a setting where people from the various disciplines can come together to discuss patients. Quite often the so-called "difficult to manage" patients are really ones that need this kind of coordinated approach, whereas a piecemeal, uncoordinated treatment approach can contribute to behavioral problems rather than solving them.

Mental health professionals have the opportunity to look at the overall picture and try to deal with some of the psychological and social aspects of the disease, in concert with the patient's family and friends, with nursing, social work, clergy, internists, and various medical specialists. Among other things, the mental health member(s) of the HIV illness care team can direct attention to the critical issue of "bedside manner" in the care of persons with AIDS (PWAs). Often, when a medical team arrives at an HIV-infected patient's room, somebody peeks in, says, "Hi, how are you doing?" and then closes the door and the conference takes place in the hallway outside. Or they huddle in one corner of the patient's room and nobody comes within 10 feet of the patient. Patients know what the doctor/patient relationship is supposed to be like, so they know that doctors usually

TABLE 4. The HIV/AIDS Care Team

Medical specialists	Psychiatry
Internal medicine/family practitioner	Consult liaison
Infectious disease	Neuropsychopharmacology
Pulmonary medicine	Medicolegal
Oncologists	Hospital counsel
Neurology	Patient advocate
Nursing	Community liaison
Intensive care (if needed)	Support services
Infection control	Housing
Visiting nurses	Financial support
Human services	Case management and coordination
Social work	
Psychology	
Clergy	
Staff education and support	

come over, palpate something, listen to something, and get rather close to them. This altered behavior around PWAs reinforces the "leper" concept and again makes the whole medical process very distressing to the patient, perhaps even more so than the diagnosis itself. Sitting down with the patient, spending time talking, touching them, and providing reassurance can do much to reduce the isolation and secondary distress of HIV illness. This is not meant to suggest that just lending an ear and a hand is enough to take care of the needs of the HIV patient, but that attention to bedside manner and our own fears and inhibitions should be an important part of diagnosing HIV-related neuropsychiatric disorders and the subsequent treatment planning process.

THE SPECTRUM OF HIV-RELATED ORGANIC BRAIN DISEASE (OBD)

Diagnostic Considerations

When we talk about neuropsychiatric problems in HIV-infected patients, it is important to keep in mind that there are many potentially treatable processes (Table 5). Everything is not just the result of HIV-1 infecting the nervous system; much of what we see in persons with HIV illness affecting behavior and cognition is secondary treatable disease of the CNS. Frequently, successful treatment of the underlying infectious, cancer, or inflammatory processes will lead to significant improvements of cognitive and behavioral functioning. Obviously, secondary brain infections are not easy to treat in immunocompromised patients, and HIV patients often will have serious reactions to the treatments. Unfortunately, progressive multifocal leukoencephalopathy and encephalitis related to herpes viruses, are not likely to resolve. Yet, even CNS lymphomas can respond to chemotherapy and radiation therapy, albeit again HIV patients are less likely to respond than would a nonimmunosuppressed patient.

The discovery of HIV could directly infect the nervous system before demonstrably affecting the peripheral immune system[21–23] has been a great turning point in terms of the

TABLE 5. Potentially Treatable Causes of CNS Dysfunction in HIV Illness

Infections
Toxoplasmosis
Crytococcosis
Herpes encephalitis
Progressive multifocal leukoencephalopathy (papillomavirus)
Mycobacterium tuberculosis (disseminated TB)
Atypical mycobacterial infection
Cancers
Primary brain lymphoma
Burkitt's lymphoma
Disseminated Kaposi's sarcoma
? Other sarcomas
Other
Anoxia due to pneumonia or cardiovascular compromise
Drug-related neurotoxicities
Nutritional deficiencies
Depression
Psychosis
Debilitation/cachexia

involvement of psychiatry in the treatment of AIDS patients. Until that point, psychiatrists were mostly involved secondarily, being called in when a patient's behavior was unmanageable or when a patient started threatening suicide or refused to be involved in a research study or an invasive diagnostic procedure, and rarely seen as primary partners in the care of HIV-spectrum patients. The discovery of a set of NP problems related to this virus has thrust psychiatrists into a major role in the care of AIDS and HIV spectrum patients. Progressive encephalitis, or what some call the AIDS or HIV dementia complex,[24] has become a central focus of psychiatric clinical care as well as psychiatric research.

Subacute encephalitis in adults, acute encephalopathy in children, and vascular myelopathy of the spinal cord, can all occur in the absence of secondary infections or cancers. According to the HIV disease classification system shown in Table 2, once one has any signs of encephalopathy or dementia, one would have class IVB HIV disease. The dilemma with this nosology is that in the absence of secondary opportunistic disease, such a patient does not have AIDS in the classic sense, so it might be better to call these CNS disorder HIV-associated organic brain disease (OBD).

HIV-associated OBD can be difficult to diagnose in the initial stages, just as any incipient dementia is very difficult to diagnose. Often mild changes in personality, memory, and behavior will be attributed to other causes. Occasionally, the early manifestations of HIV-associated organic brain damage will predate any other signs or symptoms of HIV-related illness.[26] However, if an individual shows a major change in cognition, behavior, or personality, that should be a tip-off that something has happened to the underlying immune system and should be a signal to bring back in the diagnostic team to evaluate whether any of the treatable infections or neoplasms listed in Tables 5 and 6 might be developing. One clinical principle here is that one must be prepared to do a large-scale

TABLE 6. Incidence of HIV-Related Neurological Disorders

Disorder	Patients with CNS involvement (%)
HIV-related dementia (encephalopathy, ADC)	
Asymptomatic[a]	8–15
ARC/AIDS[b]	27–50
HIV-related meningitis	17
Secondary viral encephalitis	7–10
Progressive multifocal leukoencephalopathy	1–3
Cerebral toxoplasmosis	8–20
Cryptococcal meningitis	6–25
Primary CNS lymphoma	1–8
Inflammatory demyelinating neuropathy	6
Sensory neuropathy	14
Cranial neuropathies	2
Metabolic encephalopathy	3
Cerebrovascular accident	1–2

[a]CDC category II or III, Walter Reed stages 1–4.
[b]CDC Category IV, Walter Reed stages 5–7.

workup of such patients on short notice, rather than simply writing off a change in behavior or cognition to a relentless progression of HIV dementia. At times, the patient's therapist might think the primary problem is depression, but even these patients should be carefully evaluated, since they may respond to adequate therapy and help in dealing with the underlying HIV diagnosis.

While the early organic mental changes typically involve difficulty in learning and remembering and slowing of information processing, occasionally psychotic episodes and motoric and coordination changes are present as early problems. As HIV-related OBD progresses, however, the disease becomes more and more fixed, sharing some features both of subcortical and (usually later) cortical dementias.[27,28] Such advanced phases are more easily differentiated from depression, personality problems and other functional changes than are the early changes.

A variable course of HIV-related OBD is common, steady progression being more the exception than the rule. The course of the impairment tends to parallel the course of the underlying immunodeficiency with exacerbations of the HIV-related organic brain disease occurring when secondary infections develop or the level of T-helper lymphocytes falls.[29]

Whereas the diagnosis of organicity might not be difficult in patients with more advanced disease, the documentation of early stages of HIV associated organic mental disorder can be challenging. Yet the importance of a reasonably high index of suspicion is suggested by a recent study which noted that 44% of persons who were HIV positive, but who did not have ARC or AIDS, had mild cognitive test abnormalities[30] and case reports of dementia as the presenting clinical syndrome in HIV seropositive persons.[31]

Documentation of cognitive decline can require extensive neuropsychological testing, such as the Halstead–Reitan Battery.[32] The tests most likely to show early changes are those which assess abstraction (e.g., Category Test[33]), complex perceptual-motor skills (e.g., Tactual Performance Test[34]), tests of learning and memory, and speeded information processing (e.g., Paced Auditory Serial Addition or PASAT[34]).

Since many clinicians work in settings in which extensive neuropsychological assessments may not be available, or their costs prohibitive, we suggest that at least a screening battery be considered. As will be seen, this battery assesses simple attention (Digit Span[36]), cognitive speed and flexibility (Digit Symbol; Trail Making[37]), motor speed and coordination (Grooved Pegboard[38]), and memory (figures from Wechsler Memory Scale[39]—or something similar). A self-report cognitive functions inventory[40] is also suggested. It will be appreciated that brief batteries such as these, while representing distinct improvements over unsystematic clinical observations, nevertheless are limited by their brevity and can be considered only modestly sensitive to the presence of cognitive disturbance. If there is reason to suspect significant neurocognitive impairment from any of the screening instruments, it is suggested that the clinician obtain in-depth neuropsychologic evaluation.

A complete neurologic examination should be performed on patients suspected of having organic mental complications. It is important at this point to look for focal signs that might suggest malignancy or underlying secondary infection in the nervous system. Examination for peripheral neurological problems will detect peripheral neuropathies. Asking patients if they are having any symptoms of peripheral neuropathy, such as pain, tingling, or sensory deficits, is helpful in directing attention for neurological evaluation. Peripheral neuropathies are often overlooked, yet they can produce much misery and discomfort. These and other neurological complications of HIV infection might well turn out to be more common as patients start to survive longer with AZT, acrosolized pentamidine prophylaxis, and other life-prolonging treatments. One of the more promising drugs of HIV that was being developed, dideoxycytidine (DDC), will probably be dropped from clinical trials because it produces a very high percentage of painful peripheral neuropathies. At least in those patients who are *now* on receiving this agent, such neuropathies seem to be more the rule than the exception. This is very unfortunate because DDC was to be the successor to AZT as a treatment modality for the underlying immune deficiency of AIDS. Regrettably, at the time of this writing, there are not many other promising drugs coming along without the serious side effects of AZT or DDC.

A lumbar puncture with examination of the CSF is an important laboratory diagnostic tool for further assessment of patients with significant neuropsychiatric impairment. In addition to routine analyses (cells, protein, sugar), one should look for infectious agents and level of CSF antibodies to HIV that might represent intracranial synthesis of antibodies.[41] It may be that levels of specific viral antigens, such as p24 or gp120, might correlate better with the degree of NP impairment than the HIV antibody test.[42]

Meticulous psychiatric assessment is vital in these patients. Indeed, current research efforts increasingly are using standardized, structured diagnostic interviews, such as the Schedule for Affective Disorders and Schizophrenia (SADS),[43] the Diagnostic Interview Schedule (DIS),[44] and the Structured Clinical Interview for DSM-III-R (SCID).[45] In conducting a clinical or standardized psychiatric interview, it should be borne in mind that the interviewer will be required to decide whether or not the "psychiatric symptoms" are better explained by underlying medical illness. This decision may be difficult in seriously ill patients. "Alternative" symptoms have been suggested as diagnostic criteria when it appears that physical illness may be the source of the usual criterion symptom.[46] For example, in the diagnosis of major depression, depressed facies can be substituted for weight loss, social withdrawal or decreased talkativeness for sleep disturbance, pessimism or brooding for fatigue, and lack of mood reactivity used in place of slowed thinking or difficulty concentrating. Although these alternatives have not been validated, they may provide useful guidelines. Clearly, we need to develop more rigorous criteria and structured psychiatric evaluation instruments for use in HIV study patients. Fortunately, these efforts now are begin made, especially for the SCID.

Treatment Approaches

Psychotropic agents can be valuable in the treatment of the neuropsychiatric and psychiatric complications of HIV infection. These problems, and even some of the spatial integration difficulties, may respond to antidepressant or psychostimulant agents. It is important to be very careful in titrating such medication. Patients with HIV infection can resemble geriatric patients in their reactions to antidepressants; they may respond to lower dosage levels and may have severe anticholinergic side-effects, including anticholinergic psychosis at lower drug dosage levels than one might expect in younger individuals (see Chapter 16, this volume). Thus, while tricyclics can be efficacious, it is best to stay away from those more with anticholinergic activity. Desipramine and trazodone, being less anticholinergic, represent reasonable choices. Alprazolam (Xanax) might also be useful in treating mild to moderate depression in HIV positive individuals. The sedative side effects of alprazolam may pose difficulty for anergic patients, however.

In reviewing the literature, we did not find any references to the use of monoamine oxidase (MAO) inhibitors in patients with AIDS or HIV infection. At the same time, there are increasing numbers of anecdotal reports of MAO inhibitors being used in such patients with good response. These agents might be worth considering in patients who do not respond well or cannot tolerate tricyclics and related compounds. Clinical observation and one systematic study suggests that psychostimulants (methylphenidate and dextroamphetamine) might have some value in HIV patients with anergy related to depression, organic illness, or both.[47]

There is not much experience in the long-term treatment of HIV-related OBD with psychostimulants; mostly, in the context of a terminal illness, patients have been prescribed low doses of psychostimulants to get them to be more attentive, to think more clearly, to become more engaged in the treatment process, and perhaps to determine their wishes for terminal care options. Such patients might respond for several weeks, during which time the family and significant others can work with the patient and clinical care team, and important decisions can be made, such as those regarding the use of terminal life-support measures in anticipation of the next major exacerbation of illness. After a brief duration of treatment (e.g., several weeks), the stimulants are usually stopped and the patient generally regresses to his preintervention state.

There is considerable overlap between some of the symptoms of HIV infection and those generally used to screen for depression.[48] As can be seen in Table 7, at least four of the symptoms assessed on the CES-D used to screen for depression have their corresponding HIV-related symptoms, and at least two of these could reflect HIV-associated organic mental disorder. It is frequently difficult, sometimes impossible, to arrive at a precise

TABLE 7. Overlap of HIV-Related and Depression Symptoms

HIV-related symptom	CES-D item
Weight loss	Poor appetite
Night sweats	Sleep restless
Fatigue	Could not "get going"
CNS deficit	Trouble keeping mind on what I'm doing
	Talked less than usual

diagnosis in some of these patients. The definitive diagnosis may require observing the course of illness and the evolution of symptoms. Acute psychosis can also occur in these patients. The psychotic illness can resemble schizophreniform disorder, acute paranoid disorder, brief reactive psychosis, depression with psychotic features, and even a peculiar kind of euphoria perhaps with features of *la belle indifference*. The latter type of patients are anergic, but they also deny any problems; the future is very bright, they really do not need to be in the hospital. This is very much like the euphoria seen in multiple sclerosis—and may involve a similar mechanism—disconnection because of multiple white matter lesions.

For frankly psychotic episodes, the high-potency neuroleptics are recommended, again because of their tendency to produce fewer anticholinergic side-effects. It should be kept in mind that the patient can respond to very low dosages, e.g., 1 or 2 mg of haloperidol (Halodol) bid, or equivalent.

Anxiety, obviously, can be a major symptom in many HIV-infected patients. Anxiety is usually not an issue in demented or psychotic patients, but in the HIV-infected patient without significant neuropsychiatric symptoms anxiety tends to be a major component.[49] If pharmacotherapy for anxiety is indicated, most clinicians tend to use the intermediate half-life anxiolytic agents to reduce hangover symptoms, while providing the patient long enough lasting relief. Some colleagues recommend the use of morphine for patients with HIV disease and significant anxiety, because the morphine both sedates and treats the diarrhea that very often accompanies HIV illness.[50] It is still unclear whether in the long run morphine will turn out to be a useful therapy for HIV patients, but the opiates are being used in some inpatient studies and increasingly prescribed by liaison–consultant psychiatrists seeing patients with HIV-related conditions. Morphine can also be used in agonal patients with severe pain; in some cases the addition of chlorpromazine or dilantin can enhance or replace opiate analgesia.

BRAIN IMAGING IN HIV-ASSOCIATED ORGANIC MENTAL DISORDER

Patients with more advanced ARC/AIDS, particularly those presenting with neurological symptoms, will usually display pathology on brain computed tomography (CT). Data from some of the larger series indicate that about three fourths of such patients will have abnormal CT, the commonest findings being sulcal enlargement, ventricular dilatation, and, occasionally, discrete lesions suggestive of toxoplasma or lymphoma.[51]

Recently, magnetic resonance imaging (MRI), also known as nuclear magnetic resonance (NMR), has shown promise in earlier detection of brain changes, perhaps even in otherwise asymptomatic HIV-positive persons. While MRI is probably more sensitive than CT,[51–53] it may be less specific (e.g., an area of HIV encephalitis might look similar to a toxoplasma lesion). In one recent study, MRI abnormalities were reported in 68% of AIDS and 50% of ARC patients who were asymptomatic on routine neurological examination (see Chapter 12, this volume).

The meaning of MRI lesions is not clear. Certainly, secondary complications (abscesses, tumors) will be visualized in those patient whose disease is advanced. Lesions in less advanced cases might represent HIV encephalitis, with the MRI picking up presence of increased tissue water as occurs in inflammation. MRI may be an important tool not only in detecting early CNS pathology, but also in monitoring outcome. The case studies described in Chapter 12 illustrate this point. Large trials are in progress at the time of this writing to determine whether AZT reverses neurobiological and clinical signs in patients with HIV-associated NP disturbances.[54] In at least several small series of patients, reversal of NP abnormalities during AZT treatment was associated with reversal of PET scan abnormalities[55] and decline in CSF HIV antigen levels.[42]

CONCLUSIONS

In summary, AIDS and related HIV syndromes are neuropsychiatric diseases even as much as they are infectious and immunological diseases. In the early days of AIDS research and treatment, psychiatrists, psychologists, and other mental health caregivers came on the scene mostly as an afterthought, providing support or understanding to victims of a catastrophic illness or to manage the occasional behavioral or neuropsychiatric complications. The studies reviewed here and our ongoing work indicate a true primary role of psychiatry in the diagnosis and treatment of these patients. With the retrovirus now being definitively shown present in the brain, and the work of Pert and others having shown that there are receptors on cells in the brain that are identical to those on lymphocytes which bind HIV,[57] we have to start thinking of this disease as a CNS infection. While the precise pathogenesis of HIV infection of the nervous system remains unclear, there is little doubt that many HIV-seropositive individuals are at risk of eventually developing an organic mental disorder. In the late stages of this disorder, the AIDS dementia complex or, as we prefer to call it, HIV associated organic brain disease, is well recognized and rather easily diagnosed. But we cannot yet predict what proportion of HIV seropositive person will have brain infection nor what proportion of those individuals will go on to develop clinically significant HIV-related OBD.

As for the precise mechanism of neuronal injury, there is very little known about it at this time. It is obvious that the earlier the process is recognized the more the potential for treatment with AZT or other agents as they become available. It is possible that in some patients the brain disease will continue to develop despite improvement or stabilization of the immune system. Many of the treatment studies now ongoing have been modified to take into account the possibility that there can be an independent HIV disease process in the CNS of HIV-infected persons. Therefore, halting the immune deficiency may not be enough. For a therapeutic agent to be effective and to be widely useful, it will also have to halt the CNS disease process. What is evident is that understanding and developing improved treatments for the neuropsychological manifestations of HIV infection will require the joint efforts of psychiatrists, neuroscientists, and infectious disease and immunological experts. The remaining chapters in this section describe the major areas of clinical research and experience related to the CNS aspects of HIV infection.

REFERENCES

1. Centers for Disease Control: Revision of the case definition of acquired immunodeficiency syndrome for national reporting—United States. *MMWR* 36:15, 1987.
2. Barre-Sinoussi F, Chermann JC, Rey F, et al: Isolation of a T-lymphotropic retrovirus from a patient at risk for acquired immune deficiency syndrome (AIDS). *Science* 220:868–871, 1983.
3. Gallo RC, Salahuddin M, Popovic M, et al: Frequent detection and isolation of cytopathic retroviruses (HTLV-III) from patients with AIDS and at risk for AIDS. *Science* 224:500–503, 1984.
4. Levy JA, Shimabukuro J: Recovery of AIDS-associated retro-viruses from patients with AIDS or AIDS-related conditions and from clinically healthy individuals. *J Infect Dis* 152:734–738, 1985.
5. Centers for Disease Control: Revision of the CDC surveillance case definition for acquired immunodeficiency syndrome. *MMWR* 36(suppl):3S–15S, 1987.
6. Siegal FP, Lopez C, Fitzgerald PA, et al: Opportunistic infections in acquired immune deficiency syndrome resulting from synergistic defects of both the natural and adaptive components of cellular immunology. *J Clin Res* 78:115–123, 1986.
7. Polk BF, Fox R, Brookmeyer R, et al: Predictors of acquired immunodeficiency syndrome developing in a cohort of seropositive homosexual men. *N Engl J Med* 316:61–66, 1987.
8. Bowen DL, Lane HC, Fauci AS: Immunopathogenesis of the acquired immunodeficiency syndrome. *Ann Intern Med* 103:704–709, 1985.
9. Centers for Disease Control: Classification systems for human T-lymphotropic virus Type III/lymphadenopathy associated virus infections. *MMWR* 35:334–339, 1986.
10. Cooper DA, Gold J, MacLean P, et al: Acute AIDS retrovirus infection: Definition of a clinical illness associated with seroconversion. *Lancet* 1:537–540, 1985.
11. Price RW, Brew B, Sidtis J, et al: The brain in AIDS: Central nervous system HIV-1 infection and AIDS dementia complex. *Science* 239:586–592, 1988.
12. Phair JA, Ostrow DG, Chmiel J: The Chicago natural history study of HIV infection. *Proc Ann Meet Am Psychiatric Assoc* 101; 1987 (abst).
13. Moss AR, Bacchetti P, Osmond D, et al: Seropositivity for HIV and the development of AIDS or ARC: Three year follow-up of the San Francisco General Hospital cohort. *Br Med J* 296:745–750, 1988.
14. Ostrow DG, Solomon SL, Mayer KH, et al: Classification of the clinical spectrum of HIV infection in adults, in American Medical Association AIDS Advisory Panel (eds): *ADIS: Information on AIDS for the Practicing Physician.* Chicago, American Medical Association, 1987, pp 7–15.
15. Lui K, Darrow WW, Rutherford GW: A model-based estimate of the mean incubation period for AIDS in homosexual men. *Science* 240:1333–1335, 1988.
16. Ostrow DG: Psychiatric consequences of AIDS: An overview. *Int Rev Neurosci* 32:647–659, 1987.
17. Radloft LS: The CES-D Scale: A self-repr depression scale for research in the general population. *App Psychol Measurement* 1:385–401, 1977.
18. Ostrow DG, Monjan A, Joseph J, et al: HIV-related symptoms and psychological functioning in a cohort of homosexual men. *Am J Psychiatry* 146:737–742, 1989.
19. Volberding PA: The clinical spectrum of the acquired immunodeficiency syndrome: Implications for comprehensive patient care. *Ann Intern Med* 103:729–733, 1985.
20. Ostrow DG, Grant I, Atkinson H. Assessment and management of the AIDS patient with neuropsychiatric disturbances. *J Clin Psychiatry* 49(suppl):14–22, 1988.
21. Levy JA, Shimabukuro J, Hollander H, et al: Isolation of AIDS-associated retroviruses from cerebrospinal fluid and brain of patients with neurological symptoms. *Lancet* 2:86–88, 1985.
22. Navia BA, Cho E-S, Petito CK: The AIDS dementia complex. II. Neuropathology. *Ann Neurol* 19:525–535, 1986.

26. Shaw GM, Harper ME, Hahn BH, et al: HTLV-III infection in brains of children and adults with AIDS encephalopathy. *Science* 227:177–182, 1985.
27. Navia BA, Jordan BA, Price RW: The AIDS dementia complex. I. Clinical features. *Ann Neurol* 19:517–524, 1986.
28. Benson DF. The spectrum of dementia. A comparison of the clinical features of AIDS dementia and dementia of the Alzheimer's type. *Alzheimers Dis Assoc Disord* 1:217–220, 1987.
29. Goethe KE, Mitchel JE, Marshall DW, et al: Neuropsychological and neurological function of human immunodeficiency virus seropositive asymptomatic individuals. *Arch Neurol* 46:129–130, 1989.
30. Grant I, Atkinson JH, Hesslink JR, et al: Evidence for early central nervous system involvement in the acquired immunodeficiency syndrome (AIDS) and other human immunodeficiency virus (HIV) infections: Studies with neuropsychologic testing and magnetic resonance imaging. *Ann Intern Med* 107:828–836, 1987.
31. Beckett A, Summergrad P, Manschraeck T, et al: Symptomatic HIV infection of the CNS in a patient without clinical evidence of immune deficiency. *Am J Psychiatry* 144:1342–1343, 1987.
32. Reitan RM, Wolfson D: The Halstead–Reitan neuropsychological test battery, in Wedding D, Horton AM Jr, Webster J (eds): *The Neuropsychology Handbook.* New York, Springer, 1986, pp 135–160.
33. Halstead WC: *Brain and Intelligence.* Chicago, University of Chicago Press, 1947.
34. Reitan RM, Davison, LA: *Clinical Neuropsychology: Current Status and Applications.* New York: Hemisphere, 1974.
35. Gronwall DMA. Paced auditory serial-addition task: A measure of recovery from concussion. *Percep Motor Skills* 44:367–373, 1977.
36. Wechsler DA: A standardized memory scale for clinical use. *J Psychol* 19:87–95, 1945.
37. Reitan RM: The validity of the Trail Making test as an indicator of organic brain damage. *Percept Mot Skills* 44:367–373, 1958.
38. Adams K, Rennick PM, Schoff K, et al: Neuropsychological measurement of drug effects: Polydrug research. *J Psychedelic Drugs* 7:151–160, 1975.
39. Wechsler DA: *The Measurement and Appraisal of Adult Intelligence,* Baltimore, Williams & Wilkins, 1958.
40. Broadbent D, Cooper PS, Fitzgerald P, et al: The cognitive failure questionnaire (CFQ) and its correlates. *Br J Clin Psychiatry* 21:1–16, 1982.
41. Resnick L, DiMarzo Veronese F, Schupbach J, et al: Intra-blood–brain barrier synthesis of HTLV-III specific IgG in patient with neurologic symptoms associated with AIDS or AIDS-related complex. *N Engl J Med* 313:1498–1504, 1985.
42. de Gans J, Lange JMA, Derix MMA, et al: Decline of HIV antigen levels in cerebrospinal fluid during treatment of patients with low dose zidovudine. *AIDS* 2:37–40, 1988.
43. Endicott J, Spitzer RL: A diagnostic interview: The schedule for affective disorders in schizophrenia. *Arch Gen Psychiatry* 35:837–844, 1978.
44. Robins LN, Helzer J, Croughan J, et al: The NIMH Diagnostic Interview Schedule, Version IIIR. Bethesda, Alcohol, Drug Abuse and Mental Health Agency, 1981.
45. Spitzer RL, Williams JBW, Gibbon M, et al: A Structural Clinical Interview of DSM III-R. New York State Psychiatric Institute, 1988.
46. Endicott J: Measurement of depression in patients with cancer. *Cancer* 53(suppl):2243–2249, 1984.
47. Fernandez F, Adams F, Levy JK, et al: Cognitive impairment due to AIDS-related complex and its response to psychostimulants. *Psychosom Med* 29:38–46, 1988.
48. Ostrow DG: Models for understanding the psychiatric implications of AIDS, in Bridge P (ed): *Psychological, Neuropsychiatric, and Substance Abuse Aspects of AIDS.* New York, Raven Press, 1988, pp
49. Miller D: Taking the anxiety out of AIDS. *Stress Med* 2:259–265, 1986.
50. Busch KA: AIDS and psychiatry. *Curr Clin Briefs* 8:3–5, 1987.
51. Post MJD, Sheldon JJ, Hensley GT, et al: Central nervous system disease in acquired immunodeficiency syndrome: Prospective correlation using CT, MR imaging, and pathologic studies. *Radiology* 158:141–148, 1986.
52. Levy JD, Cottingham KL, Campbell RJ, et al: Progressive multifocal leukoencephalopathy and magnetic resonance imaging. *Ann Neurol* 19:399–401, 1986.
53. Delapaz R, Floris R, Brant-Zawadski M: Magnetic resonance imaging of central nervous system complications of AIDS, in *Annual Meeting of the Society of Magnetic Resonance in Medicine, London, August 1985* (abst).

54. Schmidt FA, Bigley JW, McKinnis R, et al: Neuropsychological outcome of zidovudine (AZT) treatment of patients with AIDS and AIDS-related complex. *N Engl J Med* 319:1573–1578, 1988.
55. Yarchoan R, Berg G, Brouwers P, et al: Response of human-immunodeficiency-virus-associated neurological disease to 3′-azido-3′-deoxythymidine. *Lancet* 1:132–135, 1987.
56. Pert CB, Hill JM, Ruff MR, et al: Octapeptides deduced from the neuropeptide receptor-like pattern of antigen T4 in brain potently inhibit human immunodeficiency virus receptor binding and T-cell infectivity. *Proc Natl Acad Sci USA* 83:9254–9258, 1986 (abst).

10

Diagnosis and Treatment of Acute Psychological Problems Related to HIV Infection and Disease

DAVID MILLER

INTRODUCTION

Human immunodeficiency virus (HIV) infection and disease are as much social issues as medical issues. A distinguishing characteristic of the response of the health care establishment to patients and their social milieus is the imperative to change the ways in which people act. Such imperatives for change include the motivating of safer sexual and drug-use practices and of increased public tolerance and understanding of those (groups) directly affected.

Given this circumstance, the diagnosis and treatment of acute psychological problems related to HIV infection and disease must necessarily include a perspective not only on the patient, but on the wider and complicating spheres of his or her social context.[1,2] For example, it is clear from the reports of many patients that a fear of disease progression is frequently matched by a fear of the negative reactions of others (loved ones, colleagues, peers) to their infection or diagnosis.[3] Recent evidence of the reactions of health staff to persons with AIDS adds substance to such anxieties in some areas.[4,5] Examining the veracity of such latter fears may, for example, lead a clinician to diagnose a paranoid reaction on the one hand, or a justifiable avoidance and anxiety disorder on the other.

Of equal importance is the clinicians' necessary understanding that they, too, are bound by their professional context as they tackle the management of AIDS-related phenomena. Typically, they are a staging post in the clinical conveyor belt that has many professional and nonprofessional detours both preceding and following their intervention.[6,7] This places acute and chronic demands on the psychologist or psychiatrist—there is a need to refine his/her knowledge and understanding of (retro)virology, immunology, general medicine, oncology, dermatology, neurology, pharmacology, and so on. Further, the clinician is required to develop and maintain effective channels of communication with individuals, departments, and other agencies. They need to develop an understanding of frequently diverse subcultures and life-styles, while staying up to date with the moun-

DAVID MILLER • Academic Department of Genitourinary Medicine, The Middlesex Hospital Medical School, London W1N 8AA, England.

tainous literature, rapid developments in field, and tragically escalating caseloads. Patients are frequently the best teachers, but having a vocabulary in common, and the time to use it, is vital if both parties to the clinical contract are to benefit. Finally, the good clinician must necessarily maintain some time away from work, in order to be fit for work!

This chapter is confined to acute psychological phenomena, their diagnosis and management. The discussion will focus on two groups—those with human immunodeficiency virus (HIV) infection and those without. For each group, presenting symptoms/syndromes are described. Assessment protocols are then provided and treatment regimens (behavioral, psychosocial, and pharmacological) are suggested. There is minimal reference to neuropsychiatric issues in this discussion as they are covered specifically in Chapters 3–6 (this volume).

DIAGNOSIS AND TREATMENT OF THOSE WITH HIV INFECTION AND DISEASE

Responses to a diagnosis of HIV infection or disease across all cultures are reportedly similar to responses seen to other life-threatening illnesses.[6,8–11] There are distinguishing characteristics in HIV, however, associated with the often frequent additional HIV-related burdens of stigma, rejection, marginalization, prejudice, cultural and legal oppression, political apathy, and fear of contagion. As familiar reactions including shock, withdrawal, despair, anxiety, bargaining, avoidance, anger, and denial are expected and considered to be normal in such circumstances, the clinician is faced with making a judgment of the balance between an expected spectrum of psychological phenomena and formally classifiable and treatable psychological problems.[12] This can be difficult, particularly in view of the young mean age of many patient groups.[13] Frequently, patients in developed countries will not have endured life-threatening or catastrophic situations before and their reactions cannot be determined as being typical or otherwise.

Problems in diagnosis may also arise from the cognitive effects associated with acute distress, such as memory impairment, distractability, and disorientation.[14] These may be easily misclassified as indications of potential neurological damage associated with HIV infection, although temporary impairment in cognitive functioning is a demonstrated correlate in some persons with acute retroviral illness.[15]

A sense of history is therefore required in making initial clinical judgments, particularly if conclusions made will lead to formal interventions beyond the purely supportive.[16] This need has become even more pressing in recent times with apparently growing options and criteria for potential prophylaxis against disease onset.[17,18] For example, the onset, duration, and phenomenology of presenting symptoms must be examined in the light of coincidental and contextual factors including intercurrent diseases. There are likely to be significant differences in the reactions of those who are informed of their HIV seropositivity for the first time and those who have known of their HIV status for a longer period and who may be experiencing bad news (i.e., a diagnosis) after a period of preparation and acceptance. It is noteworthy that for those who remain unaccepting of their infection/disease, the appearance of new or repeated infections frequently evokes a similar intensity of catastrophic reaction as that seen at the time of initial diagnosis.[12]

Recent evidence has also suggested that the intensity of psychological distress is to some extent determined by clinical staging of illness: Those with AIDS-related complex (ARC) appear to experience greater psychosocial morbidity than do those who are asymptomatic and those who have frank AIDS.[19,20] Some clinical reports suggest that a sense of relief may accompany a diagnosis of AIDS in those who have been chronically ill but not previously diagnosable,[2,16] or with a diagnosis following enrollment in previously inaccessible treatment trials.

Increasingly it is recognized that all psychiatric assessments must exclude the possibility of intercurrent central nervous system (CNS) infections and/or neoplasms, in addition to the possibility of direct CNS damage associated with HIV neurotropism, in reaching formal psychiatric diagnoses.[21,22] Similarly, a history of alcohol/drug use and/or acute physical (especially cranial) trauma must also be excluded as a cause of possible organic manifestations.

Acute Psychological Syndromes

It is important that although the symptoms and syndromes described below are frequently acute presentations, they may also become chronic. Where appropriate intervention is delayed or absent, chronicity may be more likely and formal interventions will ultimately be more complicated because of the broad social consequences that such unaddressed presentations can generate.[6,9,23]

Much of the psychosocial disturbance seen after personal HIV infection or disease is identified will reflect two prominent foci of patient concern—fear for the future course of the disease and fear over the potential reactions of others. The range of phenomena seen at this time are usually to be expected in the context of a perceived "death sentence" and have been characterized as manifestations of "situational distress" or "adjustment reaction."[11]

Additionally, it may be helpful to consider clinically presenting psychosocial phenomena as characteristics of the processes of uncertainty and adjustment reportedly endured by many people with HIV.[12] These two vitally complementary processes are always dynamically linked. They appear as a tension that informs all levels or stages of health and disease expression as people struggle to live with HIV.[24]

Shock and Denial

Despite the universal recognition of the potential for HIV in many social groups, and the closeness of many persons to others with HIV infection or disease, the gap between intellectual acceptance and emotional acceptance is usually significant. Shock should always be considered in the process of counselling or structuring clinical interventions after diagnoses or laboratory results have been relayed. Shock can contribute to diagnostic and management problems because it can interfere with cognitive and behavioral functioning. Commonly in persons in shock, reassurance and health information are only partly taken in, and behaviors including withdrawal, aggression, and cathartic release can appear.[2]

Denial can be an adaptive response in many cases since it can function to reduce internal stress. However, shock and denial can be problematic since they may create confusion at a time when vital personal decisions are required. Occasionally, pathological denial resulting in repeated frantic calls to physicians or counsellors for "second opinions," or ecstatic commitment to alternative or complementary (and frequently unproven) healing regimes, may be seen. Cognitive correlates of shock, such as distractability, poor short-term memory, and disorientation may endure until the shock of HIV infection or disease is overcome.

Shock can be immediate or delayed, and may recur with the advent of new or repeated diagnostic events and circumstances (some patients maintain that they prefer to stay away from hospitals where they were initially diagnosed because the associations with trauma are too strong to endure and can precipitate new episodes of distress). Especially when life issues such as career, domestic responsibilities, and commitments are of immediate concern for the patient, the news may be blocked out while their physical and emotional stamina lasts. Some patients have appeared to make optimal responses to their diagnoses over many months, only to face the original trauma of their status once they have developed stamina-draining infections or illnesses. The management of serious opportunistic or neoplastic disease is then complicated by the rapid appearance of shock and associated psychological symptoms that surface unexpectedly.[2,16]

Anxiety

Anxiety is a ubiquitous feature in the life of the HIV-infected person.[1–3,6,8–12] The person with HIV may present with a number of autonomic nervous system (ANS) features, such as diarrhea, nausea, sweating, tremor, visual disturbances, dizziness, skin rashes, and lethargy. These may be misinterpreted by the patient as being symptomatic of HIV-related illness, compounding the anxiety. Once again, astute clinical judgment may be required to tease out the cognitive effects of anxiety from those of genuine neurological impairment. The appearance of panic attacks, experienced by some acutely and chronically highly anxious patients, is considerably discomforting and may contribute to expressed fears of mental decline.[2,12,14]

Complications arise in accurate diagnosis at correlative anxiety features in those who have resorted to alcohol and/or recreational or prescribed drugs in an attempt to manage their anxiety symptoms, especially when sleeplessness is an enduring feature.[1,3,6,10]

Some of the reasons for the development of anxiety in this population are listed in Table 1. Many of these anxieties are successfully manageable by providing appropriate information, unhurried support, reassurance, and practical interventions (e.g., concerning the issues of infectiousness, terminal illness management, medical/dental care, confidentiality, financial management, and relationship support and therapy). Other anxieties are less directly manageable, however, because of the prevailing uncertainties associated with prognoses, impact of experimental or prophylactic treatments and their side-effects, and social stigmatizing and understanding of the infection and of those infected.

Depression

Depressive reactions are a further common acute manifestation, for reasons given in Tables 1 and 2. The behavioral and cognitive effects of depression can produce considerable functional handicaps for people with HIV. Like the other common acute symptoms, depression significantly alters the nature of the person's relationships with those they are

TABLE 1. Some Reasons for AIDS-Related Patient Anxieties

Prognosis in the short and long term
Infection risk to and from other people
Social, occupational, domestic, and sexual hostility and rejection
Abandonment, isolation, and physical pain
Inability to alter circumstances
How to maximize future health
Ability of loved ones/family members to cope
Availability of appropriate medical/dental/welfare management
Being identified as homosexual/drug user/sex worker/unfaithful
Loss of privacy/confidentiality
Loss of dignity with increasing physical dependence
Future social and sexual unacceptability
Declining ability to cope
Loss of physical and financial independence

close to or with whom they interact daily.[2,11,12] Depression, particularly when associated with worsening physical health, also interferes with perceptions of, adaptation to, and acceptance of, the new health circumstances, and the range of possible environmental support.[25]

A prominent symptom of depression in those recently diagnosed is withdrawal. It is necessary to consider the withdrawal associated with the shock of diagnosis when making a formal diagnosis of depression, however. For example, the shock of diagnosis may not coincide with the cognitive deficits associated with depression, and will not last as long as in the depressed patient.[14] A functional and social retreat will restrict the patient's exposure to positive intervention and reinforcement from physicians, counsellors and peers, family, and work colleagues. Withdrawal may be motivated as much by anxiety over the possible rejecting responses of others[3] as by the sense of helplessness that HIV generates with the recognition of an absence of a cure, the constant associations drawn with health decline and death, uncertainty over the impact of drug and other treatment regimens, and of future life being predicated mainly on HIV.[12] Importantly, withdrawal interferes greatly with the process of acceptance of the situation, largely because of the reduced opportunities for discussion and modeling of adaptive responses.[12,24,25] Without such influences, the corrosive effects of uncertainty, fear, self-blaming, and self-recrimination may flourish. Indeed, the assault of the diagnosis on the self-esteem of the patient may lead to precipitate impulsive actions of self-harm (suicidal actions are discussed below). It is interesting that, even with thousands of people with HIV infection and disease (including AIDS) living actively and successfully in most societies, many newly diagnosed patients will automatically conjure up self-images characterized by wasting decline and disfigurement, sometimes generated as "evidence" of punishment for prior "misdeeds" or "moral worthlessness." A number of health-worker surveys indicate that health staff may hold or endorse such naive and deplorable sentiments.[4,5]

Other Psychological Issues and Phenomena

An acute and high level of concern for physical health becomes a major preoccupation for many recently diagnosed people. For some, however, this is manifested as an obsessive preoccupation with bodily checking for emerging signs of disease. Blemishes or marks and pre-existing skin marks, moles, freckles, and glands will be minutely scrutinized, counted, and perhaps prodded and poked. Such self-scrutiny may involve particular bodily areas or parts (e.g., cervical lymph nodes) or cover the whole body. Checking may occur only when undressing occurs (e.g., when bathing or showering) or may be a random spontaneous occurrence. Frequency varies widely across cases, from perhaps once daily, to eight or nine or more times daily in total bodily checking, and perhaps five or six times hourly in those concentrating on specific areas. Any variation in numbers of freckles counted, for example, will provoke acute distress. The latter group may also present classically in the manner of patients presenting with dysmorphophobia,[14] i.e., of those with obsessive ruminations about particulars of their bodily appearance.

For those with obsessive ruminations alone, the presentations involve an involuntary dwelling on images and thoughts of HIV disease in others and perhaps the self. Often, the appearance of obsessive preoccupations coincides with a poverty of action or involvement on the part of the patient who has perhaps stopped work or withdrawn socially. They thus have no distractions from the lure of obsessional self-concern. Obsessive disorders can thus occur alone or as part of a reactive depressive pattern. In others, the obsessions occur despite attempts at distractions.[3,6] It is important to consider a predisposition toward obsessive states as a possible feature of the premorbid personality.

For many people, the recognition of personal vulnerability to HIV constitutes a traumatic complication in the context of pre-existing psychological difficulties.[1,2,26] The extra stress associated with becoming identified as having HIV infection or disease can lead to the expression of previously manageable or controlled symptomatology, in much the same way that AIDS and HIV have become a vehicle for the expression of sexual guilt in many of the non-HIV-infected "worried well."[27,28] For example, it is not uncommon for people fearful of or suspecting the presence of HIV disease to resort to the use of alcohol, recreational drugs, or, in some cases, high-risk activity associated with a risk of physical injury or death as a means of coping.[6,29] In such situations, and with those with previously established alcohol/drug dependencies,[30] the expression, diagnosis, and management of HIV-related psychological disturbance may be very complicated and require active intervention from more than one agency. Similarly, the diagnosis received may lead to a renewed expression of the traumas associated with previous painful or emotionally scarring life events, such as rejection experienced when "coming out" as a gay man, divorce, the death of loved family members or peers.[2,3,6,10–12]

For these reasons, it is important to become familiar with coping strategies that have been adopted by the patient in the past.[1,6,9,12,16] Those that have been successful may be of use again, and discussion of them may also stimulate an awareness that current difficulties can be faced and may encourage motivation to try. A summary of acute psychological phenomena seen in those with HIV is given in Table 2.

Although for many persons such reactions may be quite transitory, for some they will come to characterize their life with HIV. Although it has yet to be empirically determined, it is possible that vulnerability to these effects and indeed the whole process of adjustment to life with HIV will, to some extent, be determined by the patient's previous experience of severe illness or life trauma, either in themselves or in loved ones, and the success of their personal management at those times. Other equally important mediators of reactions to life with HIV or AIDS include personality and temperament; social, familial, and occupational resources, support; and flexibility.[1,6,9] Generally speaking, greater difficulties tend to be faced by those with unresolved emotional concerns about their sexuality or life-style to that point, who may be socially isolated, with poor or uncertain accommodation, irregular or unsatisfying employment, and little spare money.[16] Access to reliable and sympathetic medical and social services is increasingly recognized as a pivotal element in determining quality of care, and thus quality of life, for those with HIV.

Researchers have recently analyzed coping responses of recently diagnosed people with AIDS in greater detail.[31] They found that the style of coping adopted by patients was predictive of their psychological, and thus physical, well-being: Those showing avoidance had the greatest levels of concern regarding personal health, existential issues, friends, and their self. They also had the highest levels of depression, the lowest measured self-esteem, and were much less likely to receive social or practical support because they were seen as less attractive or motivated by support-givers—they seemed less receptive (they were avoiding it).

On the other hand, those who adopted an active–cognitive coping style, by building "mental defenses" and relying on the establishment of positive thinking alone, often

TABLE 2. Acute Psychological Phenomena Seen in People with HIV

Shock
Of diagnosis and possible death
Over loss of hopes for good news
Fear and anxiety
Uncertain prognosis and course of illness
Of disfigurement and disability
Effects of medication and treatment
Of isolation and rejection
Of infecting others and being infected by them
Of others' abilities to manage possible illness
Of loss of cognitive, physical, social, and work abilities
Depression
Over "inevitability" of decline
Over absence of a cure
Over the virus controlling future life
Over limites imposed by ill-health and rejection by others
From self-blame and recrimination over being exposed to HIV
Anger and frustration
Over inability to overcome the virus
Over new and involuntary health/lifestyle restrictions
At being "caught out" and the uncertainty of the future
Guilt
Over past lifestyle exposing one to HIV
Over possibly having unwittingly infected others
Obsessive problems
Relentless searching for new bodily diagnostic "evidence"
Faddism over health and diet regimes
Preoccupations with illness and death, and avoidance of new infections

developed obsessive and ruminative thoughts and attitudes (what elsewhere has been referred to as "the tyranny of positive thinking."[12] This was overcome if cognitive strategies led on to the takeup of active–behavioral coping strategies: Such persons had better mood states, fewer major concerns, higher perceived quality of life, and greater self-esteem independent of medical status.[31]

Conceptual issues associated with acute presentations include the issue of personal control.[1] The absence of a cure for HIV infection, despite growing sophistication in management of HIV-related opportunistic infections and neoplasms, emphasizes a feeling of entrapment for many patients. Some have described the total frustration that follows from being unable to plan ahead, even for tomorrow where illness is critical.[12] This can lead to a sense of helplessness and motivational inhibition which, in the longer term, can become a correlate of chronic depression. Control is also undermined by the often intense hospital and clinical involvement that many are required to endure (sometimes called "medicalization"). Vulnerability to and frustration with this process—with its attendant uncertainties regarding information about drugs, outcomes, and simply what might happen next—may be expressed as anger, or as a series of impulsive decisions, medical noncompliance, even physically dangerous pursuits: Each may be the vehicle for expressing a desire for mastery and resumption of personal control in the face of this most deskilling individual circumstance.[6,8,12] Medical noncompliance manifested as not reporting symptoms or not taking prescribed medication in the face of physical deterioration ("passive suicide"[32]) may be a final means of asserting personal control in those with terminal disease who wish to avoid prolonged, undignifying, and painful decline, especially where neurological deterioration is feared.

Self-esteem is a further conceptual issue with concrete significance. It is undermined by the physical, occupational, sexual, and recreational restrictions associated with HIV illness and infection. The person with HIV, aware of the often major limitations and decisions that require confrontation in the process of adaptation for survival, may feel reduced personal and social worth.[2,3] The pitiable assaults of few noisy and frankly bigoted public commentators, politicians, religious and even medical authorities, frequently asserting prejudice, unprofessionalism, and inhumanity in the guise of prophetic morality or even social safety, can encourage sometimes bitter social and self-recrimination over past lifestyles and behaviors and present circumstances. Additionally, the physical effects of severe disease, including physical wasting and the appearance of widespread, and, in particular, facial, Kaposi's sarcomas and other opportunistic diseases (e.g., molluscum contagiosum, seborrhoeic dermatitis), can create irreversible self-image problems. Even where such physical effects are not apparent the realization that they might become so can lead to anticipatory grief and self-image disorders. Self-assertion can be undermined or eliminated at a a time when it may be most needed.

The issue of suicidal activity or planning must be acknowledged in persons with HIV. Suicidal responses have followed where positive results have been identified from HIV-antibody testing without consent or pre-counseling.[33] It appears that along with contextual variables, like social, emotional, and practical support, the manner in which news of infection or disease is presented is important in determining the likelihood of impulsive suicidal activity.[1,33] Clinical experience suggests that even where the intention for suicide or the making of contingency plans for this is not openly suggested, those who are socially and culturally isolated or fearful present a heightened risk of suicidal activity, particularly during the initial shock after diagnosis and where follow-up support and counselling is not offered or available. A recent analysis of suicide rates in New York City for the year of 1985 concluded that men with AIDS were 36 times more likely to commit suicide than men without this diagnosis, and 66 times more likely to do so than the general population.[34]

Amongst the 23% of USAF personnel identified as HIV-positive who had psychiatric consultations up to 1987, 25% were diagnosed with depression, 22% with adjustment disorders, and 4% with major depression.[35] Of 147 who were reevaluated 11 months after identification of infection, eight had attempted suicide, of whom one was successful. This is an attempted suicide rate of 5% in those identified as being HIV-positive in this population.[35] Retrospective case control analysis revealed the following predictive factors: (a) multiple psychosocial stresses; (b) perceived social isolation; (c) perceiving oneself as a victim; (d) reliance on denial as the central and only defense; (e) substance abuse; and (f) perceived unavailable social support. A prior history of psychiatric illness was also implicated as a predictive variable. It is of interest to notice the close fit between these predictors and those identified in the context of general psychiatry as presenting a risk for suicidal activity.[14]

A study of 218 HIV-positive persons (CDC groups II and III) compared to 60 noninfected persons "at risk" and 50 HIV-negative heterosexual subjects at "low risk" of infection concluded that homosexual men and substance misusers had a higher psychiatric morbidity, including a history of attempted suicides, than heterosexuals.[36] Importantly, however, a prior psychiatric history and a history of attempted suicide were better predictors of current psychiatric morbidity or suicidal activity than diagnosis of HIV infection.[36] A San Francisco study revealed that among AIDS-related suicides in San Francisco not associated with IV drug use, 30% died within one month of a diagnosis of AIDS, 46% died 12 or more months following their diagnosis (median time between diagnosis and suicide as 8 months).[37]

Clinical experience suggests that determination of suicide is a complex and frequently misleading process, and that suicide attempts can be active (taking tablets or jumping from a window[38]) or passive, involving a nonreporting to medical authorities of the appearance of patient-recognized symptoms of HIV disease. Thus, even where the intention for suicide or the making of contingency plans for this is not openly suggested, it seems wise to consider and even to raise the issue, especially in the isolated or alone, during the initial time after HIV identification.

ASSESSMENT AND INTERVENTION

Assessment

Assessment of presenting psychological and psychosocial problems in the context of HIV are to some degree mediated by

1. The life-threatening significance of HIV infection and/or disease
2. The possible presence of intercurrent infection/disease(s) in many patients

3. Psychosocial constraints and previous patient experience of life-threatening situations and interventions
4. The availability of formal health care and informal support

In order to clearly understand the appropriateness of the patient's presentation, it is necessary to assess the background to the presentation. It is necessary to do a formal examination, to rule out the possible significance of intercurrent disease processes, and to assess the nature of the psychosocial support available to the patient in their own milieu. Important aspects of such a background assessment include a consideration of the manner of diagnosis and the patient's reaction to this, the role of loved ones, especially spouses and/or lovers and family.

In performing a formal examination, it is necessary to differentiate between organic and psychogenic syndromes. A resume of issues to consider is presented in Table 3. These issues can then be used as the basis for further history-taking as seems appropriate.

In view of the increasingly reliable reports of central nervous system (CNS) disease and organic mental disorders (OMD) as causative processes in acute psychological and psychiatric presentations,[21,22] it will be necessary to exclude such processes in order to effectively differentiate signs of psychosocial distress from genuine CNS presentations (see Table 3; and Chapters 3–5, this volume).

TABLE 3. Preliminary Formal Psychosocial Examination Issues

At presentation
Nature of presenting symptoms, onset, and duration
Circumstance and nature of medical diagnosis, and sequence of responses, including history of HIV status
Assessment for presence of possible neurological signs and history
Reported changes in mental status, consciousness, sensorium
Reported changes in primary relationships, and at work, socially, recreationally, and circumstances of changes;
Reported changes in sleep, eating, weight, drinking and smoking, inability to make decisions and communicate with others, and vulnerability to emotional display
Background issues
Primary relationships: nature, duration and character, quality of support provided and required, complicating issues (e.g., sex, illness, work)
Family relationships: character and quality, tolerance or understanding of patient's lifestyle, degree of communication, complicating issues (e.g., divorce separation, children)
Social support structure: friends, colleagues, involvement in and understanding of patient's lifestyle and illness, social HIV experience, nature and quality of involvements
History of previous psychiatric/psychological issues and treatments, including alcohol and drug use
Previous coping mechanisms and present options available, responses made to offers of support, including (para)medical interventions
Present range of (para)medical care provision and providers
Prior knowledge of, and attitudes to, HIV/AIDS, personal acknowledgment of risk (including steps taken to reduce HIV exposure risk)
Challenges to coping abilities, including issues of denial, resignation, anger, depression, hysteria
Verifications
Reliable other person(s)
Prior medical records and health care professionals/providers
Laboratory/clinical assessments: CT scan, blood tests for intercurrent processes (i.e., HIV may not be causing primary illness), spinal tap, acute infections, CNS neoplasms, acute trauma (especially neurological)

Further important assessment issues include the manner in which the patient was diagnosed and has been followed up, and familial support and occupational resources available to the patient to help in coming to terms with the diagnosis. Regarding the former, clinical experience indicates that the quality of immediate postdiagnostic adjustment can largely be determined by the level and quality of preparation of the patient has received in advance of the news.[4,33] In the context of HIV antibody screening, anecdotally verified suicides have followed positive results delivered in the context of no precounseling, or when the patient has been previously unaware that his/her blood has been tested and there is a lack of adequate follow-up counseling and professional support in place. People are left in a state of acute shock, without advice or support, and under the impression that they will one day (probably soon) die of AIDS. On the other hand, when adequate pre- and post-test counseling is provided, and it is the patient who makes the decision to be tested, vulnerability can be adequately assessed beforehand by the counsellor or physician, the trauma of a positive result can be shared, and management directed at redeveloping a sense of personal control is immediately accessible.[16,17,33]

The social milieu of the person with HIV is of paramount importance. Where the patient self-identifies with a community including known people or friends with AIDS, modeled responses may already have been adopted. Where friends or loved ones have developed AIDS or died, the patient's fears for his or her own future may become intensified, leading to an exacerbation of presenting symptoms.[9] Mounting concern over the impact of the diagnosis on loved ones, family, and friends may contribute to increased trauma, especially where loved ones and friends over-identify with the patient's experience and lead the patient to fear for the ability of others to cope with the circumstances.[12,39]

Associated with the pressures on relationships is the issue of the stigma of HIV/AIDS. These pressures can lead to family estrangement, or family being kept out of the news of diagnosis and even treatment, or, where family are directly involved, to the development of a conspiracy of avoidance in which the true nature of the diagnosis is never discussed with outsiders.[12] The pressures of such conspiracies can themselves be counterproductive and divisive, particularly where children are involved and where planning for the future becomes advisable or necessary.

Longer-term adjustment also required consideration of the patient's actual knowledge of HIV infection and disease,[1,6,12] and his/her level of experience with the management of the disease within his/her own community. Linked with this is the person's experience with peer-group professional and community AIDS agencies, and their level of involvement with other medical and paramedical care providers.

Intervention

Once the individual's psychosocial issues and needs and coping resources have been defined, the stage is set for intervention. Perhaps the first step in effective formal intervention is careful resource planning based on clinical needs identified elsewhere. Because of the wide range of personal and social issues already highlighted in psychological management of HIV, it is possible and necessary to identify specific resources and personnel in advance of the need for them. For example, in the context of hospital-based management, the clinical service shopping list for psychosocial backup suggested in Table 4 is desirable.

TABLE 4. Suggested Services for Backup of Psychosocial Management

Hospital	Community
Support groups	Social services personnel
Drug dependency services	Homosexual support agencies
Gynecologist/obstetrician	Hemophilia support agencies
Social worker	Drug advice/support agencies
Religious chaplain	General practitioners
Surgeon	Legal/citizens advice service
Dentist	"Buddy" services
Physicians	Telephone crisis counselors
Neurologist/neuropsychologist	Rape counseling services
Dietician/nutritionist	Police service personnel
Pediatricians	Clergy
Venereologist	Marital/sexual therapists
	Financial support services
	Hospice facilities
	Heterosexual support agencies

Other important aspects of intervention include:

1. *Access to services:* It goes without saying that no services will work if they are unable to be reached by their intended consumers. Recent American studies have shown that access to services is a major influence on decision-making about termination in HIV-infected mothers. Also, it should be obvious that access is also measured by levels of sensitivity, acceptance, and consistency in personal management and where such qualities are found to be lacking, patients will usually vote with their feet!

2. *Time:* Time for ventilation of distress, to be heard, or perhaps simply to give a sense of structure to someone whose life seems to them to be chaotic at that time. The opportunity to have time to ventilate anxieties can be especially valuable for those who are socially isolated or who have been 'hiding' or 'bottling up' their health worries for fear of social, occupational or familial rejection.

3. *Information-giving:* News of infection or disease will, because of the often immediate patient extrapolation of diagnosis to death from AIDS, need to be placed in a perspective of potential for management.[2,6,40] Information/advice should therefore be discussed and/or made available on (a) known facts about the condition(s) motivating psychosocial morbidity; (b) available treatment options and available experimental/ research regimes; (c) "health boosting" and infection-control measures under the patient's control, such as safer sex techniques, advice on healthy eating, sleeping, recreation, and exercise regimes; (d) who to tell and what to say, especially in the first few days; and (e) the range of community support, advice, and information agencies which may be able to offer complementary practical and emotional assistance and advice in the short and long term.

4. *Behavioral/cognitive/brief analytic psychotherapeutic support:* This is useful either for individuals, families, or groups.[2,3,6,8–12,14,16,24,39–42] The question of which form of therapeutic intervention is the best for particular populations or issues remains

dogged by a lack of good outcome studies on treatment effectiveness.[7] Rarely, for example, have behavioral or cognitive approaches to managing HIV-related psychosocial and other difficulties systematically been evaluated. Nevertheless, anecdotal reports and increasingly frequent empirical reports[21,22] testify to the value of such interventions, particularly when emphasis is also placed on the management of practicalities arising from illness or the threat of it.[12] Such interventions may be short- or long-term, or perhaps simply episodic, depending on the patient's needs. Characteristically, psychotherapeutic support involving loved ones nominated by the patient will, after the acute presentation, be provided on a short-term basis as needs arise over time.[1,2,6,11]

Group-based interventions have proven therapeutic for people with HIV infection and disease and their loved ones.[1,12,41] Such groups can provide powerful and effective coping models (from "veteran" members), together with information updates on therapeutic advancements, social contacts, and, crucially, a regular opportunity to meet other people without the otherwise constant pressure of keeping secret one's health status. Such groups may also develop a "personal awareness" orientation in which attitudes towards lifestyle, sexuality, illness, and adjustments advised or made are consciously examined as a means of developing a perspective of personal mastery over infection or illness.

5. *Pharmacological interventions:* Any pharmacological prescriptions for those with HIV must be managed with extreme care. The potential for suicide has been mentioned: Take-home prescriptions of dangerous drugs should be in amounts that are insufficient to cause damage if taken all at once. Some persons with AIDS may have a reduced tolerance for side-effects of, for example, tricyclic and tetracyclic antidepressants at conventional psychotropic doses.[1,2,6] The mechanisms of this reduced tolerance remain largely unknown, although in some people it may be overcome by a slowly graduated dosage up to the therapeutic window.[43] The additional propensity of some antidepressants to induce leukopenia must also be borne in mind, with weekly or fortnightly white blood cell (WBC) counts recommended.

Considerable caution in the use of anxiolytics and hypnotics is also advised, in view of the respiratory depression associated with them, particularly in pulmonary infections such as *Pneumocystis carinii* pneumonia (PCP). Some patients may also present with preexisting benzodiazepine or other drug dependencies, placing the physician in a prescription dilemma. With both anxiolytic and antidepressant medication, it is also necessary to consider the possibility of exacerbating presenting conditions that may be due to underlying OMDs.[1] With such drugs, short-term empirical ameliorative intervention will often enable the patient to resume previous coping strategies more effectively.

Full discussions of the use of psychotropic medications, and rationales for them, are given elsewhere.[21,43] It is important, however, that the possibility of a reduced drug tolerance in this population is not used as an invitation to undertreat, when careful, appropriate management may produce very considerable benefits.[32,43]

6. *Referral to community and statutory out-patient services:* Voluntary peer-group agencies, where they are available, can help people with HIV in many ways: By providing models of coping behavior, peer support groups, "buddy" services, and other forms of home or financial help and guidance that lie beyond the scope of many statutory agencies. This is not to say that hospital/clinic involvement stops at the clinic door: Facilitation of psychosocial and medical needs requires a fine meshing of all potentially helpful resources. The provision of mental and physical health workers necessitates a continued,

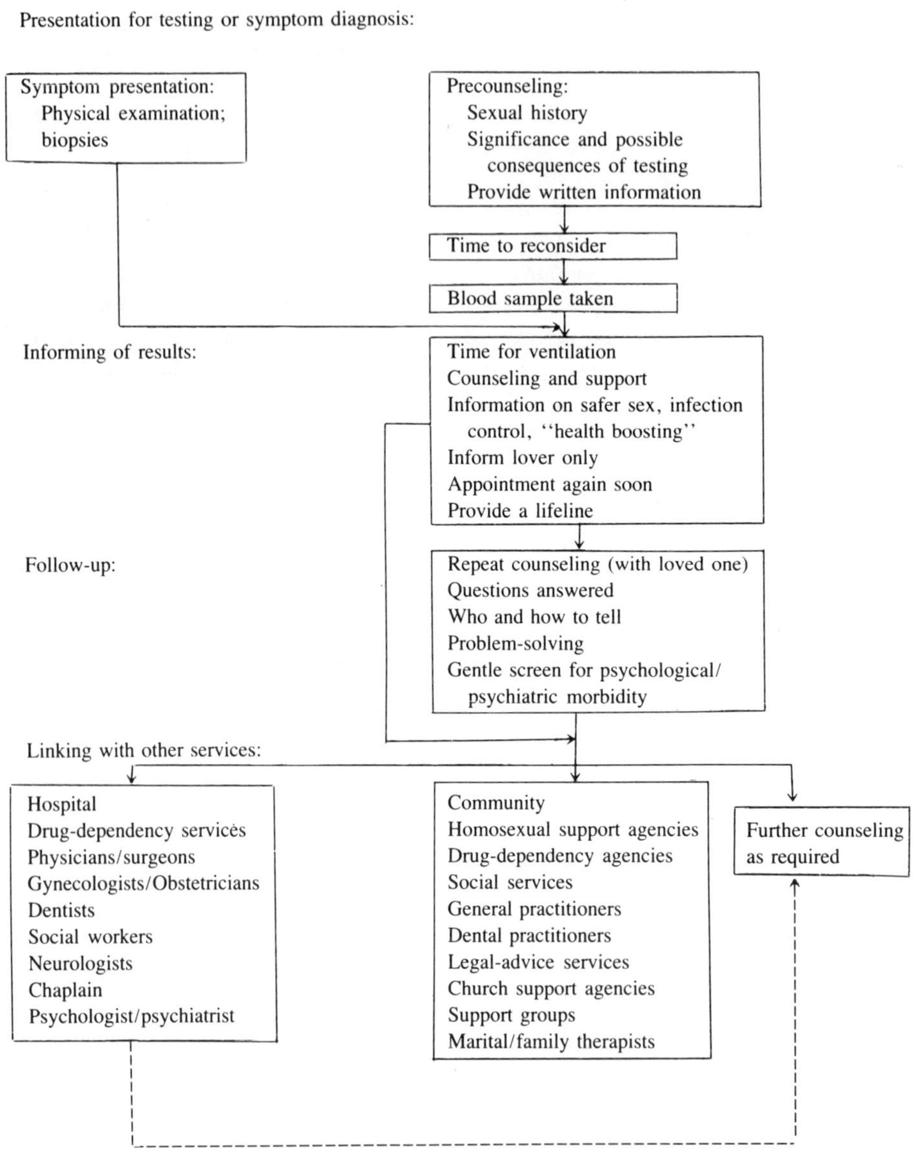

FIGURE 1. Structure for counseling and intervention.

TABLE 5. A Program to Meet Psychosocial Needs of HIV-Affected Persons[a]

Care of persons with HIV
Provison of in- and out-patient longitudinal care coordinated by a primary physician
Patient participation in all treatment and management decision-making, as they desire
Sensitive and hopeful provision of accurate medical information as fully as desired by the patient
Full provision of in- and out-patient medical, domestic and community care in coordination with the full range of community-based services, including peer-support voluntary services; all personnel to have an informed and sympathetic understanding of psychological, psychiatric, and psychosocial needs
Provision of information about measures to enhance personal control, quality of life and health, including safer sex, "health boosting," and lifestyle risk-reduction
Routine (informal) assessment for psychological/psychosocial distress and referral to appropriate professionals and services as required
Early accurate diagnosis of CNS disease, OMD, and functional psychiatric disorders and optimal medical treatment, individual/family/group supportive psychotherapy as desired and access as appropriate to experimental treatment
Care of loved-ones and close care-givers of HIV patients
Routine (informal) screening of needs for information, involvement in decision-making and management (at the discretion of the patient), and psychological/psychosocial support; appropriate service provision on an individual/group basis; provision of services for (post) bereavement support

[a] After Wolcott, Fawzy, and Pasnau (1985).

trusting liaison, both within and without the hospital, not least in order to preserve the confidentiality of the person with HIV. This is especially the case where pre-morbid psychological states are reactivated in the light of the HIV diagnosis, e.g., substance abuse. Such community and statutory services or agencies may be required repeatedly as new or old diseases emerge during the course of life with HIV. A plan for such provision is shown in Fig. 1.

Finally, a program outline designed to meet psychosocial and psychiatric needs of HIV-affected persons[6] is summarized in Table 5. This program incorporates necessary and desirable elements of longitudinal care relevant to all persons affected directly by HIV.

ASSESSMENT AND TREATMENT OF THOSE WITHOUT HIV INFECTION: THE WORRIED WELL

Perhaps one of the most conspicuous and clinically disruptive psychiatric disorders featuring concern about HIV in noninfected persons concerns the appearance of hypochondriasis. A number of recent reports[27,28,44,45] have described patients suffering the conviction that they have symptoms of HIV infection, despite remaining infection-free as verified by oft-repeated serological testing and clinical assessment. This group have been called the "worried well," and it is important to distinguish them from those persons who may present with anxieties about their possible exposure to, or symptoms of, HIV infection, but who are appropriately reassured that they do not have HIV infection after a discussion of their sexual/lifestyle history and negative clinical and/or antibody or antigen status. With the worried well, negative clinical and serological findings will usually be of very short-term benefit, and patients will return with the renewed conviction that the doctor has "got it wrong" or "missed something."

Some reports have used the term "AIDS phobia" to describe this clinical population, but this is misleading as it suggests diagnostic and therapeutic options of little direct use to this patient group.[28] However, it should also be noted that the term "worried well" is not of diagnostic utility. Rather, it specifies a spectrum of consistently seen presenting and background phenomena to which diagnostic and therefore treatment decisions can appropriately be applied.

Presenting Phenomenology

Striking consistencies have been found in the presentations within this patient group. Such consistencies have allowed reliable markers of vulnerability to be specified, and include:

1. Often multiple somatic symptoms misinterpreted by the patient as "clear evidence" of HIV infection or disease, such as sweating, swollen glands, skin rashes and blotches, gastrointestinal upsets with associated, clinically insignificant, loss of weight, muscle aches and pains, shortness of breath, dizziness, mouth ulcers, sore throats, and fatigue. Such symptom constellations usually match expected sequallae of chronic, high-level anxiety.
2. Often chronic, high-level anxiety, producing the physical disturbances described above, and often associated with panic attacks. Panic attacks can be sparked off by media reports of HIV/AIDS, or by intrusive thoughts about the subject.
3. Obsessive ruminations about having HIV or AIDS, about physical decline, and having "passed" the infection to loved-ones, children. Such thoughts may be associated with compulsive rituals such as checking of body areas for signs of emerging HIV disease, palpating bodily areas, repeatedly washing potential sources of infection, and repeated demands on physicians and health workers for clinical examinations and reassurance.
4. Depression is frequently a primary feature, although it may be unclear whether depression preceded the obsessive disorder or followed it. Reported depression may follow due to the doctor's apparent inability to diagnose their HIV disease, or because of the "inevitability" of decline, and the impact of their supposed infection/disease on loved-ones.
5. Many patients present as a risk for suicide, often with suicide being cited as "the only way out" from the tremendous guilt and stress associated with the commonly help belief that they have AIDS, and that they have passed it on to those they love. Related to this is a significant degree of substance abuse, typically alcohol or prescribed drugs, used to help with sleep or anxiety.

Background Features

Patients in the worried well group also have striking consistencies in their background features. In a recent series of 19 persons,[28] most were found to have a history of difficulties in postadolescent sexual adjustment, leading to a low-risk adult sexual history usually involving covert and guilt-producing sexual expression (especially if sex occurred outside of a "marriage," for example, or involved undisclosed homosexuality or bisexuality). The frequently covert and guilt-producing sexual expression coincided with a fear of all sexually transmitted disease (venereophobia), and so was usually of a very-low-risk nature and would subsequently lead to a high level of "bargaining" about future sexual expressions ("If you can only prove I don't have AIDS, I will be so relieved—I promise I will never be unfaithful again . . .").

A further consistency in patients' backgrounds is the significant incidence of previous psychiatric or psychological morbidity requiring formal intervention. In the series referred to, 53% have a previously diagnosed psychiatric problem, such as depression, eating disorders, or anxiety.[28] This group also features high levels of dependency where established domestic relationships exist, and where they do not, patients had a significant level of social isolation along with difficulties in making friends or maintaining personal relationships.

Intervention

Optimal treatment of the worried well depends on the primary diagnosis. For example, where the primary diagnosis is one of chronic depression, treatment of the depression may lift the symptoms effectively. In other cases, the primary diagnosis is one of hypochondriasis, featuring an underlay of morbid health preoccupations which are "rational" consequences of obsessional thoughts. People in this category have been successfully treated by tackling a central presenting feature which frequently obstructs any prospect of long-term benefit—reassurance. This approach posits that reassurance distracts the patient and the physician from the underlying anxiety-provoking issues responsible for their vulnerability. Where reassurance has been a prominent feature of intervention, beneficial effects are relatively short-term. Therefore, within the context of a strictly defined behavioral contract, the following intervention is made[28]:

1. Prevention of reassurance, as reassurance helps the patient avoid the real problems
2. Offer correct explanations for somatic problems and symptoms, and limit discussion of symptoms to the very end of each session
3. Work to change thoughts and attributions regarding the causes of somatic and cognitive difficulties
4. Change behaviors, away from constant checking and demands for reassurance, to nonchecking of bodily 'symptoms' and nonattentiveness to somatic changes and sensations. Patients must be offered alternative activities to distract them from their previous anxiety-maintaining habits.

This must be a collaborative process between patient and therapist, especially where symptoms and etiological issues are being reinterpreted. Although presenting symptoms may resolve within a few sessions by such an approach,[28] it is important to recognize the need to offer follow-up discussion to such patients, especially where unresolved conflicts over sexuality and other life issues may possibly generate future vulnerability without adequate intervention. It is also important to recognize the team-centered approach that this group necessitates, especially where late identification of suicidal intent may require psychiatric admission. A checklist of presenting and background features in the worried well is presented in Table 6.

TABLE 6. Checklist of Presenting and Background Features in the Worried Well

Presenting features
Acute, high-level anxiety with multiple, anxiety-related somatic features
Intervention-resistant ideas/beliefs that such symptoms are related to HIV infection
Frustration and depression at the inability of doctors to successfully "diagnose" HIV infection and disease
Repeated dwelling on thoughts/images of HIV infection, disease, and decay
Prominent fears that infection has been passed on to loved-ones, children
Obsessive–compulsive features, including bodily checking, washing, and/or repeated questioning of health staff
Conspicuous guilt over sexual and/or lifestyle activities seen as leading to "infection"
Expressed or covert suicidal ideation/planning, sometimes with a history of unsuccessful attempts
Background features
History of covert and usually low-risk sexual expression, in the context of guilt, stress, and "venereophobia"
Poor post-adolescent sexual adjustment
Previous psychiatric/psychological history (e.g., depression, eating disorders), or high level of physician attendance
Often multiple negative HIV test results
High dependency in close relationships and poor social networking

CONCLUSION

This chapter has considered a range of psychological phenomena associated with HIV infection and disease, particularly shortly after an HIV-related diagnosis. Meeting the clinical challenge of such phenomena requires a multi-level and multi-disciplinary approach, incorporating hospital, clinic, and community statutory and voluntary agencies. Planning and maintaining such resources entails a recognition of the escalating demands that increased expertise brings, both on the service and its providers. So much psychological dysfunction rests on an absence of confidence. In many ways, it is our job as clinicians to transfer our diagnostic and management confidence to the patient so they may learn to master the appalling uncertainty associated with the continuing emergence of clinical disease. In HIV/AIDS, our patients remain our teachers, giving us the inspiration and confidence to understand more. Our combined efforts signify our recognition of that debt.

REFERENCES

1. Wolcott DL: Psychosocial aspects of acquired immune deficiency syndrome and the primary care physician. *Ann Allergy* 57:95–102, 1986.
2. Miller D: Psychology, AIDS, ARC and PGL, in Miller D, Weber J, Green J (eds): *The Management of AIDS Patients*. London, Macmillan Press, 1986, p 131.
3. Christ GH, Weiner LS: Psychosocial issues in AIDS, in DeVita VT, Hellman S, Rosenberg SA (eds): *AIDS: Etiology, Diagnosis, Treatment and Prevention*. Philadelphia, JB Lippincott, 1985, p 275.
4. Kelly JA, Saint Lawrence JS, Hood HV, et al: Nurses' attitudes towards AIDS. J Contin Ed Nurs 19:78–83, 1988.
5. Gordin FM, Willoughby AD, Levine LA: Knowledge of AIDS among hospital workers: Behavioral correlates and consequences. AIDS 1:183–188, 1987.
6. Wolcott DL, Fawzy FI, Pasnau RO: Acquired immune deficiency syndrome (AIDS) and consultation–liaison psychiatry. *Gen Hosp Psychiatry* 7:280–292, 1985.

7. Carballo M, Miller D: HIV counselling: Problems and opportunities in defining the new agenda for the 1990s. *AIDS Care* 1:117–123, 1989.
8. Dilley JW, Ochitill HN, Perl M, et al: Findings in psychiatric consultations with patients with acquired immune deficiency syndrome. *Am J Psychiatry* 142:82–86, 1985.
9. Morin SF, Charles KA, Malyon AK: The psychological impact of AIDS. *Am Psychol* 39:1288–1292, 1984.
10. Nichols SE, Ostrow DG: *Psychiatric Implications of Acquired Immune Deficiency Syndrome.* Washington DC, American Psychiatric Press, 1984.
11. Nichols SE: An overview of the psychological and social reactions to AIDS, in Gluckman JC, Vilmer E (eds): *Acquired Immunodeficiency Syndrome: International Conference on AIDS, Paris, 23–25 June, 1986.* Paris, Elsevier, p 261.
12. Miller D: *Living With AIDS and HIV.* Basingstoke, Macmillan Press, 1987.
13. Piot P, Plummer FA, Mhalu FS, et al: AIDS: an international perspective. *Science* 239:573–579, 1988.
14. Carnwath T, Miller D: *Behavioural Psychotherapy in Primary Care: A Practice Manual.* London, Academic Press, 1986.
15. Cooper DA, Gold J, Maclean P, et al: Acute AIDS retrovirus infection; definition of a clinical illness associated with seroconversion. *Lancet* 1:537–540, 1985.
16. Miller D, Green J: Counselling for HIV infection and AIDS, in Pinching AJ (ed): *Clinics in Immunology and Allergy,* Vol. 6, (3): *AIDS and HIV Infection.* London, WB Saunders, 1986, p 661.
17. Miller D, Pinching AJ: HIV tests and counselling: Current issues. *AIDS* 3 (suppl 1):S187–S193, 1989.
18. Fischl MA: State of antiretroviral therapy with zidovudine. *AIDS* 3 (suppl 1):S137–S143, 1989.
19. Temoshok L, Mandel JS, Moulton JM, et al: A longitudinal psychosocial study of AIDS and ARC in San Francisco: Preliminary results, in *Annual Meeting of American Psychiatric Association, Washington DC, May 13, 1986.*
20. Tross S, Holland J, Hirsch D, et al: Psychological and social impact of AIDS spectrum disorders, in *International Conference on AIDS, Paris, June 23–25, 1986.*
21. Maj M: Psychiatric and mental health aspects of HIV infection and AIDS. *Psychol Med.* In press.
22. World Health Organization: *Report of the Consultation on the Neuropsychiatric Aspects of HIV Infection,* Geneva, 14–17 March, 1988.
23. Deuchar N: AIDS in New York City with particular reference to the psycho-social aspects. *Br J Psychiatry* 145:612–619, 1984.
24. Miller D: Psychosocial problems associated with HIV infection and disease, in Miller D, Weber J, Green J (eds): *The Management of AIDS Patients,* ed 2. London, Macmillan Press, in press.
25. Zich J, Temoshok L: Perceptions of social support in patients with ARC and AIDS. *J Appl Soc Psychol* 17(3):193–215, 1987.
26. Atkinson JH, Grant, I, Kennedy CJ, et al: Prevalence of psychiatric disorders among men infected with human immunodeficiency virus. *Arch Gen Psychiat* 45:859–864, 1988.
27. Miller D: The worried well: Phenomenology, predictors of psychological vulnerability and suggestions for management, in Temoshok L, Baum A (eds): *Psychological Perspectives on AIDS: Etiology, Prevention and Treatment.* New York, Lawrence Erlbaum, in press.
28. Miller D, Acton TMG, Hedge B: The worried well: Identification and management. *J Roy Coll Phys Lond* 22(3):158–165, 1988.
29. Holland J, Tross S: The psychosocial and neuropsychiatric sequelae of the immunodeficiency syndrome and related disorders. *Ann Intern Med* 103:760–764, 1985.
30. DesJarlais DC, Friedman SR: HIV infection among intravenous drug users: Epidemiology and risk reduction. *AIDS* 1(2):67–76, 1987.
31. Namir S, Wolcott DL, Fawzy FI, Alumbaugh MJ: Coping with AIDS: Psychological and health implications. *J Appl Soc Psychol* 17(3):309–328, 1987.
32. Miller D, Riccio M: Functional psychiatric syndromes associated with HIV1 infection and disease. Submitted for publication, 1990.
33. Miller, D, Jeffries DJ, Green J, et al: HTLV-III: Should testing ever be routine? *Br Med J* 292:941–943, 1986.
34. Marzuk PM, Tierney H, Tardiff K, et al: Increased risk of suicide in persons with AIDS. *JAMA* 259(9):1333–1337, 1988.
35. Rundell J, Thomason R, Zajac D, et al: Psychiatric diagnosis and attempted suicide (AS) in HIV infected USAF personnel. Paper presented at the *Fourth International Conference on AIDS,* Stockholm, 12–16 June, 1988.

36. Gala C, Merkin S, Pergeuni A, et al: Psychiatric history among homosexuals and drug addicts infected with HIV. Poster presented at the *Fifth International Conference on AIDS,* Montreal, 4–9 June, 1989.
37. Engelman J, Hessol NA, Lifson AR, et al: Suicide patterns and AIDS in San Francisco. Paper presented at the *Fourth International Conference on AIDS,* Stockholm, 12–16 June, 1988.
38. Halstead S, Riccio M, Harlow P, et al: Psychosis associated with HIV infection. *Br J Psychiat* 153:618–623, 1988.
39. Church J, Kocsis AE, Green J: Effects on lovers of caring for HIV infected individuals related to perceptions of cognitive, behavioral and personality changes. Paper presented at the *Fourth International Conference on AIDS,* Stockholm, 13–16 June, 1988.
40. Green J, McCreaner A (eds): *Counselling in HIV Infection and AIDS.* Oxford, Blackwell Scientific, 1988.
41. Miller, R, Bor R: *AIDS: A Guide to Clinical Counseling.* London, Science Press, 1988.
42. Jacoby-Klein S, Fletcher W (III): Gay grief: An examination of its uniqueness brought to light by the AIDS crisis. *J Psychosoc Oncol* 4(3):15–25, 1986.
43. Schmidt U, Miller D, Ikkos G, et al: Dilemmas in psychiatric management of HIV infection and disease, in Miller D, Weber J, Green J (eds): *The Management of AIDS Patients, 2nd ed.* Basingstoke, Macmillan Press, in press.
44. Miller D: Predictors of chronic psychosocial disturbance arising from the threat of HIV infection: Lessons from heterosexual, bisexual and homosexual worried well patients. Poster presented at the *Third International Conference on AIDS,* Washington D.C., 1–6 June, 1987.
45. Jager H, Hualla T: AIDS phobia: Irrational and pathologic anxiety in HIV seronegative persons. Poster presented at the *Fourth International Conference on Aids,* Stockholm, 12–16 June, 1988.

11

Diagnosis and Treatment of Neurologic Disorders in AIDS and Other Sexually Transmitted Diseases

JUSTIN C. McARTHUR, JAMES ASHE, and DOUGLAS JABS

INTRODUCTION

This chapter provides an overview of the range of neurological problems that may develop in association with AIDS and other sexually transmitted diseases. The first section is devoted primarily to those occurring in acquired immune deficiency syndrome (AIDS), excluding the AIDS dementia complex. The second section is devoted to the diagnosis and treatment of neurological problems associated with other sexually transmitted diseases.

DIAGNOSIS AND TREATMENT OF NEUROLOGICAL PROBLEMS ASSOCIATED WITH AIDS

It has become clear over the past 2 or 3 years that the human immunodeficiency virus (HIV) has neurotropic properties and that nervous system invasion may occur at an early stage of infection.[1] Current estimates predict that up to 70% of patients with AIDS will develop clinical signs of the AIDS dementia complex (ADC), and fully 90% of these individuals may show pathological evidence of subacute encephalitis at autopsy.[2,3] While it is clear that ADC is the most frequent single neurological complication of AIDS, other important disorders are discussed in this section. Recognition of these disorders in patients with HIV infection is critical for several reasons: (1) they are potentially treatable if timely diagnosis is made, (2) they may occur concurrently with ADC and complicate the man-

JUSTIN C. McARTHUR and JAMES ASHE • Department of Neurology, The Johns Hopkins University School of Medicine, Baltimore, Maryland 21205. DOUGLAS JABS • Department of Ophthalmology, The Johns Hopkins University School of Medicine, Baltimore, Maryland 21205.

TABLE 1. Neurological Disorders in AIDS

Disorder	Prevalence in AIDS (%)	Treatment
Central nervous system		
AIDS dementia complex	20–70	Symptomatic
HIV-related meningitis	5–10	Symptomatic
Cryptococcal meningitis	10	Amphotericin B or Fluconazole
Progressive multifocal leukoencephalopathy	2	None
Other fungal infections	1–2	Amphotericin B or Fluconazole
Tuberculous meningitis	<2	Appropriate Rx
Bacterial meningitis	<2	Appropriate Rx
Neurosyphilis	Rare	Appropriate Rx
AIDS related myelopathies	20[a]	Symptomatic
Herpes simplex encephalitis	~2	Acyclovir
CMV encephalitis	<1	DHPG[b] (Ganciclovir)
CMV retinitis	5–20	DHPG
Cerebral toxoplasmosis	10	Pyrimethamine + sulfadiazine
Peripheral nervous system		
CMV radiculitis	Rare	DHPG (Ganciclovir)
Herpes zoster radiculitis	3	Acyclovir
AIDS-related neuropathies	30[a]	Symptomatic, plasmapheresis

[a] Prevalence unknown; etiology speculative.
[b] 9-(1,3-Dihydroxy-2-propoxymethyl)guanine.

agement of this entity, (3) the disorders can mimic ADC and lead to an inaccurate diagnosis of ADC with delay in appropriate therapy, and (4) some of the conditions may occur during the earlier stages of HIV infection and may therefore be indicators for the subsequent development of AIDS. Table 1 summarizes the prevalence and possibilities for treatment of these disorders.

HIV-Related Meningitis

Clinical Features

An acute febrile syndrome, with myalgias, arthralgias, and rash, not unlike infectious mononucleosis, develops in a proportion of individuals within days or weeks of the primary exposure to HIV, representing the initial response to the virus.[4] Meningitis is recognized in perhaps 5–10% of patients with HIV infection, usually developing in the early stages of disease and predating ARC or full-blown AIDS.[5] In some individuals, meningitis occurs at the time of seroconversion, apparently indicating that nervous system involvement can be an early manifestation of HIV infection. Although only a small fraction of infected individuals develop symptoms of meningitis, it may be subclinical and therefore unrecognized in some. The clinical features of HRM include fever, meningismus, headache, and cranial neuropathies, most frequently involving cranial nerve VII and mimicking idiopathic facial palsy (Bell's palsy) (Fig. 1). Rarely an acute encepha-

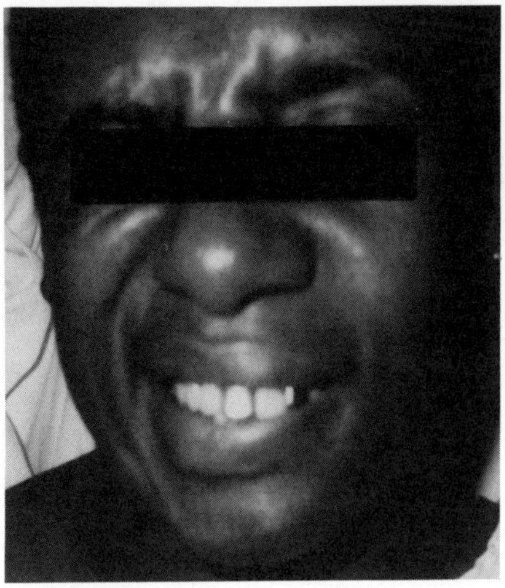

FIGURE 1. Cranial neuropathy. This 30-year-old homosexual man was HIV-seropositive but asymptomatic until a transient left facial weakness developed in association with a mild CSF pleocytosis.

lopathy can occur, and in one patient who was profoundly encephalopathic, the encephalogram (EEG) showed loss of normal activity, slow activity and repetitive slow-wave complexes compatible with a viral encephalitis.[6]

Diagnosis

The diagnosis can be established by lumbar puncture. A predominantly mononuclear cerebrospinal fluid (CSF) pleocytosis with 10–300 WBC/mm^3 is seen and the CSF protein may be elevated. In our experience, the CSF pleocytosis may persist for several months or longer even after symptoms have receded. In an ongoing prospective study of homosexual men with seroconversion, 2 of 8 (25%) asymptomatic individuals had a CSF pleocytosis and 3 of 7 (43%) had HIV isolated from CSF by culture techniques.[7] Other investigators have also isolated HIV by culture from the CSF.[5] Specific HIV antibodies and p24 antigen may appear in the CSF of patients with HRM.[8] The distribution of CSF T-cell subclasses in HRM differs from other acute meningoencephalitides. Specifically, CD4 (helper/inducer) cells are reduced and CD8 increased, resulting in an inversion of the CD4 : CD8 ratio.[9] Typically neither CT nor MRI is abnormal, although they may be helpful in excluding cerebral toxoplasmosis, CNS lymphoma, or herpes simplex encephalitis, conditions which might be confused with HRM. In these disorders areas of focal abnormality should be demonstrable. Other diagnostic considerations include neurosyphilis and fungal or lymphomatous meningitis. CSF cytology, cryptococcal antigen, fungal culture, and VDRL should therefore be performed in all patients with suspected HRM. If available, HIV isolation should be attempted, or CSF frozen for testing for HIV antibody or antigen.

Treatment

In most individuals, treatment is only symptomatic, with analgesics/antipyretics. The symptomatic phase usually lasts no longer than a few weeks at most. In patients with cranial neuropathies and facial weakness who have inadequate eye closure, corneal protection with artificial tears and eye patching is important.

Implications

Because HIV-related meningitis probably reflects the initial invasion of the central nervous system by HIV,[10] recognition of the syndrome has implications for staging the extent of HIV infection. It is not yet clear, however, whether the occurrence of HRM is predictive of the later development of the AIDS dementia complex. Prospective neuropsychological studies are underway under the auspices of the Multicenter AIDS Cohort Study (MACS) to follow homosexual men at risk for the development of AIDS. The significance of the early CNS invasion with HIV is that the blood–brain barrier may segregate virus from systemic antiviral medications and create a persistent unchecked reservoir of infection. To effectively block viral replication, therefore, antiviral drugs must adequately penetrate the brain parenchyma. An example exists with the treatment of syphilis. Meningitis is also seen in 25% of cases of secondary syphilis and incomplete or inadequate penicillin therapy may produce clearance of systemic infection but fail to sterilize the brain adequately. This allows persistence of the latent neural infection and a delayed development of active neurosyphilis: meningovascular syphilis, general paresis, or tabes dorsalis. Applying this paradigm to AIDS, the use of antivirals with inadequate brain penetrance might permit continued replication of HIV within the nervous system despite systemic clearance.[10] Meningitis may also occur in other retrovirus infections. For example, visna virus, which is both morphologically and genomically similar to HIV, is associated with a subclinical meningitis in experimentally infected animals.[11]

AIDS-Related Myelopathies

There are increasing numbers of reports of myelopathies associated with HIV infection; however, neither the breadth of clinical manifestations nor the full spectrum of pathological changes has been well characterized (Table 2). Some of the clinicopathologic presentations may reflect the direct effect of HIV infection. Others may result from the immune disturbance permitting infection with agents like the herpes group of viruses.

Diagnostic and therapeutic strategies are as yet limited in the AIDS related myelopathies. First, clinical syndromes have not yet been well defined. Second, they often occur in association with other neurological manifestations such as peripheral neuropathy and/or

TABLE 2. AIDS-Related Neuropathies and Myelopathies

Neuropathies	Myelopathies
Painful sensory	Vacuolar myelopathy
Inflammatory demyelinating	Gracile tract degeneration
Cranial	Herpes group myelitis
Multiple mononeuropathy	Other retroviruses
Herpes group radiculitis	Nutritional deficiencies
Nutritional deficiencies	Toxic
Compression	
Toxic	

AIDS dementia complex. Other CNS opportunistic infections are also frequent concurrent events. Third, the spinal cord is relatively inaccessible and difficult to evaluate or image. However, even with these caveats, it may be possible to recognize distinct clinical syndromes.

Vacuolar Myelopathy

This manifests with progressive spastic paraparesis and loss of proprioception in the legs with relative sparing of the upper extremities, and is often accompanied by AIDS dementia complex. Spinal cord involvement of this type has been identified in 20% of a sample of patients with AIDS dying in New York City and New Jersey.[12] Clinical manifestations in that group included spastic paraparesis and sensory ataxia and in 14/20 of the cases there was an associated dementia. The pathological features included a noninflammatory vacuolation (spongy change) in the spinal white matter, particularly in the lateral and posterior columns of the thoracic spinal cord. The changes were similar to those that occur with vitamin B_{12} deficiency (subacute combined degeneration) and the authors postulated that nutritional or metabolic factors might have been important. It was also speculated that primary HIV infection might have played an etiologic role as immunohistochemical stains for herpes group viruses and for *T. gondii* were negative in seven of the spinal cords examined. In another series, one patient with AIDS with a progressive spastic paraparesis showed similar pathological features including vacuolar degeneration of the lumbar cord.[5] HIV was isolated from the CSF before death and directly from the spinal cord at autopsy.

Other investigators have described similar pathological changes[13,14] and some have commented on the possibility of neurotoxicity related to the use of sulfonamides for treatment of P. carinii pneumonia.[14] The etiology of the vacuolar myelopathy associated with AIDS remains conjectural, and whether this entity is a direct effect of HIV alone, or involved interaction with other viruses or nutritional/toxic factors remains to be uncovered.

Gracile Tract Degeneration

The clinical counterparts of this newly described pathological syndrome include painful paresthesias and dysesthesias in the feet and lower extremities. There is only minimal weakness. The disorder progresses in parallel with AIDS dementia and is accompanied by selective degeneration of the gracile tract in the posterior columns. It is discussed in detail in the peripheral neuropathy section. In four patients with AIDS who developed painful dysesthesias and paresthesias in the feet, a discrete degeneration localized to the gracile tract of the posterior columns was found at autopsy.[15] While the etiology of this syndrome remains speculative as with vacuolar myelopathy, direct infection of dorsal root ganglion cells by HIV could lead to a "dying-back" process within centrally and peripherally directed axons.[16]

Other Viral Infections

Other infectious agents, typically viruses, may also produce spinal cord damage in the setting of the immunoincompetency caused by HIV infection. For example, there are scattered reports of myelopathies produced by herpes simplex and cytomegalovirus.[17–19] Occasionally myelitis can develop months after shingles, and may reflect either reactivation of herpes zoster within the cord or vasculitis within the blood vessels supplying the cord (personal observation).

Human retroviruses other than HIV have been implicated in the development of myelopathies. For example, antibodies to HTLV-I were present in a high proportion of patients (59%) with tropical spastic paraparesis (TSP), a progressive myelopathy occurring both endemically and epidemically in many tropical areas.[20] A variety of nutritional factors, both toxic and deficiency conditions have been associated with the development of epidemic forms of TSP, however, it now seems plausible that HTLV-I may be a causative factor for endemic TSP. HTLV-I has also been linked to the development of spastic paraparesis in nontropical areas.[21] HTLV-I has now been isolated by culture from the CSF of a patient with a progressive myelopathy in Japan, however, it remains to definitively identify HTLV-I within the spinal cord. In a sample of intravenous drug users from New York City 9% had evidence of HTLV-I antibodies and 41% were HIV seropositive.[22] Concurrent infection with both HTLV-I and HIV may also be common among homosexually active men. Some of the neurological disorders described with AIDS may thus result from HTLV-I infection either acting as a primary pathogen, or a copathogen with HIV. Active research is under way into the potential pathogenic roles of human retroviruses in neurological disorders.[23]

Diagnosis

A patient presently with progressive spinal cord dysfunction must be adequately evaluated to exclude spinal cord compression from degenerative bony disease, disc protrusion, or epidural lymphomatous deposits. Most patients with cord compression will have back pain and a sensory level; in this situation, careful consideration for myelography and/or spine CT must be given. MRI has become a useful tool for ruling out structural lesions, and as experience with the technique grows it may eventually supplant myelography.

Examination of the spinal fluid in patients with vacuolar myelopathy or gracile tract degeneration may show a mild pleocytosis and slightly elevated protein. HIV has been isolated from the CSF of patients with vacuolar myelopathy.[5] With herpes group infections the virus can sometimes be isolated from the CSF and CSF serologies may be helpful. There is as yet relatively little information about electrophysiological studies such as somatosensory evoked potentials (SSEPs), that one might expect to be a sensitive tool for detecting ascending sensory tract dysfunction. SSEPs have been examined in asymptomatic HIV-positive men, and found to be abnormal.[24] This preliminary report implies that spinal cord dysfunction may in fact occur relatively early and antedate other neurological symptoms and full-blown AIDS. Myelography and spine CT are usually normal with these AIDS-related myelopathies. As MRI techniques become more sophisticated, particularly with the use of high Tesla strength devices, changes within individual fiber tracts within the spinal cord may be identifiable.

Treatment

A detailed prospective study is under way in Baltimore and Chicago to delineate the clinical characteristics of the various myelopathic syndromes occurring in the setting of

HIV infection. However, besides eliminating nutritional deficiencies, such as vitamin B_{12} and E deficiency, treatment is symptomatic. For example, spasticity may respond to antispasticity agents, baclofen (Lioresal) or valium (Diazepam). Paresthesias and dysesthesias may similarly be alleviated by careful use of tricyclic antidepressants or carbamazepine (Tegretol) (see section on painful sensory neuropathy).

AIDS-Related Peripheral Nerve Disorders

As with the AIDS-related myelopathies, involvement of the peripheral nervous system may occur in diverse ways (see Table 2). Not only do discrete clinical syndromes exist, but the basic pathogenic mechanisms differ for the various neuropathic disorders, suggesting important therapeutic implications.

Painful Sensory Neuropathy

Painful sensory neuropathy (PSN) is a clinical syndrome that may overlap with gracile tract degeneration, since a proportion of cases with PSN will demonstrate this pathological feature (see previous section: AIDS-related myelopathies). Painful acral dysesthesias and paresthesias are common symptoms occurring in up to 30% of patients with AIDS. This has been termed painful sensory neuropathy (PSN) or distal symmetrical sensory neuropathy. Snider et al. (1983) reviewed the neurologic complications in 50 AIDS patients and reported 8 with PSN.[25] This manifestation appears to be distinguishable from one other type of described neuropathy, an inflammatory demyelinating polyneuropathy (IDP). PSN typically occurs later in the course of infection with HIV, usually in association with profound immunoincompetency and multiple opportunistic infections (Table 3). Electrophysiologic studies have revealed evidence of distal axonal degeneration with secondary demyelination or loss of large myelinated fibers.[26]

As has been discussed above, there is speculation that PSN may reflect direct infection of dorsal root ganglia neurons by HIV and possibly other retroviruses. Nutritional and toxic factors may also be of importance in its production, as similar features can occur in diverse nutritional deficiencies in man[27] or experimentally in animals.[28] Most of the patients who develop this complication are wasted and malnourished and have been treated with multiple antimicrobials. However, comparison of patients with painful sensory neuropathy and a group of 23 patients without PSN dying with AIDS showed no discernible differences in diet, weight, or nutritional status.[15]

Treatment. Pain-modifying agents such as amitriptyline (Elavil) 10–25 mg qhs or carbamazepine (Tegretol) 100–200 mg bid may provide some relief. Careful increases in dosage can be made, but many of these patients develop AIDS dementia concurrently and are therefore highly susceptible to delirium provoked by these psychoactive drugs. Blood counts and liver function tests should be monitored regularly in patients receiving carbamazepine. Vitamin B-group supplements should be used and mechanical irritation from bed sheets limited by use of bed cradles. In bed-bound patients care should be taken to avoid compressive neuropathies and skin ulcers. A recent preliminary report of 3 patients with AIDS dementia and peripheral neuropathy treated with azidothymidine (AZT) suggested an improvement in both clinical and electrophysiological parameters of the neuropathy.[29] Larger-scale studies are underway with AZT and other antiviral agents.

TABLE 3. Clinical and Pathological Features of AIDS-Related Neuropathies

	Painful sensory	Inflammatory demyelinating
Prevalence	30%	<1%
Onset	Late: full-blown AIDS	Early: asymptomatic seropositive
Symptoms	Pedal paresthesias, dysesthesias, "burning feet"	Weakness, sometimes acute GBS[a] or CIDP[b]
Signs	Abnormal vibratory sensation, hyperpathia, bsent ankle reflexes, accompanying AIDS dementia	Weakness, areflexia, Later wasting
NCV/EMG	Axonal degeneration, secondary demyelination	Marked slowing compatible with primary demyelination
CSF	Protein: 40–60 mg/dl Cells: 5–10 WBC/mm^3	Protein: 50–200 mg/dl Cells: 10–40 WBC/mm^3
Pathology	Dying-back axonopathy (gracile tract degeneration)	Internodal demyelination Macrophage infiltration
Pathogenesis	HIV infection of dorsal root ganglia neurons? Nutritional/toxic factors?	Immunopathogenic
Prognosis	Poor—usually develops in preterminal stages of AIDS	Good—not necessarily predictive of poor outcome
Treatment	Symptomatic	Plasmapheresis (steroids)

[a]GBS, Guillain Barré syndrome.
[b]CIDP, chronic inflammatory demyelinating neuropathy.

Inflammatory Demyelinating Polyneuropathies

A number of possibly immune phenomena have been described in association with HIV infection, including inflammatory demyelinating polyneuropathies (IDP)[26] and thrombocytopenia.[30] Both occur at relatively early stages of HIV infection, before profound immunoincompetency, and probably result from immunopathogenic mechanisms rather than direct viral infection.[26,31]

Our group and others[32,33] have identified patients with HIV infection who develop inflammatory demyelinating polyneuropathies, disorders which are considered to be immunopathogenic (see Table 3). In our patients, neurological symptoms antedated the development of constitutional symptoms and ARC, and with a median follow-up period of 20 months, only one of eight reported patients had developed AIDS. Their neuropathic presentations took two forms, either an acute demyelinating neuropathy (Guillain-Barré syndrome) or a more chronic course with predominantly motor weakness, chronic inflammatory demyelinating neuropathy (CIDP).[26] There were CSF changes that distinguished this group of patients from HIV-seronegative patients with IDP including the presence of a CSF pleocytosis (mean 23 WBC mm^3). This contrasts to a mean of 1.8 WBC mm^3 in a group of HIV-seronegative patients with inflammatory demyelinating neuropathies.[34] CSF ratios of T-helper (T4) and T-suppressor (T8) lymphocytes were inverted, in contradistinction to patients with IDP not associated with HIV infection.[9] The CSF total protein was usually markedly elevated (mean 178 mg/dl). Electrophysiologic studies were usually indicative of primary demyelination with profound slowing of nerve conduction velocities. With time, secondary axonal loss with evidence of denervation may develop.

Nerve biopsies performed in five disclosed mononuclear–macrophage infiltration and internodal demyelination—typical of inflammatory demyelinating polyneuropathy. Most patients recovered either spontaneously or with corticosteroids or plasmapheresis.

The pathogenesis of the demyelinating process is unclear even though circulating antiperipheral nerve antibodies have been preliminarily identified in some patients.[35] These may represent an epiphenomenon rather than the primary cause of the neuropathy, since they appear to be present only in low concentrations and stain the axon rather than the myelin sheath.

The significance of recognition of this potentially immunopathic disorder is, first, that infection with HIV (and possibly co-viruses) may disturb the host immune system in such a way as to trigger autoimmune phenomena. Second, the development of IDP is not necessarily predictive of a worse outcome than in patients without IDP, in fact the rate of progression to AIDS is comparable to that of patients without IDP. Third, plasmapheresis can generally be safely used and appears to be effective although controlled trials have not been performed. Fourth, the materials that come into contact with the bloodstream during pheresis are disposable, and thus there should be no chance of transmission of HIV by subsequent phereses in other patients provided that adequate precautions are followed.

Treatment. On the premise that immunopathic mechanisms cause IDPs, a variety of immunomodulatory therapies have been tried (Tables 3 and 4). Our group's experience suggests that corticosteroids or plasmapheresis may be effective, if the neurological illness is sufficiently severe to require treatment. Corticosteroids are likely to suppress cell-mediated immunity further and thus plasmapheresis is the preferred initial therapy. In patients with acute IDPs, 5 plasmaphereses are performed, usually within the first 10 days

TABLE 4. Diagnostic Approach to Patient with Suspected Neuropathy

Workup	Diagnostic study	Implication
Blood studies	Vitamin B_{12}, vitamin E	Replacement therapy
	VDRL	Appropriate antibiotics
	Thyroid studies	Replacement therapy
	CD4 (T helper) count	Degree of immunosuppression
	Serology HIV, HTLV-I	Serostatus
CSF studies	Cells	10–50 WBC/mm^3 with IDP
	Total protein	50–200 mg/dl with IDP
	VDRL	+ with neurosyphilis
	Oligoclonal bands	Intrathecal antibody synthesis
	IgG index	
	Myelin basic protein	Myelin breakdown in CNS
	HIV culture	+ with PSN and AIDS dementia
	Other viral cultures	CMV, herpes simplex, zoster
Electrodiagnostics	NCV	Marked slowing with IDP
	EMG	Axonal degeneration with PSN
	SSEPs	Posterior column dysfunction
Nerve biopsy	Microscopy	Internodal demyelination, macrophage infiltration with IDP, dying-back axonopathy with PSN
	HIV culture	Unknown utility

of hospitalization exchanging a total of 200–250 ml of plasma/kg body weight. Each exchange is 2–3 liters. In patients with CIDPs, plasmapheresis is individualized based on the initial response. Some patients' symptoms seem to be controlled with monthly pheresis.

Multiple Mononeuropathy

Multiple mononeuropathy is an uncommon subtype of AIDS-related peripheral neuropathy and perhaps may be a variant of the HIV-related IDPs. Lipkin and colleagues described 12 homosexual men with constitutional symptoms consistent with ARC who developed a predominantly sensory neuropathy.[36] The clinical findings were multifocal in 8 of the 12, and symmetrical in the remainder and occasionally affected the cranial nerves. In 4 of 6 nerve biopsies performed, inflammatory cells were seen without definite vasculitis and the authors postulate that this was possibly "an immune-mediated" disorder. Four of the 12 patients under study later developed AIDS. CSF-demonstrated elevated protein and a pleocytosis and electrodiagnostic studies were indicative of a multifocal process or axonal degeneration. It remains to be determined whether this is a distinct subtype of neuropathy or should be more appropriately categorized with one of the previously described types of HIV-related neuropathy.

Because of the relative rarity of this entity and the unclear pathogenesis, there is little information regarding therapy. Occasionally patients appear to undergo a spontaneous remission. Both steroids and plasmapheresis have been used in small numbers of patients.

Herpes Zoster Radiculitis

Herpes zoster nerve root infection (radiculitis) typically presents with a painful dermatomal shingles eruption (Fig. 2). It is caused by the reactivation of herpes zoster lying dormant in dorsal root ganglia neurons, and affects patients with HIV infection with increased frequency because of their impaired cellular immunity. In a small cohort of homosexual men with ARC, 26% developed shingles during a 4-year period of observation.[37] Typically, pain or paresthesias may precede the development of the rash by up to several days. The eruption may develop in a dermatomal distribution over the trunk or face or in a limb. Dissemination over the body can occur. When the eruption affects a limb, muscle weakness may develop as a result of involvement of the spinal cord by the viral infection spreading centrally into the spinal cord from the dorsal root ganglia. Rarely as ascending myelitis is seen with development of upper motor neuron signs and a spastic paraparesis.[38] Examination of the CSF shows a moderate pleocytosis and occasionally herpes zoster will be isolated by culturing the CSF. Herpes zoster IgM may be elevated in the CSF.

Treatment. Because of the relative insensitivity of herpes zoster to acyclovir (Zovirax) compared with herpes simplex, high doses of intravenous acyclovir are necessary for treatment (30 mg/kg per day). The severe pains that often accompany herpes zoster infection may persist—post herpetic neuralgia, requiring pain-modifying agents such as amitriptyline (Elavil) or carbamazepine (Tegretol).[39] A topical preparation of capsaicin

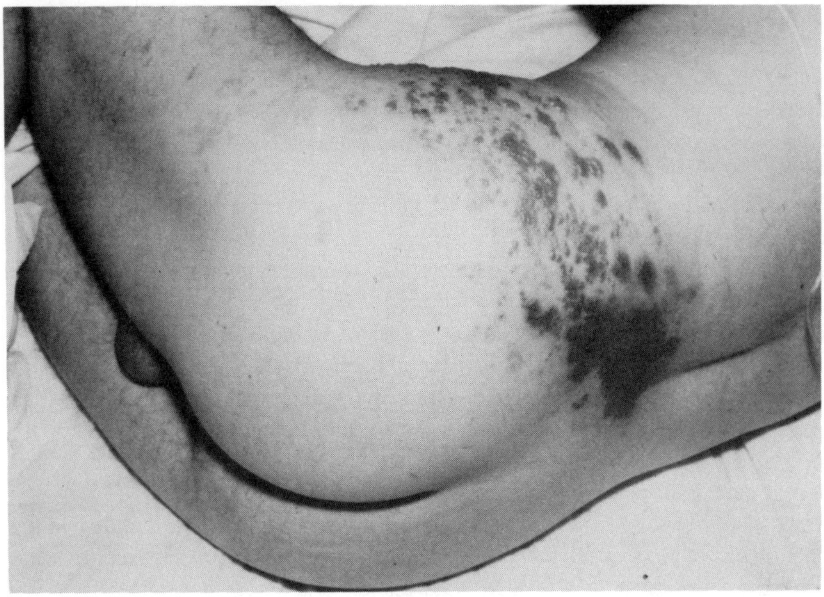

FIGURE 2. Herpes zoster. A typical vesicular eruption is present over the lower thoracic dermatomes.

(Zostrix) has recently been licensed for use in post-herpetic neuralgia. Experience with this agent, particularly in the setting of HIV infection, is limited.

Other Peripheral Nerve Disorders

Recently, CMV has been identified as the cause of both root and spinal cord damage in the setting of AIDS with descriptions of a progressive cauda equina syndrome, involving lumbar and sacral roots and presenting with sacral parethesias, sphincter disturbance and leg weakness.[18] There was a brisk CSF pleocytosis and immunostaining demonstrated inclusions typical of CMV within endoneurial and endothelial cells of the dorsal root ganglia in one autopsied case. There is as yet no effective anti-CMV agent available for treatment although DHPG is being used experimentally for suppression of CMV retinitis and may eventually prove useful for other CMV CNS infections.[40]

Poliomyelitis or coxsackie infection can cause a flaccid asymmetric weakness, and is usually accompanied by fever and a CSF pleocytosis. To date, neither has been reported with AIDS.

Cranial Neuropathies

These are uncommon, affecting 2–3% of patients with AIDS (see Fig. 1). Occasionally cranial neuropathies will occur with HIV-related meningitis.[41] Multiple cranial neuropathies may be a manifestation of chronic inflammatory polyneuropathy or of the multiple mononeuropathy syndrome. Rarely lymphomatous meningitis may present with cranial neuropathies. Treatment is discussed in the separate sections.

Other Neuropathies

Nutritional deficiencies, particularly of B-group vitamins and vitamin E, should be considered in any patient presenting with a neuropathy (see Table 1). In patients with AIDS, malnutrition, weight loss, and diarrhea are common and may lead to vitamin deficiencies. Vitamin supplements are reasonable adjuncts in cachexic patients, particularly if a neuropathy is present. Similarly, the patient who has suffered profound weight loss, and who may be bed-bound, is susceptible to nerve compression.

The most common symptom complexes are (1) ulnar nerve compression at the elbow producing pain and parethesias in the forearm and 4th and 5th digits, sometimes with weakness in the intrinsic hand muscles; (2) common peroneal nerve compression at the fibula head resulting in a foot drop with numbness over the lateral lower extremity and dorsum of the foot; and (3) tarsal tunnel syndrome with compression of the tibial nerve at the ankle usually causing pain and paresthesias limited to the sole of the foot. These are recognizable clinically and can be confirmed with NCVs. Treatment consists of appropriate padding and limb positioning to avoid further trauma.

Many patients with AIDS receive numerous antimicrobial drugs, either alone or in combination, as well as experimental agents such as AZT or DHPG. Neuropathies have been linked to a number of antimicrobials agents, including metronidazole (Flagyl),[42] nitrofurantoin,[43] and possibly sulfonamides.[14] Some of the neuropathic symptoms seen in AIDS may thus result from antimicrobial use and further study is needed of the potentially harmful interaction of certain drugs and vitamin deficiencies.

Opportunistic Infections in AIDS

Opportunistic infections of the nervous system are common in the setting of HIV infection and reflect the underlying impairment of cell-mediated immunity produced by infection and lysis of CD4 lymphocytes. Individuals with AIDS may have multiple concurrent opportunistic infections and a wide range of organisms have been identified (See Table 1).

Cerebral Toxoplasmosis

Clinical Features. Infection with *T. gondii,* an obligate intracellular protozoan, causes necrotic and inflammatory abscesses, which are often multifocal and scattered throughout the cerebral hemispheres. Levy and colleagues[41] reported cerebral toxoplasmosis in 28% of patients with AIDS, making toxoplasmosis the most common opportunistic infection in their experience. The typical clinical presentation is subacute in tempo, with fever, altered mentation, seizures in 15%, and focal neurological signs developing over a few days.[44]

Computed tomography (CT) scans usually demonstrate multiple contrast-enhancing lesions, surrounded by edema.[45] While the appearance is characteristic of an intracranial abscess, it can be mimicked by lymphoma, metastatic tumor, or even by the lesions of multiple sclerosis. Magnetic resonance imaging (MRI) is more sensitive than CT in the detection of cerebral toxoplasmosis and often demonstrates lesions that are not apparent on CT or that might be more easily biopsied.[46] MRI should be used when brain biopsy is

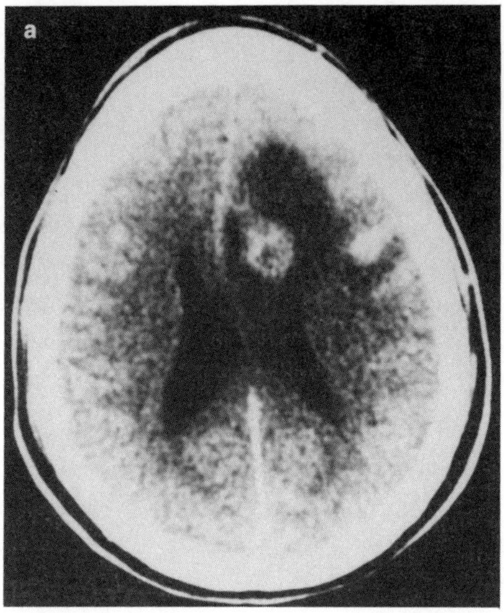

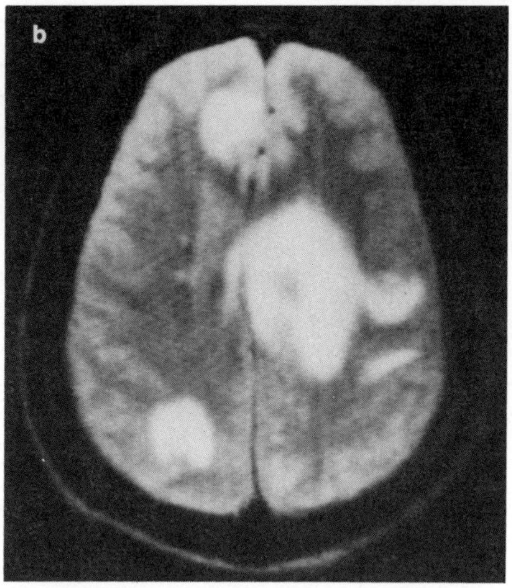

FIGURE 3. Toxoplasmosis. (a) A 34-year-old homosexual man presented with fever, headache, and right-sided hemiparesis. CT scan demonstrated two contrast-enhancing lesions in the left hemisphere with surrounding edema. (b) MRI scan performed at the same time shows several abnormal areas of high signal intensity that are not evident on CT.

planned, or when CT is negative but clinical suspicion of toxoplasmosis is strong (Fig. 3a, b). The CSF is often abnormal, with elevated total protein and a modest pleocytosis, however, lumbar puncture should not be performed when evidence of mass effect from a large focal lesion is present. Occasionally cytopathological study of the CSF will demonstrate the tachyzoites of *T. gondii* (personal observation).

Serological tests are insensitive, as there is usually a failure of appearance of specific IgM, however, a fourfold or greater rise in IgG, assayed by Sabin–Feldman or agglutination, is predictive of active toxoplasmosis.[47] The majority of patients with AIDS and cerebral toxoplasmosis will have detectable serum *Toxoplasma* IgG.[44] The Sabin–Feldman test for *Toxoplasma* IgG was positive in CSF in 8 of 12 patients and may be helpful particularly when a biopsy material may fail to demonstrate the organism in approximately 50%, however, a peroxidase–antiperoxidase technique is sensitive for demonstrating the tachyzoites.[47]

Treatment. First-line treatment is with a combination of pyrimethamine (Daraprim) and sulfadiazine given with leucovorin to prevent bone marrow suppression.[44] Many centers now start treatment empirically based on a typical clinical and radiologic presentation with multifocal lesions, reserving biopsy for atypical or refractory cases. Biopsy is also considered when serum antitoxoplasma IgG is negative, or when there is only a single cerebral lesion. Prompt initiation of antimicrobial therapy is critical because this can lead to clinical and radiologic improvement in up to 70% of patients. Recrudescence is common, occurring in 30%, and mortality directly from cerebral toxoplasmosis approaches 40% in those with this diagnosis.[44] Side effects of treatment are frequent, including nausea and vomiting, pancytopenia and rash. This usually results from the sulfadiazine and clindamycin (Cleocin) may be a useful substitute. Trimetrexate and other experimental folate antagonists which may be useful in treatment of toxoplasmosis and *P. carinii* infection are under study. Steroids may be used if there is marked mass effect, and standard anticonvulsants are effective for seizure control.

Looking to the future, the more widespread use of MRI may permit earlier detection and treatment of cerebral toxoplasmosis. The use of CT-guided stereotactic biopsy of focal cerebral lesions may allow for the safe differentiation from other CNS disorders. New antimicrobials will hopefully combine effective treatment with fewer side effects than conventional drugs.

Cryptococcosis

Clinical Features. C. neuformans, a ubiquitous yeast, produces CNS infection in 11% of patients with HIV infection[41,48] and in a proportion may be the first recognized opportunistic infection. Meningitis is the most common presentation (18 of 27 patients) with headache, meningismus, altered mentation, or nausea. This constellation of symptoms can mimic HIV-related meningitis, cerebral toxoplasmosis or even AIDS-related dementia.

The CSF may have normal cellular and protein constituents—in one series the leukocyte count was normal in 11 of 17 (65%), and protein was normal in 5 of 16 (31%). The CSF India ink was positive in 14 of 17 (82%), with uniformly positive cultures (18 of 18) and cryptococcal antigen detectable in both CSF and serum.[48] The assay of cryptococcal antigen is therefore highly predictive for cryptococcal meningitis. Occasionally with a particularly acute presentation, the cryptococcal antigen will be falsely negative, because too few fungal cells are present within the CSF. When clinical suspicion is high, the CSF should be centrifuged and the pellet of cells tested (Charache P: personal communication). MRI and CT are usually normal in cryptococcal meningitis, although they may be necessary to exclude toxoplasmosis and other conditions.

Treatment. Antifungal therapy is only of moderate efficacy in cryptococcal meningitis, and is poorly tolerated. The median survival after diagnosis of cryptococcal meningitis is 9 months. The mainstay of antifungal therapy is amphotericin B, which can cause renal impairment, chills, and fevers. Either amphotericin B alone (0.4–0.6 mg/kg per day) or a combination of amphotericin B (0.3 mg/kg per day) and flucytosine (Ancobon) (15 mg/kg per day) is used. This latter combination permits a lower dose of amphotericin B to be given, however, flucytosine may cause diarrhea and bone marrow suppression. While use of these antifungals may suppress the infection and lead to clinical improvement, it is extremely unusual for complete clearance to occur, and relapse is frequent. During successful treatment, both the serum and the CSF cryptococcal antigen titers can be expected to fall. Suppressive treatment with amphotericin B administered once or twice weekly via an indwelling Hickman catheter may maintain clinical response. The administration of amphotericin B via an intrathecal route, or into the ventricles through an indwelling Ommaya reservoir, does not seem justified by any difference in outcome in the small numbers reported to date.

Progressive Multifocal Leukoencephalopathy

Clinical Features. In 2–3% of patients with AIDS, PML will develop, which typically presents with a progressive accumulation of focal neurological deficits—aphasia, hemiparesis, or ataxia.[49] The disorder is caused by the reactivation of a papovavirus under conditions of immunoincompetence, most commonly JC or SV 40 viruses.[50] Prior to the description of AIDS, PML was seen most frequently in patients with lymphoma, leukemia, or receiving immunosuppressive drugs for treatment of rheumatoid arthritis or sarcoidosis, or following organ transplantation. The reactivated papovavirus affects the hemisperhic white matter, especially the occipital lobe, and causes patchy foci of demyelination, which may become confluent. Giant atypical astrocytes and oligodendrogilia with markedly enlarged nuclei are seen and inflammatory infiltrates may appear. Electron microscopy may reveal intranuclear papovavirions.

Diagnosis is usually made by recognition of a typical clinical course with CT scans demonstrating multiple hypodense areas within the white matter.[45] Typically, the lesions do not enhance with intravenous contrast and do not cause mass effect. Biopsy may be necessary to differentiate PML from cerebral toxoplasmosis, other opportunistic infections, or CNS lymphoma.

Treatment. There is no effective treatment although antiviral agents such as adenosine arabinoside have been tried. The neurological disorder often progresses inexorably to death over weeks or a few months.

CMV Retinitis

Clinical Features. CMV retinitis is the most common ocular infection in patients with AIDS an has been reported to occur in from 4–38% of AIDS patients, overall CMV retinitis appears in approximately 20%.[51–54] CMV retinitis is recognized by its characteristic ophthalmoscopic appearance of retinal necrosis admixed with hemorrhage (Fig. 4). It is important to distinguish CMV retinitis from cotton wool spots, which are microinfarcts of the nerve fiber layer of the retina, are noninfectious in origin, and may be related to immune complex deposition. A retinal microangiopathy consisting of cotton wool spots with or without intraretinal hemorrhages occurs in 40–92% of AIDS patients but generally does not interfere with vision.[55] It is occasionally difficult to make a clear-cut clinical distinction between very early CMV retinitis and cotton wool spots; therefore, careful ophthalmic follow-up may be required. It is generally possible to culture CMV from either the blood or urine of patients with active CMV retinitis.[56] Untreated, CMV retinitis is a progressive disease that can lead to blindness.

Treatment. The only currently available form of treatment for CMV retinitis is an investigational antiviral agent 9-(1,3-dihydroxy-2-propoxymethyl)guanine, also known as DHPG.[40] Several open-labeled studies have demonstrated the efficacy of DHPG in suppressing CMV infection.[57–59] Treatment consists of an initial induction phase in the hospital for approximately 2 weeks giving the drug either bid or tid. intravenously. Subsequently maintenance therapy, using a once daily intravenous infusion five days every week, must be continued. In AIDS patients, discontinuation of maintenance DHPG

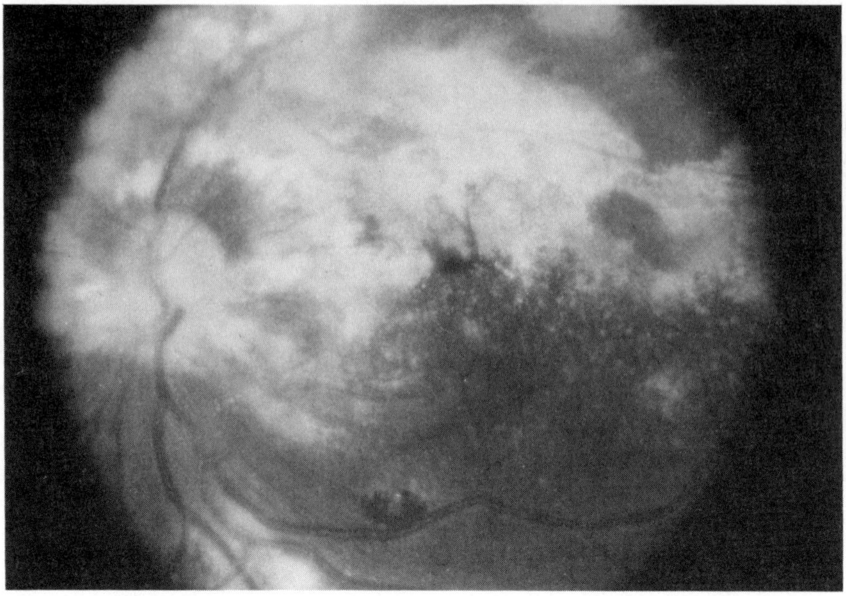

FIGURE 4. CMV retinitis. This 28-year-old homosexual developed sudden complete loss of vision in both eyes. There are extensive areas of hemorrhagic inflammation.

has almost universally resulted in the relapse of active CMV retinitis. Because of this relapse, maintenance treatment with DHPG must be maintained lifelong. Currently, no oral form of the drug is available.

The most significant side effect of DHPG is leukopenia, which occurs to a mild degree in most patients given DHPG. If severe leukopenia develops (the absolute neutrophil count falls to less than 500 cells/mm^3), then DHPG treatment must be temporarily interrupted. DHPG-induced leukopenia is reversible, and the drug can be reinstituted upon recovery of the white count.

Other Opportunistic Infections

There are scattered reports of other opportunistic infections including aspergillus and candida cerebral abscesses.[41] Multiple concurrent infections are sometimes recognized.[60] Atypical mycobacterial infections are also common and in the setting of disseminated mycobacterium avium intracellulare, CNS involvement is common, although it may not be identified antemortem.

Viral Infections in AIDS

Members of the Herpes group of viruses can produce direct damage to the CNS through infection. Herpes simplex I and II, herpes zoster, and CMV have all be identified as occasionally causing encephalitis in patients with AIDS.[41,61,62] Concurrent herpes simplex and CMV encephalitis and retinitis have been reported.[63]

These viral infections often present as a focal or diffuse encephalitis with change in mental status, fever, and seizures. CSF pleocytosis is common, particularly with herpes simplex encephalitis. Poorly defined areas of enhancement on CT or bright signal areas on MRI correspond to the areas of infection and damage. Often a diagnostic biopsy is necessary to distinguish these viral infections from cerebral toxoplasmosis. Both herpes simplex and herpes zoster encephalitis have been treated with intravenous acyclovir (Zovirax) 30 mg/kg per day. DHPG may prove useful in the treatment of CMV encephalitis.

Neoplastic Involvement of the Nervous System

Involvement of the nervous system by neoplasms is an infrequent manifestation of HIV infection. However, as previously discussed, presentation with a focal intracerebral lesion may result in a diagnostic dilemma, and may require biopsy for definition.

Primary CNS Lymphoma

These are classified as large-cell lymphomas, and are of similar histological appearance to those observed in immunosuppressed renal allograft recipients.[64] Epstein–Barr virus is thought to be linked with their development and in one homosexual with primary CNS lymphoma, EB virus genomes were identified in lymphoma tissue by in situ hybridization.[65] The exact prevalence of this complication of HIV infection is unknown, since some primary lymphomas are clinically silent, and may only be detected incidentally at autopsy. Our experience, and that of other groups, suggests that the CT findings are not specific, and that enhancement mimicking infection may be present. CSF cytopathology may demonstrate atypical lymphomatous cells.

Treatment. Corticosteroids are of occasional benefit, although their use is complicated by the additional immunosuppression. The response to radiation therapy appears to be poor.[41]

Systematic Lymphoma

The Centers for Disease Control (CDC) have included non-Hodgkins' lymphoma, occurring in a patient seropositive for HIV, as one of the diagnostic criteria for AIDS since 1985.[66] Complications related to lymphomatous nervous system involvement are rare but have included cranial neuropathies, lymphomatous meningitis, epidural cord compression and cerebral metastasis.[41]

Kaposi's Sarcoma

In patients with disseminated systemic Kaposi's sarcoma, a range of neurologic manifestations may be uncommonly observed. The peripheral nervous system can be involved directly; severe dysesthesias from local infiltration of peripheral nerves in the feet has been described by our group (personal observation). The central nervous system may rarely be the site of KS, which may have a preponderance for hemorrhage, particularly in the setting of thrombocytopenia.[41]

NEUROLOGICAL COMPLICATIONS IN SEXUALLY TRANSMITTED DISEASES

Neurosyphilis

Though involvement of the nervous system by syphilis was first described in the 16th century, it was not until the nineteenth century that its diverse manifestations were documented both clinically and pathologically. Because of its ability to mimic other conditions, neurosyphilis (NS) remains a prominent consideration in the differential diagnosis of neurological and psychiatric disease in the population at risk for AIDS. With the continued high incidence of syphilis in the community, the prevention, recognition and treatment of NS assumes great importance.

Syphilis was so named after the protagonist in a 16th century poem by Frascastorius who was afflicted by the condition. Its appearance in Western Europe was coincident with the return of Columbus's sailors, who are thought to have introduced it from the West Indies causing an epidemic known as the great pox in the late 15th century. Others exonerate Columbus from blame and hold that the sudden emergence of the disease in the Middle Ages resulted from temperature-induced minor genetic variation in organisms causing nonvenereal treponemal diseases elsewhere.[67,68]

Epidemiology

Syphilis is the third most frequently reported communicable disease in the United States. Having shown a steady increase since 1977, the incidence of new cases of syphilis in the population has declined slightly. A total of 69,888 new cases were reported in 1984, representing an incidence of 29.8 per 100,000 of the population. There is wide geographical variation in incidence from 0.6 in 100,000 in Vermont to 76.4 in 100,000 in Florida.[69] Precise figures for the incidence and prevalence of neurosyphilis do not exist, however, in the Oslo study, neurosyphilis developed in 5–10% of those subjects whose primary syphilitic infection was not treated.[70] Since an estimated 50,000 cases of syphilis remain undetected each year,[69,71] the annual incidence of neurosyphilis can be estimated at 2–5 per 100,000 of the population. To put this in perspective, it is similar in incidence to other neurological illness such as amyotrophic lateral sclerosis. The incidence of neurosyphilis is higher in caucasians than in blacks or orientals,[72] and febrile illness and pregnancy seem to be protective against the development of neurosyphilis.

Pathogenesis

Syphilis is caused by *Treponema pallidum,* which was first isolated in 1905.[73] Like HIV, transmission requires intimate contact, almost invariably sexual. If untreated, 25-30% of those who contract a primary infection will develop direct involvement of the nervous system which usually occurs within 3–18 months.[74]

Neurosyphilis always begins with a meningitis which is either asymptomatic or associated with a flulike illness, and as discussed earlier, may serve as a parallel for the acute atypical meningitis occurring with HIV infection. It may undergo spontaneous remission, continue as asymptomatic syphilitic meningitis or progress to other forms of neurosyphilis. The effect of the organism on various parts of the nervous system has been used as the basis for the description of distinct clinical syndromes. The meninges are the first to be involved and more persistent infection may involve the blood vessels causing meningovascular syphilis. Chronic infection of the parenchyma of the brain and spinal cord is responsible for general paresis and tabes dorsalis respectively. Though neurosyphilitic syndromes may occur at any stage after infection their peak incidence varies (Fig. 5).

Diagnosis

The diagnosis of neurosyphilis may be considered on the basis of symptoms and clinical signs (which may be minimal or absent). It is then confirmed by serology and analysis of CSF. Incidentally positive serology may be the only indication that a patient is at risk of neurosyphilis. Isolation of the organism, which is the gold standard for diagnosis in other infectious diseases, is unrealistic and usually impossible in cases of neurosyphilis.

Serological Tests. These tests detect treponemal and non-treponemal antibodies stimulated by the organism in the course of infection. The most commonly used non-treponemal tests are the Venereal Disease Research Laboratory (VDRL) and the rapid plasma reagin (RPR) tests. They detect antibodies to lipoidal antigens (reagins) thought to be the result of interaction between *T. pallidum* and the host tissue. The standard trepenemal test is the fluorescent treponemal antibody absorption test (FTA–ABS), which

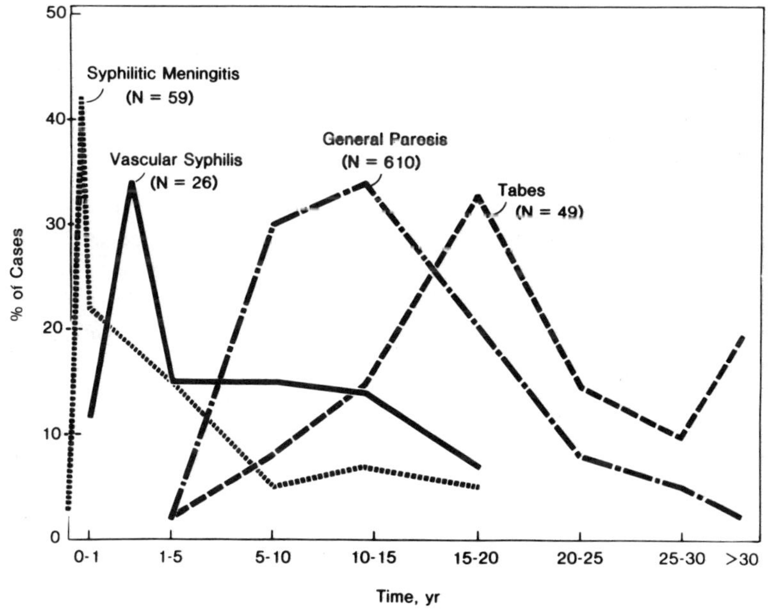

FIGURE 5. The time course of the development of the different clinical syndromes of neurosyphilis. (From Simon.[75a])

identifies antibodies specific for *T. pallidum.* Other treponemal tests such as the microhemagglutination assay for *T. pallidum* (MHA-TP) and the *T. pallidum* hemagglutination test (TPHA) are also used.

The VDRL usually becomes positive during primary infection. The titer reaches a peak during the first year after which there is a slow decline and it is unreactive in up to 25% of cases of late syphilis.[75] The quantitative nature of the VDRL and RPR makes them useful in assessing response to treatment. It will be rendered nonreactive with adequate treatment though the speed of and degree to which this occurs depends on the length of previous infection.[76] False-positive results may be seen transiently in association with pregnancy and acute infections.[77] More longlasting false seropositivity is seen with autoimmune disease, old age,[78] and narcotic addition.[79] Nevertheless, in up to 50% of cases,[77] the cause of the spurious result is unknown. The VDRL titer may be used as a guideline as it is usually $< 1:8$ with false-positive results.

FTA–ABS is the first test to become positive in primary infection, remains so for life, and is not affected by treatment. It is positive in 96–100% of cases of neurosyphilis[80,81] and will also be positive in nonvenereal treponemal disease such as yaws and pinta. False positive results have been reported though less frequently than with nontreponemal tests. Borderline results should be rechecked.

MHA–TP remains reactive for life, is unaffected by treatment and is positive in 93.5–100% of cases of symptomatic late syphilis.[82]

CSF Tests. In addition to the measurement of opening pressure, cell count, protein and glucose, the VDRL should be performed on the CSF. The CSF VDRL has reported sensitivities in neurosyphilis ranging from 10 to 89%.[83,84] Its specificity, however, approaches 100%. Because of low specificity and difficulty in interpretation, the CSF FTA–ABS is not recommended for routine use.[85]

Clinical Syndromes

Neurosyphilis always begins as a meningitis and persistent infection affecting specific areas of the brain and spinal cord accounts for the well known clinical syndromes. The syndromes themselves are not mutually exclusive and there may be overlap between them. The full-blown syndromes may now have become supplanted by "modern" neurosyphilis. They tend to occur within specific intervals after primary infection (see Fig. 5). Why one syndrome rather than another should occur in any particular person is not known.

Asymptomatic Neurosyphilis. This group is composed of those who have evidence of neurosyphilis on analysis of CSF but have no signs or symptoms of the disease. Some authors have included within this category those in whom abnormal pupils were the only sign of central nervous system involvement.[86] The existence of subclinical infection emphasizes the importance of CSF examination in the management of syphilis.

Syphilitic Meningitis. Meningitis occurs in up to 35% of untreated cases and is generally asymptomatic.[74] The signs and symptoms are dependent on the intensity of meningeal inflammation, its site and duration. In symptomatic cases, the typical presentation of infectious meningitis—headache, neck stiffness, and photophobia—is less common than expected. Nevertheless, symptoms of increased intracranial pressure due to disruption of CSF flow are not uncommon. Predominant involvement of the meninges over the vertex of the brain may present with seizures, hemiplegia, or sudden alteration in level of consciousness. Chronic inflammation at the base of the brain may cause cranial nerve involvement—II, III, VI, VII, and the auditory division of VIII being the most common.[86] Pupillary abnormalities are relatively frequent because if III involvement, however, the Argyll-Robertson pupil, characterized by small irregular pupils responding to accommodation but not to light, is rare in this syndrome. There is a focal form of meningeal neurosyphilis that leads to the formation of gumma. These gummata are comprised of granulation tissue, the result of intense localized inflammatory response of the meninges. They enlarge and compress underlying brain. Presentation is with symptoms and signs of a space-occupying lesion. Definitive diagnosis can only be made by biopsy and surgical excision is the only effective form of treatment.

Meningovascular Syphilis. This syndrome was first described by Budd in 1842 and generally occurs within 5 years of primary infection. It is characterized pathologically by endarteritis and vessel thrombosis with areas of encephalomalacia. The middle cerebral artery is most commonly involved, though any intracranial vessel may be affected. The presentation is with a stroke, the symptoms and signs of which obviously depend on the vessel involved. The strokes may be characterized by a stuttering course in 25% of cases. The stroke may have been preceded by a prodrome of headache, malaise, and personality change for weeks or months. In the past, meningovascular syphilis was a frequent cause of stroke in young age groups and should still be considered today. Angiographic[81] and CT findings[88] are nonspecific. If the inflammatory process predominantly affects the spinal cord, a radiculomyelopathy can result. The CSF is abnormal in all cases.[89]

Paretic Neurosyphilis. This chronic meningoencephalitis leads to a general deterioration in mental function. It was first described in psychiatric patients by Haslam in 1798. Earlier this century when syphilis was more prevalent in the general population and treatment inadequate, general paresis accounted for 10% of psychiatric hospital admissions.[86] The first clinical pathological descriptions appeared in 1822 and emphasized generalized brain atrophy particularly in the frontal and temporal lobes. This is seen microscopically as a diffuse loss of neurons with gliosis. The organism *T. pallidum* has been found in some brains, and though most frequently seen in the frontal grey matter, may have a patchy distribution.

Its presentation may mimic many known psychiatric diseases. The initial symptoms are usually of mild dementia. Then follows a psychotic state which may take many forms: agitated depression, mania, or paranoia. The well described "delusions of grandeur" were seen in 20% of a series by Merritt.[86] The manifest psychosis eventually degenerates into a state of profound dementia. Corticospinal tract signs are seen with degeneration of the motor cortex thus accounting for the "paresis." Other neurological signs include leonine paralytic facies, tremor at rest, pupillary disturbances and dysarthria. Without treatment, the average life expectancy from time of diagnosis is two years.

Tabes Dorsalis. This literally means wasting of the back. It was first adequately described by Romberg who did not make the association with syphilis. This was later provided by Erb and Fainnier. It is characterized by degeneration of the posterior columns and the dorsal roots of the spinal cord. More common in males than females, the average incubation is 21 years.[86]

Presenting symptoms can include ataxia, sensory loss, disturbance of bladder, and sexual dysfunction. "Lightening pains" which are severe and intermittent, occurring particularly in the legs are seen in 75% of cases. "Visceral crises" which are bouts of sudden agonizing epigastric pain associated with nausea and vomiting and unresponsive to most medications occur in one fifth. Though abnormalities of vibration and proprioception are typical, pain and temperature loss also occur. There is a generalized hypotonia of the limbs and abdominal wall. Reflexes are asymmetrical and frequently absent. Charcot joints and perforating ulcers on the legs are seen. Optic atrophy occurs in 15–20% and pupillary disturbances are very common; some degree of abnormality is seen in 90%, one half of whom have the classic Argyll–Robertson pupil.[90]

Cranial nerves may be involved early, most commonly affected being III and VI followed by the auditory division of cranial nerve VIII. Hyperalgesia in the trigeminal distribution is not uncommon. Involvement of the facial nerve is rare.

"Modern" Neurosyphilis. The above descriptions of clinical syndromes are strongly based on texts written before penicillin became widely available and thus represents the true natural history of the disease. It has been postulated that because of the widespread use of antibiotics in the community for unrelated conditions, these syndromes are seen less often.[91,92] Rather, patients are much more likely to present with less dramatic symptoms and signs, the result of partially treated condition. In reviewing 365 cases of neurosyphilis described since 1965, Hotson found that new onset seizures and neuro-ophthalmological findings were the most common forms of presentation, occurring in a total of 50% of patients.[91] Syphilis should be considered in young adults with new onset seizures and a positive FTA. Neuro-ophthalmological findings may include optic neuritis, progressive optic atrophy, abnormal extraocular movements and pupillary disturbances.[93]

Treatment

The question of who should receive treatment is perhaps more important than the specific regime used. For practical purposes, a nonreactive serum FTA is incompatible with the diagnosis of neurosyphilis.[94] The potential for neurosyphilis exists in patients with a positive serum FTA who have a history of untreated, or partially treated, syphilis of more than 1 year's duration. Neurosyphilis can also develop in those found incidentally to be seropositive with no history of previous syphilis infection, whether neurological symptoms and signs exist or not. CSF examination should be performed in all such cases to exclude neurosyphilis. The importance of CSF examination cannot be overemphasized, as it has therapeutic implications. In the aforementioned groups, any increase in protein, a lymphocytic pleocytosis, or a reactive CSF VDRL is indicative of neurosyphilis and should be treated appropriately. In populations at risk for AIDS, other causes of an abnormal CSF such as HIV-related meningitis may cause confusion.

Penicillin is the drug of choice for *T. pallidum* infections. Any effective regime used in neurosyphilis must achieve treponemicidal levels within the CSF. Of the current CDC recommendations for the treatment of neurosyphilis, two regimens fulfill this criterion:

1. Aqueous crystalline penicillin G 12–24 million units IV/day for 10 days followed by benzathine penicillin G 2–4 million units IM weekly for 3 doses.[95]
2. Aqueous procaine penicillin G 2–4 million units IM daily plus probenecid 500 mg by Po qid both for 10 days followed by benzathine penicillin G 2–4 million units IM weekly for 3 weeks.[96]

The use of benzathine penicillin alone does not achieve adequate CSF levels,[95] has been associated with treatment failures,[97] and is not to be recommended. Following therapy, the CSF should be examined at 6-month intervals for 24 months or until normal. A rising cell count is an indication for retreatment.

Patients with suspected penicillin allergy should have the allergy confirmed, since no data exist for the efficacy of drugs other than penicillin in the treatment of neurosyphilis. Doxycyline, a tetracycline derivative, has been used because of its CSF penetration.

Genital Herpes

The incidence of genital herpes has increased more than that of any other sexually transmitted disease in recent years. The estimated yearly incidence of new cases in the United States is 724,000, with a cumulative prevalence of 20 million infected people.[98] Its tendency to recur and the lack of a specific cure make genital herpes a major health issue.

Pathogenesis

Herpes simplex virus has two antigenically distinct serotypes: herpes simplex 1 (HSV1) and herpes simplex 2 (HSV-2). HSV-1 causes most orolabial infections while HSV2 is responsible for the majority of genital infections.[99] Transmission of HSV-2 usually requires sexual contact with a person who has active genital ulceration or, more rarely, one who is asymptomatically shedding the virus. Following virus replication at the site of infection, it is transported intra-axonally to autonomic and sensory nerve ganglia in the lumbosacral area.[100] Subsequent centrifugal spread of virus along sensory nerves may lead to more extensive vesicular eruption on the skin in primary infection. Once the primary infection has resolved, the virus remains latent in the ganglia but becomes reactivated intermittently causing recurrences. The mechanisms of latency and reactivation are unknown. Active inflammation of the meninges, spinal cord, and nerve roots usually during primary infection leads to the neurological complications of meningitis, myelitis, and radiculitis, respectively.

Neurological Complications

Although symptoms and signs of meningeal irritation have been reported in 36% of women and 13% of men with primary infection,[101] and the occurrence as aseptic meningitis with HSV2 has been established,[102] the actual incidence of aseptic meningitis with genital herpes is unknown. The prognosis in the reported cases is excellent, unlike the encephalitis associated with HSV-1 infection.

Sacral radicular paresthesias are common in primary infection and may occur as a prodrome in recurrences. Frank sacral radiculitis with urinary retention and CSF evidence of inflammation is rare,[103,104] although it does occur more commonly with herpes proctitis than with perineal lesions.[105] These patients may have constipation and urinary retention.[106] More extensive root involvement with weakness, altered sensation, and diminished or absent reflexes in the lower limbs has also been described but is even less common.[107] Transverse myelitis with or without radicular involvement has been reported.[108,109] It must be emphasized that serious neurological complications are rare with genital herpes.

Diagnosis

In a patient with primary genital herpes who develops symptoms of meningitis, urinary retention, lumbar radiculitis, or transverse myelitis, CSF should be examined for protein, glucose, cells, viral culture, and complement-fixing antibodies to herpes simplex virus. Even without significant titers to herpes simplex within the CSF, the coincidental appearance of an acute neurological problem with primary genital herpes in the presence of an inflammatory CSF is circumstantial evidence in favor of the diagnosis.

Treatment

Intravenous and oral acyclovir has been effective in reducing the length of virus shedding and in decreasing the duration of symptoms in primary infections.[110,111] This agent has also been used in preventing infection in immunocompromised hosts, for example, patients undergoing bone marrow transplantation. It would seem the obvious choice in neurological involvement but no data exist to support this.

Gonorrhea

In 1984, there were 878,556 new cases of gonorrhea diagnosed in the United States.[63] The only neurological complication is gonococcal meningitis, which occurs in the context of disseminated gonococcal infection. Since the organism was first isolated from the CSF of a patient in 1909,[112] about 25 further cases have been identified.[113] Presentation is with headache, photophobia, nausea, and vomiting. The CSF has the typical characteristics of bacterial infection with a polymorphonuclear leukocytosis, low glucose, and elevated protein. The treatment of choice is very-high-dose penicillin IV for at least 2 weeks.

ACKNOWLEDGMENTS. This work was supported by National Institutes of Health AI72634 and NS26643. This chapter, originally submitted in 1987, has not been updated since.

REFERENCES

1. Johnson RT, McArthur JC: AIDS and the brain. *Trends Neurosci* 9:91–94, 1986.
2. Navia BA, Jordan BD, Price RW: The AIDS dementia complex: I. Clinical features. *Ann Neurol* 19:517–524, 1986.

3. Navia BA, Cho E-S, Petito CK, et al: The AIDS dementia complex. II. Neuropathology. *Ann Neurol* 19:525–535, 1986.
4. Cooper DA, Gold J, Maclean P, et al: Acute AIDS retrovirus infection: Definition of a clinical illness associated with seroconversion. *Lancet* 1:537–540, 1985.
5. Ho DD, Rota TR, Schooley RT, et al: Isolation of HTLV-III from cerebrospinal fluid and neural tissues of patients with neurologic syndromes related to the acquired immunodeficiency syndrome. *New Engl J Med* 313:1493–1497, 1985.
6. Carne CA, Tedder RS, Smith A, et al: Acute encephalopathy coincident with seroconversion for anti-HTLV-III. *Lancet* 2:1206–1208, 1985.
7. McArthur JC, Farzadegan H, Cornblath DR, et al: Cerebrospinal fluid abnormalities in homosexual/bisexual men with and without neuropsychiatric symptoms, in *Third International Conference on Acquired Immunodeficiency Syndrome (AIDS) June 1-5, 1987, Washington, DC* (abst).
8. Goudsmit J, de Wolf F, Paul DA, et al: Expression of human immunodeficiency virus antigen (HIV-Ag) in serum and cerebrospinal fluid during acute and chronic infection. *Lancet* 2:177–80, 1986.
9. McArthur JC, Sipos E, Chupp M, et al: Immunocytochemical staining of blood and cerebrospinal fluid mononuclear cells in AIDS-spectrum disorders. *Neurology (NY)* 37(suppl 1):319, 1987.
10. Black P: HIV, AIDS, and the brain. *N Engl J Med* 313:1538–1539, 1985.
11. Nathanson N, Georgsson G, Palsson PA, et al: Experimental visna in Icelandic sheep: The prototype lentivirus infection. *Rev Infect Dis* 7:75–82, 1985.
12. Petito CK, Navia BA, Cho E-S, et al: Vacuolar myelopathy pathologically resembling subacute combined degeneration in patients with the acquired immunodeficiency syndrome. *N Engl J Med* 312:874–879, 1985.
13. Singh BM, Levine S, Yarrish RL, et al: Spinal cord syndromes in the acquired immune deficiency syndrome. *Acta Neurol Scand* 73:590–598, 1986.
14. Goldstick L, Mandybur TI, Bode R: Spinal cord degeneration in AIDS. *Neurology (NY)* 35:103–106, 1985.
15. Rance N, McArthur J, Cornblath DR, et al: Gracile tract degeneration and sensory neuropathy in patients with AIDS. *Neurology (NY)* 38:794–796, 1988.
16. Spencer PS, Schaumburg HH: Central-peripheral distal axonopathy: The pathology of dying-back polyneuropathies. *Prog Neuropathol* 3:253–295, 1976.
17. Britton DB, Mesa-Tejada R, Fenoglio CM, et al: A new complication of AIDS: Thoracic myelitis caused by herpes simplex virus. *Neurology (NY)* 35:1071–1074, 1985.
18. Eidelberg D, Sotrel A, Vogel H, et al: Progressive polyradiculopathy in acquired immune deficiency syndrome. *Neurology (NY)* 36:912–916, 1986.
19. Tucker T, Dix RD, Katzen C, et al: Cytomegalovirus and herpes simplex virus ascending myelitis in a patient with acquired immune deficiency syndrome. *Ann Neurol* 18:74–79, 1985.
20. Gessain A, Borin F, Vernant JC, et al: Antibodies to human T lymphotropic virus type I in patients with tropical spastic paraparesis. *Lancet* 2:407–409, 1985
21. Osame M, Usuku K, Izumo S, et al: HTLV-I associated myelopathy, a new clinical entity. *Lancet* 1:1031 1032, 1986.
22. Robert-Guroff M, Weiss SH, Giron JA, et al: Prevalence and antibodies to HTLV-I, -II, -III in intravenous drug abusers from an AIDS epidemic region. *JAMA* 255:3133–3137, 1986.
23. Johnson RT, McArthur JC: Myelopathies and retroviruses. (Editorial.) *Ann Neurol* 21:115–118, 1987.
24. Jakobsen J, Trojaborg W, Helweg-Larsen S, et al: A Cross sectional population study of AIDS in Denmark: Neurological and electrophysiological report, in *The Second International Meeting of the Peripheral Neuropathy Association on America, Hilton, South Carolina, November 4–8, 1986.* (abst).
25. Snider WD, Simpson DM, Nielson G, et al: Neurological complications of acquired immune deficiency syndrome: Analysis of 50 patients. *Ann Neurol* 14:403–418, 1983.
26. Cornblath DR, McArthur JC, Kennedy PGE, et al: Inflammatory demyelinating peripheral neuropathies associated with human T-cell lymphotropic virus ype III infection. *Ann Neurol* 21:32–40, 1987.
27. Fisher M: Residual neuropathological changes in Canadians held prisoners of war by the Japanese. *Can Serv Med J* 11:159–199, 1955.
28. Spencer PS, Schaumburg HH (eds): *Experimental and Clinical Neurotoxicology.* Baltimore, Williams & Wilkins, 1980.

29. Yarchoan R, Brouwers P, Spitzer AR, et al: Response of human immunodeficiency-virus-associated neurological disease to 3′-azido-3′-deoxythymidine. *Lancet* 1:132–135, 1987.
30. Morris L, Distenfeld A, Amorosi E, et al: Autoimmune thrombocytopenic purpura in homosexual men. *Ann Intern Med* 96:714–717, 1982.
31. Stricker RB, Abrams DI, Corash L, et al: Target platelet antigen in homosexual men with immune thrombocyopenia. *N Engl J Med* 313:1375–1380, 1985.
32. Miller RG, Parry G, Lang W, et al: Aids-related inflammatory olyradiculoneuropathy: Prediction of response to plasma exchange with electrophysiologic testing. *Muscle Nerve* 8:626, 1985.
33. Mishra BB, Sommers W, Koski CK, et al: Acute inflammatory demyelinating polyneuropathy in the acquired immune deficiency syndrome. *Ann Neurol* 17:131, 1985.
34. Cornblath DR, Griffin JW, Tennekoon G: CSF myelin basic protein in peripheral neuropathies. *Ann Neurol* 20:370–372, 1986.
35. Kiprov DD, Abrams D, Pfaeffl W, et al: ARC/AIDS-related autoimmune syndromes and their treatment, in *The Second International Conference on AIDS, Paris, June 1986* (abst).
36. Lipkin WI, Parry G, Kiprov D, et al: Inflammatory neuropathy in homosexual men with lymphadenopathy. *Neurology (NY)* 35:1479–1483, 1985.
37. Janssen RS, Saykin AJ, Kaplan JE, et al: Neurologic complications of lymphadenopathy syndrome associated with human immunodeficiency virus infection. *Neurology (NY)* 37(suppl 1):344, 1987.
38. Muder RR, Lumish RM, Corsello GR: Myelopathy after herpes zoster. *Arch Neurol* 40:455–448, 1983.
39. Watson PN, Evans RJ. Postherpetic neuralgia. *Arch Neurol* 43:836–840, 1986.
40. Collaborative DHPG Treatment Study Group: Treatment of serious cytomegalovirus infections with 9-(1,3 Dihydroxy-2-propoxymethyl)guanine in patients with AIDS and other immunodeficiencies. *N Engl J Med* 314:801–805, 1986.
41. Levy RM, Bredesen DE, Rosenblum ML: Neurological manifestations of the acquired immunodeficiency syndrome (AIDS): Experience at USCF and review of the literature. *J Neurosurg* 62:475–495, 1985.
42. Coxon A, Pallis CA: Metronidazole neuropathy. *J Neurol Neurosurg Psychiatry* 39:403–405, 1976.
43. Lhermitte F, Fritel D, Cambier J, et al: Polyneurites au cours de traitements par la nitrofurantione. *Presse Med* 71:767, 1963.
44. Navia BA, Petito CK, Gold JWM, et al: Cerebral toxoplasmosis complicating the acquired immune deficiency syndrome: Clinical and neuropathological findings in 27 patients. *Ann Neurol* 19:224–238, 1986.
45. Elkin CM, Leon E, Grenell SL, et al: Intracranial lesions in the acquired immunodeficiency syndrome. *JAMA* 253:393–396, 1985.
46. Levy RM, Mills CM, Posin JP, et al: The superiority of cranial magnetic resonance imaging (MRI) to computed tomographic (CT) brain scans for the diagnosis of cerebral lesions in patient with AIDS, in *The Second International Conference on AIDS, Paris, June 1986* (abst).
47. Luft BJ, Brooks RG, Conley FK, et al: Toxoplasmic encephalitis in patients with acquired immunodeficiency syndrome. *JAMA* 252:913–917, 1984.
48. Kovacs JA, Kovacs AA, Polis M, et al: Cryptococcosis in the acquired immunodeficiency syndrome. *Ann Intern Med* 103:533–538, 1985.
49. Miller JR, Barrett RD, Britton CB, et al: Progressive multifocal leukoencephalopathy in a male homosexual with T cell immune deficiency. *N Engl J Med* 307:1436–1438, 1982.
50. Narayan O, Penney JB, Johnson RT, et al: Etiology of progressive multifocal leukoencephalopathy. Identification of papovavirus. *N Engl J Med* 289:1278–1282, 1973.
51. Freeman WR, Lerner CW, Mines JA, et al: A prospective study of the ophthalmologic findings in the acquired immune deficiency syndrome. *Am J Ophthalmol* 97:133–142, 1984.
52. Holland GH, Pepose JS, Pettit TH, et al: Acquired immune deficiency syndrome: Ocular manifestations. *Ophthalmology* 90:859–873, 1983.
53. Khadem M, Kalish SB, Goldsmith J, et al: Ophthalmologic findings in acquired immune deficiency syndrome (AIDS). *Arch Ophthalmol* 102:201–206, 1984.
54. Rosenberg PR, Uliss AE, Friedland GH, et al: Acquired immunodeficiency syndrome: Ophthalmic manifestations in ambulatory patients. *Ophthalmology* 90:874–878, 1983.
55. Newsome DA, Green WR, Miller ED, et al: Microvascular aspects of acquired immune deficiency syndrome retinopathy. *Am J Ophthalmol* 98:590–601, 1984.
56. Murray HW, Knox DL, Green WR, et al: Cytomegalovirus retinitis in adults: A manifestation of disseminated viral infection. *Am J Med* 63:574–584, 1977.

57. Palestine AG, Stevens G Jr, Lane HC, et al: Treatment of cytomegalovirus retinitis with dihydroxy propoxymethyl guanine. *Am J Ophthalmol* 101:95–101, 1986.
58. Rosecan LR, Stahl-Bayliss CM, Kalman CM, et al: Antiviral therapy for cytomeglovirus retinitis in AIDS with dihydroxy propoxymethyl guanine. *Am J Opthalmol* 100:405–418, 1986.
59. Holland GN, Sakamoto MJ, Hardy D, et al: Treatment of cytomegalovirus retinopathy in patients with acquired immunodeficiency syndrome. *Arch Ophthalmol* 104:1794–1800, 1986.
60. Levy RM, Bredesen DE, Davis RL, et al: Multiple intracranial pathologies in the acquired immunodeficiency syndrome (AIDS): A report of 20 cases, in *The Second International Conference on AIDS, Paris, June 1986*. (abst).
61. Edwards RH, Messing R, McKendall RR: Cytomegalovirus meningoencephalitis in a homosexual man with Kaposi's sarcoma. *Neurology (NY)* 35:560–562, 1985.
62. Hawley DA, Schaefer JF, Schultz DM, et al: Cytomegalovirus encephalitis in acquired immunodeficiency syndrome. *Am J Clin Pathol* 80:874–875, 1983.
63. Pepose JS, Hilborne LH, Cancilla PA, et al: Concurrent herpes simplex and cytomegalovirus retinitis and encephalitis in the acquired immunodeficiency syndrome (AIDS). *Ophthalmology* 91:1669–1670, 1984.
64. Snider WD, Simpson DM, Aronyk KE, et al: Primary lymphoma of the nervous system associated with acquired immune-deficiency syndrome. *N Engl J Med* 308:45, 1983.
65. Hochberg FH, Miller G, Schooley RT, et al: Central nervous system lymphoma related to Epstein–Barr virus. *N Engl J Med* 309:745–748, 1983.
66. Centers for Disease Control: Revision of the case definition of acquired immunodeficiency syndrome for national reporting—United States. *MMWR* 34:373–374, 1985.
67. Hollander DH: Treponematosis from pinta to venereal syphilis revisited: Hypothesis for temperature determination of disease patterns. *Sex Transm Dis* 8:34, 1981.
68. Fieldstal AH: Genetics of treponema, in Schell RF, Musher DF (eds): *Pathogenesis and Immunology of Treponemal Infection*. New York, Marcel Dekker, 1983, p 39.
69. *Sexually Transmitted Disease Fact Sheet*, ed 24. HEW Publication (CDC) 79-8195. Washington, DC, U.S. Department of Health, Education and Welfare, 1980.
70. Gjestland T: The Oslo study of untreated syphilis. *Acta Derm Venereol (Stockh)* 35(suppl 34):1–368, 1955.
71. Brown WJ: Status and control of syphilis in the United States. *J Infect Dis* 124(4):428–433, 1971.
72. Turner TB: The race and sex distribution of the lesions of syphilis in 1000 cases. *Bull Johns Hopkins Hosp* 46:159, 1930.
73. Schaudinn FR, Hoffman E: Vorlaufiger bericht uber das vorkommen von spirochaeten in syphilitischen krakheitsproducken und bei papillomen arbeien aus dem. *K Gesundkeitsamte* 22:527, 1905.
74. Moore JE: *The Modern Treatment of Syphilis*, ed 2. Springfield, Illinois, Charles C Thomas, 1943.
75. Sparling PF: Diagnosis and treatment of syphilis. *N Engl J Med* 284:642–653, 1971.
75a. Simon RP: Neurosyphilis. *Arch Neurol* 42:606–613, 1985.
76. Fiumara NJ: Serologic responses to treatment of 128 patients with late latent syphilis. *Sex Transm Dis* 6:243–246, 1979.
77. Catterall RD: Systemic disease and the biological false positive reaction. *Br J Vener Dis* 48:1–10, 1972.
78. Tuffanelli DI: Aging and false positive reactions for syphilis. *Br J Vener Dis* 42:40–41, 1966.
79. Kaufman RE, Weiss S, Moore JD, et al: Biological false positive serological tests for syphilis among drug addicts. *Br J Vener Dis* 50:350–353, 1974.
80. Larsen SA, Hunter EF, McGrew BE: Syphilis, in Wentworth B, Judson FN (eds): *Laboratory Methods for the Diagnosis of Sexually Transmitted Disease*. Washington, DC, American Public Health Association, 1984.
81. Harner RE, Smith JL, Israel CW. The FTA-ABS test in late syphilis: A serological study in 1985 cases. *JAMA* 203:545–548, 1968.
82. Larsen SA, Hambie EA, Peltidge DE, et al: Specificity, sensitivity and reproducibility among the fluorescent treponemal antibody absorption test, the microhemagglutination assay for treponema pallidum and the hemagglutination treponemal test for syphilis. *J Clin Microbiol* 14:441–445, 1981.
83. Larsen SA, Hambie EA, Wobig GH, et al: Cerebrospinal fluid test for syphilis, treponemal and nontreponemal tests, in Morreset R, et al (eds): *Advances in Sexually Transmitted Diseases* Utrecht, The Netherlands, VNU Science Press, 1985, pp 157–162.

84. Bracero L, Wormster GP, Boltone EJ: Serological tests for syphilis: A guide to interpretation in various stages of disease. *Mt Sinai J Med (NY)* 46:289–292, 1979.
85. Criteria and techniques for the diagnosis of early syphilis. DHEW Publication 98-376. Atlanta, Centers for Disease Control, 1979.
86. Merritt HH, Adams RD, Solomon HC: *Neurosyphilis.* Oxford University Press, New York, 1946.
87. Vata K, Scheibel R, Keiffer et al: Neurosyphilis and diffuse cerebral angiopathy: A case report. *Neurology (NY)* 24:472–476, 1974.
88. Godt P, Stoeppler L, Wrischer U, et al: The value of computed tomography in cerebral syphilis. *Neuroradiology* 18:197–200, 1979.
89. Fishman RA: *Cerebrospinal Fluid in Diseases of the Nervous System.* Philadelphia, WB Saunders Co, 1980, pp 225–285.
90. Merritt HH. *A Textbook of Neurology.* Philadelphia, Lea & Febiger, 1973.
91. Hotson JR: Modern neurosyphilis: A partially treated chronic meningitis (Medical Progress). *West J Med* 135:191–200, 1981.
92. Luxon L, Lees AJ, Greenwood RJ: Neurosyphilis today. *Lancet* 1:90–93, 1979.
93. Fletcher WA, Sharpe JA: Tonic pupils in neurosyphilis. *Neurology (NY)* 36:188–192, 1986.
94. Jaffe HW, Robins SA: Cerebrospinal fluid examinations in patients with syphilis. *Rev Infect Dis* 4:842–847, 1982.
95. Mohr JA, Griffiths W, Jackson R. et al: Neurosyphilis and penicillin levels in cerebrospinal fluid. *JAMA* 236:2208–2209, 1976.
96. Polnikorn N, Witoonpanich R, Varachit M, et al: Penicillin concentrations in cerebrospinal fluid after different treatment regimens for syphilis. *Br J Vener Dis* 56:363–367, 1980.
97. Tramont EC: Persistence of treponema pallidum following penicillin therapy. *JAMA* 236:2206–2207, 1976.
98. Institute of Medicine. *New Vaccine Development: Establishing Priorities.* Vol 1: *Diseases of Importance in the United States.* Appendix 1. Prospects for immunizing against herpes simplex viruses. Report by a committee at the Institute of Medicine. Washington, DC, National Academy Press, 1985.
99. Dowdle WR, Nahmias AJ, Harwell RW et al: Association of antigenic type of herpes virus hominis with the site of virus recovery. *J Immunol* 99:974–980, 1967.
100. Hill TJ: Herpes simplex virus latency, in Roizman B (ed): *The Herpes Virus,* Vol 3. New York, Plenum Press 1985, pp 175–240.
101. Corey L, Adams HG, Brown ZA, et al: Genital herpes simplex virus infections: Clinical manifestations, course, and complications. *Ann Intern Med* 98:958–972, 1983.
102. Brenton DW: Hypoglycorrhachia in herpes simplex type 2 meningitis. *Arch Neurol* 37:317, 1980.
103. Hemrika DJ, Schutte MF, Bleker OP: Elsberg syndrome: A neurologic basis for acute urinary retention in patients with genital herpes. *Obstet Gynaecol* 68(3 suppl):537–539, 1986.
104. Caplan LR, Kleeman FJ, Berg S: Urinary retention probably secondary to herpes genitalis. *N Engl J Med* 297:920–921, 1977.
105. Goodell SE, Quinn TC, Mkrtichian E, et al: Herpes simplex proctitis in homosexual men: Clinical, sigmoidoscopic and histopathologic features. *N Engl J. Med* 308:868–871, 1983.
106. Jacome DE, Yanez GF: Herpes genitalis and neurogenic bladder and bowel. *J Urol* 124:752, 1980.
107. Black D, Steward J, Melmed C: Sacral nerve dysfunction plus generalized polyneuropathy in herpes simplex genitalis. *Ann Neurol* 14:692, 1983.
108. Handler CE, Perkin GD, Fray R, et al: Radiculomyelopathy associated with herpes simplex genitalis treated with adenosine arabinoside. *Postgrad Med J* 59:388, 1983.
109. Klastersky J, Cappel R, Snoeck JM, et al: Ascending myelitis in association with herpes simplex virus. *N Engl J Med* 287:182, 1972.
110. Corey L, Fife KH, Benedetti JK et al: Intravenous acyclovir for the treatment of primary genital herpes. *Ann Intern Med* 98:914–921, 1983.
111. Bryson YJ, Dillon M, Lovett M, et al: Treatment of first episodes of genital herpes simplex virus infection with oral acyclovir: A randomized double blind control trial in normal subjects. *N Engl J Med* 308:916–921, 1983.
112. Smith D: Gonococcal meningitis. *Lancet* 1:1217, 1922.
113. Rice RJ, Schalla WO, Wittington WL, et al: Phenotypic characterization of *Neisseria gonorrhoeae* isolated from three cases of meningitis. *J Infect Dis* 153:362–365, 1986.

12

Diagnosis and Management of HIV Primary Dementia

FRANCISCO FERNANDEZ and JOEL K. LEVY

INTRODUCTION: DEMENTIA IN HIV DISEASE

Dementia is generally recognized as an acquired intellectual impairment characterized by persistent deficit in multiple areas including memory, language, cognition, visuospatial skills, personality or emotional functioning.[1] The acquired nature of dementia distinguishes it from mental retardation, whereas its persistence differentiates it from delirium. Dementia is largely a problem of elderly individuals, with approximately 20% of individuals over age 65 suffering from dementia.[2] The clinical syndrome of dementia may have multiple etiologies which may be either reversible or irreversible.[3] Table 1 presents the differential diagnosis of dementia and Table 2 lists the formal evaluation of a demented patient. In rare cases, the syndrome of dementia can occur in young individuals; however, this is the exception rather than the rule.

Individuals infected with the human immunodeficiency virus (HIV) manifest signs of the disease ranging from asymptomatic infection to fully developed acquired immune deficiency syndrome (AIDS).[4,5] Although the effects of HIV on the immune system are now well recognized, significant involvement of the central nervous system (CNS) has become evident with an alarming prevalence.[6–11] HIV-infected patients have presented with cognitive impairment, language disorders, movement disorders, psychosis, depression, delirium, and dementia. As the number of HIV-infected individuals increases, the neuropsychiatric complications of HIV will demand an increasing share of the health care professionals' time, the AIDS-related health care budget, and hospital and nursing home beds. Therefore, psychiatrists must have a working knowledge of HIV-related diseases in order to provide optimum and timely assessment and intervention with each individual. For psychiatrists, this implies that in any case in which infection may be possible (and in the future this may include anyone), a broadening of theoretical approaches will be required to include a neuropsychiatric perspective. In other words, with HIV disease, any symptoms of a psychiatric nature must be considered to be organic until proved otherwise, so that prompt medical intervention may be rendered. Physicians and other health profes-

FRANCISCO FERNANDEZ • St Luke's Episcopal Hospital, Houston, Texas 77030; Department of Psychiatry and Behavioral Sciences, Baylor College of Medicine, Houston, Texas 77030. JOEL K. LEVY • Department of Psychiatry and Behavioral Sciences, Baylor College of Medicine, Houston, Texas 77030.

TABLE 1. Etiologies of Dementia in HIV Disease

Systemic illnesses	Collagen vascular/vascular disorders
Infection	Hydrocephalus
Anemia	Seizure
Electrolyte imbalance	Anoxia
Hepatic/renal insufficiency	Cranial irradiation
Cardiomyopathy	Toxicities/drugs
Hemodynamic instability	Antiviral, antineoplastic, and immunorestorative agents
Pulmonary insufficiency	Alcohol/sedative hypnotics
Endocrinopathies	Anticholinergic agents
Addison's/Cushing's disease	Antibiotics and antifungals
Hypoglycemia	Narcotic analgesics
Thyroid and parathyroid disturbance	
Steroid treatment	
Deficiency states	
Vitamin B_{12} folate, niacin deficiency	
Malnutrition/malabsorption	
Trace elements	

sionals should be on guard for neuropsychiatric manifestations, including the cognitive decline frequently encountered in HIV-infected patients. Responding to this challenge demands an integrated, comprehensive, and systematic approach to identifying dementing illnesses in HIV disease, differentiating from among the many etiologies of dementia in HIV spectrum disorders, and developing management programs that will include the use of adjunct psychopharmacological agents. This chapter addresses the clinical features of the dementing illness associated with HIV disease which are relevant for the practice of psychiatry and offer suggestions on the management of the psychiatric complications associated with HIV primary dementia.

NEUROPSYCHIATRIC ISSUES IN HIV-RELATED ILLNESS

Psychiatric complications in HIV infection are prevalent. Many patients show evidence of a mood disturbance and organic mental disorder. Yet, investigators have noted the psychiatric consultations are requested for only a few of these patients.[12] This lack of consultation is surprising considering the high incidence of psychiatric morbidity in this population. The neuropsychiatric and psychosocial factors of HIV disorders must be jointly considered, as there is no other life-threatening disorder in which both facets are as prevalent as with HIV infection. When patients with HIV infection manifest an abnormal mental or emotional state, medical causes must be systematically reviewed for evidence of central nervous system disturbance. The onslaught of this disease complex upon the patient's mental health is multifactoral and one must consider the possible neuropsychiatric basis of these disturbances and consider them first before ruling in any of the multiple psychological/psychosocial complications as the sole source of the patient's problem.

Disorders of cognitive function in HIV disease continue to be considered a terminal

TABLE 2. Evaluation of Dementia in HIV Disease

History

GDS stage[a]	Clinical stage
1	Normal: no cognitive decline
2	Forgetfulness: subjective complaints
3	Early confusional: mild cognitive decline
4	Late confusional: moderate cognitive decline
5	Early dementia: moderately severe cognitive decline
6	Middle dementia: severe cognitive decline
7	Late dementia: global deterioration

Physical and neurological examination (for the psychiatrist)
- State of consciousness: level, variability
- Pattern of breathing
- Size and reactivity of pupils
- Eye movements and vestibular response
- Motor responses (including psychomotor)

Psychiatric (mental status)
- Cognitive: attention, concentration, memory, abstraction
- Affective: apathy, irritability, startle, lability
- Perceptual: hypersensitivity, illusions, hallucinations
- Physiological: sleep–wake, headache, weakness
- Behavioral: impulsivity, tact, activities of daily living

Clinical laboratory assessment[b]

CBC	Urinalysis
BUN, creatinine	Blood gases
FBS	CT scan of the brain
VDRL	Chest radiography
CMV, EBV, *Toxoplasma, Candida,* herpes, and cryptococcal serologies	Liver enzymes, bilirubin, ammonia
Electrolytes	Ca, P, alkaline phosphatase
Liver function tests	T4, T3 uptake, TSH
Vitamin B_{12}, folate	EEG
Serum cortisols	CSF
	Magnesium, zinc
	Toxic screen

[a]Global Deterioration Scale from Reisberg et al.[3a]
[b]Recommended battery for HIV

event, involving opportunistic infections or neoplasia in the brain, and Table 3 includes the many opportunistic infections and neoplasias which may occur. Also, the encephalopathic effects of systemic sepsis, electrolyte imbalances, multifocal leukoencephalopathy, temporal lobe dysrhythmias, and other metabolic involvements in end-stage HIV disease may secondarily alter cognitive status.

Nonetheless, ample evidence is now available that HIV itself can cause serious cognitive dysfunction early in the course of HIV infection.[10,11,13,14] Table 4 lists the neuropsychiatric signs and symptoms seen early in the course of the AIDS dementia

TABLE 3. Central Nervous System Infections and Malignancies Associated with HIV[a]

Subacute encephalitis
Atypical aseptic meningitis
Herpes simplex virus encephalitis
Progressive multifocal leukoencephalopathy
Varicella–zoster virus encephalitis or vasculitis
CMV encephalitis
Toxoplasma gondii
Cryptococcus neoformans
Candidiasis
Aspergillus
Coccidioidomycosis
Mycobacterium tuberculosis
Atypical mycobacteria
Primary or secondary CNS lymphoma
Kaposi's sarcoma

[a] Adapted from Bredesen et al.[12a]

complex. Table 5 lists the profound, later-stage disabilities of this dementing illness. The incidence of these disorders in HIV infection is unknown, given that cognitive impairment can occur at any time during infection and that exact numbers of seropositive individuals are unavailable. Some clinical studies project that most HIV-infected patients will develop an organic mental disorder some time during the course of the illness, the most common being dementia.[15]

Early indications of HIV cognitive involvement may be mild and, as such, are frequently attributed to the systemic illness or a psychological reaction to HIV infection.

TABLE 4. Early Manifestations of Dementia in HIV Disease[a]

Complaints/symptoms	Signs/findings
Memory loss	Psychomotor slowing
Impaired concentration	Memory dysfunction
Comprehension difficulties	Impairment of information processing
Conceptual confusion	Mild to moderate constructional difficulties
Apathy	Visuospatial disorganization
Depressive mood	Mild frontal lobe dysfunction
Agitation	Dysgraphia
Psychotic features	Dysarthria/dysnomia
Unsteady gait	Mild–moderate cerebellar dysfunction
Tremor	Hyperreflexia
Clumsiness	
Motor weakness	

[a] Adapted from Brew et al.[14a]

TABLE 5. Late Manifestations of Dementia in HIV Disease[a]

Global cognitive dysfunction
Mutism
Aphasia
Amnestic features
Frontal lobe disturbance
Dominant and nondominant parietal lobe signs
Organic hallucinosis
Weakness
Spasticity
Dyskinesia
Parkinsonism
Ataxia
Myoclonus
Incontinence
Seizures

[a] Adapted from Brew et al.[14a]

For instance, the dementing complaint of patients, such as forgetfulness, difficulty in attention and concentration, slowing of cognitive functions, and loss of interest in everyday activities, can often be misinterpreted as a reactive depression secondary to having contracted HIV disease. Often, these changes are viewed as "appropriate" in light of the awareness of the anticipated disability and the threat of death that HIV infection implies. Under the influence of this degenerative and destructive process, many patients will be cognizant of their own mental and physical sluggishness and personality changes, and affective symptoms may occur concomitantly. Psychosis, mania, and motor disturbances may predominate the clinical picture later. The course of the AIDS dementia complex steadily worsens with the development of moderate to severe cognitive deficits, confusion, psychomotor slowing, and seizures. Patients, at times, appear mute and catatonic. Socially inappropriate behavior and marked motor abnormalities include ataxia, spasticity, hyperreflexia, and incontinence of bladder and bowel.

The neuropathology associated with HIV–CNS involvement predominantly involves the white matter and deep gray nuclei, particularly the basal ganglia[16] and the mesolimbic system.[17] The distribution of HIV in the brain closely parallels these neuropathological changes.[18] Positron emission tomographic (PET) scans of cognitively impaired or behaviorally disturbed HIV patients reveal characteristic alterations in regional cerebral metabolic rate for glucose.[19] Subcortical hypermetabolism is a characteristic of early HIV-related cognitive impairment, commensurate with severity and progression of disease as measured by neuropsychological testing. Neurocognitive deterioration was accompanied by corresponding PET changes with hypometabolism noted in cortical and subcortical gray matter. Spectral analysis electroencephalographic (EEG) techniques have also proved useful as a possible screening test for detecting early HIV involvement of the central nervous system.[20,21] Both techniques may also have a potential role for monitoring the efficacy of treatment with AZT[20–23] and other agents.

It is unclear as to how other laboratory findings relate to HIV primary dementia. In

TABLE 6. Correlation of Peripheral Blood Findings with Neuropsychological Markers in HIV Disease[a,b,c]

	WBC	TOT-T	T4	H/S
		ARC		
TMT-A	−0.38	0.04	0.014	0.07
TMT-B	0.02	0.25	0.25	0.06
LTS	0.45	−0.48	−0.38	−0.29
CLTR	−0.64	0.19	−0.03	0.03
MMSE	0.04	−0.08	−0.16	−0.15
		AIDS		
TMT-A	0.008	0.28	0.14	0.08
TMT-B	0.07	v.39	0.21	0.13
LTS	0.23	0.10	−0.36	0.13
CLTR	−0.34	−0.37	0.13	−0.06
MMSE	0.02	0.09	−0.12	0.01

[a]From Fernandez et al.[23a]
[b]$N = 80$ (nARC = 39, nAIDS = 41); $p > 0.5$ - Pearson correlation coefficients: all nonsignificant.
[c]*Abbreviations:* WBC, white blood cell count; TOT-T, total T-cell count; T4, T4 (T-helper cell) count; H/S, helper/suppressor ratio; ARC, AIDS-related complex; AIDS, acquired immune deficiency syndrome; TMT-A, Trail Making Test Part A; TMT-B, Trail Making Test Part B; LTS, Long-term storage (from the Selective Reminding Test); CLTR, continuous long-term retrieval (from the Selective Reminding Test); MMSE, Mini-Mental State Examination.

our studies of AIDS-related complex (ARC) and AIDS patients, no significant correlations were found between neuropsychological and behavioral markers and various blood indices (Table 6). Although others have also reported no significant correlation between CD4 : CD8 ratios, McArthur and colleagues reported a significant difference in CD4 subsets between early and late demented patients.[24] Other changes, particularly the CSF–β_2-microglobulin[25] have been noted to correlate with severity of dementia suggesting that it may be an early marker for HIV–CNS impairment.

IMPORTANCE OF NEUROPSYCHOLOGICAL TESTING

The recognition of these neuropsychiatric complications may be clouded due to the fact that this symptomatology typically overlaps with the medical and psychosocial dimensions of HIV disease. Because of the possibility of confusion between the psychosocial and organic factors and the danger of misdiagnosis and potential mismanagement, the necessary order of procedure begins with a comprehensive neurobehavioral assessment. With such an assessment, diagnostic issues of organic versus functional effects will be clarified and the test results will add much to the understanding of the patient's abilities to comprehend and comply with his or her treatment. In advanced HIV spectrum disorder, including the end stage associated with severe dementia, neurocognitive assessment may be limited only to noting behavioral observations. The range of cognitive impairment is therefore wide and, thus, as with any assessment of a medically ill patient, the selection of neuropsychological evaluative instruments will have to be based on the patient's endurance and ability to respond, rather than to apply standard lengthy comprehensive batteries.

HIV-related cognitive disorder has been characterized as a subcortical dementing process.[26,27] This description suggests that fundamental functions, such as alertness, arousal, motivation, attention, and timing, will be disrupted by HIV–CNS involvement. Subcortical dementia refers to the pattern of cognitive, behavioral, and affective deficits produced by diseases affecting predominantly subcortical structures and disrupting the functions that they mediate. This description suggests that instruments that reflect memory registration, storage, and retrieval, and psychomotor speed, and rate of information processing are essential in a test battery for the HIV subcortical dementing syndrome. Speech and motor system abnormalities may also appear, but these abnormalities contrast sharply with the aphasia, agnosia, amnesia, and abnormal motor function characteristic of disorders involving predominantly the cerebral cortex. Table 7 suggests a neuropsychological testing battery for evaluating not only the effects of HIV infection but also the effects of neurotoxicity from antiviral, immunorestorative, and other chemotherapeutic agents.

Elements of this battery may be added or omitted, depending on the patient's behav-

TABLE 7. HIV Neuropsychological Screening Battery[a,b]

General
Mini-Mental State Examination[39]
Memory
Verbal Selective Reminding Test[40]
Benton Visual Retention Test[41]
Rey–Osterrieth Complex Figure[42]
Language/Speech
Controlled Oral Word Association (from Benton Multilingual Aphasia Examination)[43]
Visual Naming Test (from Benton Multilingual Aphasia Examination)[43]
Orientation
Pfeiffer Short Portable Mental Status Questionnaire[44]
Benton Temporal Orientation Test[45]
Visuospatial
Bender–Gestalt Test[46]
Raven Progressive Matrices[47]
Intellectual/Executive/Psychomotor
Digit Span, Arithmetic, Digit Symbol from the WAIS or WAIS-R[48]
Trail Making Test, Parts A and B[49]
Wisconsin Card Sorting[42]
Finger Oscillation Test[49]
Grooved Pegboard[42]
Reaction Time—Simple Auditory, Simple Visual, and Four-Choice Visual[48]
Shipley Institute of Living Scale[50]
Stroop Color Word Test[51]

[a] From Fernandez.[17a]
[b] Suggested battery for evaluating the CNS effects of HIV infection and neurotoxic effects from antivirals and chemotherapeutic agents.

ioral status. The tests suggested require approximately 2 hr to complete and, for the most part, are repeatable or have alternate forms for followup through the course of the illness. Many of the elements have age-adjusted norms. Not only may this test battery be used to determine level of impairment in cognitive areas that may be affected by HIV primary dementia, but elements of the battery are also useful for detecting the earlier prodromal cognitive changes associated with delirium, the ever-present danger that haunts many hospitalized HIV patients. Thus, neuropsychological testing can answer a number of important questions in the care of HIV patients. Issues of competency and organic versus functional diagnosis can be addressed with the documentation provided by the tests. The test results are especially helpful if a baseline evaluation had been done early in the course of the patient's disorder such that quantification of cognitive changes can be noted. Finally, these considerations all have bearing on the appropriateness and type of clinical management and pharmacotherapy selected for the treatment of the neuropsychiatric disturbances encountered in HIV disease.

MANAGEMENT OF THE PATIENT WITH HIV PRIMARY DEMENTIA

Management of demented patients involves a multilevel strategy approach:

1. Etiologic diagnosis and disease-specific management
2. Management of behaviors produced by the dementia
3. Prevention of secondary complications
4. Support of the patient's significant others and family

One should avoid thinking of dementia as a unitary syndrome of brain failure. Dementia should be recognized as a complex clinical syndrome produced and aggravated by a multitude of different disease processes. Thus, proper management depends on identifying the etiologic disorder and instituting disease-specific treatment. For example, control of the secondary infectious processes with antibiotics, correction of underlying metabolic disturbances, elimination of neurotoxic agents, and management of secondary depressive syndromes will all be important in the care of HIV patients.

Obviously, a significant amount of the disability that demented HIV patients experience is not necessarily the direct result of existent degeneration. For example, additional morbidity may be produced by a delirium or coexisting sensory impairment superimposed on the dementia; other illnesses may also add to the disability. These may go undiagnosed because of the patient's social withdrawal and lack of ability to give an accurate medical history. With specific treatment of such secondary disorders, particularly delirium or depression, the possibility of reversing this excess disability exists.

Excess disability may also arise when friends and caretakers have unrealistic expectations and do not adapt to the demented patient's diminished cognitive capacity and behavioral dysfunction. Prevention, recognition, and treatment of all causes of disability in these patients can result in remarkable and gratifying improvement. Diagnostic vigilance is needed in all cases, but especially whenever there is a sudden deterioration.

When psychoactive agents are necessary to control abnormal behavior or psychosis, the use of neuroleptics should be considered. Minor tranquilizers in demented patients should be avoided, as they tend to disinhibit these individuals, further compromising their intellectual functioning. The agents may also possibly either aggravate or unmask a delirious process. Neuroleptics in these cases are the drugs of choice. However, we have found HIV patients to have an increased susceptibility to the untoward and adverse effects associated with these agents, specifically extrapyramidal reactions.[28] Nevertheless, marked clinical improvements can be obtained with the use of oral molindone, with few significant treatment-emergent side effects.[29] For agitated delirious HIV patients, intravenous (IV) haloperidol, either alone[30] or in combination with lorazepam[31] or hydromorphone,[32] may be used with minimal, if any, side effects.

Depression may accompany HIV primary dementia and can exacerbate any of the pre-existing neuropsychological impairments.[29,33,34] The standard guidelines for the treatment of depression in HIV-demented patients should be followed, as effective therapy may reverse at least a portion of the mental status deficits. However, many neurocognitively impaired HIV patients will be unable to tolerate the anticholinergic and antihistaminic side effects of these agents. We advocate the use of the psychostimulants, either methylphenidate or dextroamphetamine, in depressed HIV patients.[33–35] These agents are effective in remitting the major signs and symptoms of depression in demented patients without serious adverse affects. Psychomotor activation, appetite stimulation, and qualitative as well as quantitative improvement in higher cortical functions and in affect occur within hours to days. Treatment with methylphenidate can be initiated with 5–10 mg (or its equivalent in dextroamphetamine or pemoline) by mouth, feeding tube, or suppository and adjusted gradually. A typical schedule would be 5–20 mg of methylphenidate administered at 7:00 AM, 10:00 AM, and 1:00 PM. More than 30 mg/day is rarely needed, but doses of 90 mg/day may sometimes be required. In cases in which methylphenidate is ineffective, patients should be crossed over to dextroamphetamine. We have noted significant clinical improvement with this crossover in methylphenidate nonresponders.[35] We are unsure why this occurs, but we suspect that there is a differential effect on central catecholamine pools. Psychostimulant treatment is effective in treating the various depressive signs and symptoms of the different etiologies and can be safely continued for several weeks or months after the patient becomes asymptomatic. Thus, methylphenidate and dextroamphetamine can be used in HIV-infected patients with organic personality disorders and organic affective disorders with marked improvements in affective, behavioral, and cognitive disturbances.

For depressed, terminally ill HIV patients, IV amitriptyline also may be used.[36] Although not FDA approved for IV use, permission for compassionate treatment may be sought from one's institutional pharmacy. The specifics of this mode of treatment include an initial infusion of 10 mg of the commercially available injectable amitriptyline (FDA approved for intramuscular use) in 100 ml of either normal saline or 5% dextrose solution over precisely 90 min at bedtime. Doses are then adjusted by 5–10 mg nightly until the patient shows improvement in target symptoms, such as insomnia, tearfulness, and dysphoria. A rapid therapeutic response, equivalent to that of ECT, is often seen. Many times, individuals on home parenteral nutrition can be treated safely at home with IV amitriptyline.

As with patients experiencing dementia of other etiologies, attention must also be directed toward the family and significant others of the demented HIV patient.[37] Education should be the primary goal, and family members should be informed about the cause of the patient's changed behavior, any available treatments, the patient's prognosis, and realistic expectations. In addition, one must make sure to provide additional support, such as Home Health Aid and Visiting Nurses, to allow the patient to be maintained at home for an extended period of time. Legal advice should be sought early in the course of the illness to help the patient and family regarding future disposition and conservatorship issues.[38] Finally, supportive therapy, either individually or through HIV-oriented support groups, may help with the anticipated feelings of loss, grief, and guilt common among the patient and the family.

SUMMARY AND CONCLUSIONS

Dementia in patients with HIV infection is a common, serious, and often frustrating problem. The literature to date has focused largely on descriptive aspects and associated neuropathology. A further discussion of clinical treatment issues is needed to facilitate the effective management of individuals with primary HIV dementia. The clinical presentation of HIV dementia, including cognitive impairment and psychomotor changes in different settings, has been discussed. The progression of dementia clearly does not correlate with systemic infection or metabolic derangements. It is usually an insidious, progressive illness which can easily be mistaken for functional psychiatric syndromes.

In the future, we must continue to elucidate other causes of morbidity in HIV patients and to develop effective management strategies, including the use of psychopharmacologic agents. There is a need to extend palliative care in managing the complex psychosocial issues associated with HIV disease, given the significant proportion of HIV-infected patients who experience symptoms of an emotional or cognitive disturbance. However, despite the potential for effective use of psychotropic agents in the management of these symptoms, there remains a significant discrepancy between the prevalence of these disturbances and the use of psychotropic agents in HIV patients. We are unsure as to why psychotropic drugs are either underused or used inappropriately in this population. It is our impression that this may be secondary to a popular and long-standing bias against medical intervention for psychological symptoms, or *psychopharmacologic Calvinism* (the notion that untreated suffering builds character). Psychotropics clearly have an enormous therapeutic potential for either the cognitively impaired or demented HIV patients. Given the demonstrated effectiveness of psychostimulants in cognitively impaired HIV patients, a judicious trial of these agents is warranted.

With cure of HIV dementia presently impossible, effective palliation of the degenerative features must involve the skillful use of all the tools in the psychiatric physician's armamentarium. Through cognitive–behavioral strategies, supportive care, and appropriate pharmacotherapy, we should be able to improve higher cortical functioning, retard progression of symptomatology, and enhance the quality of life in this significant group of patients. Given the increasing prevalence of HIV dementia, knowledge of these clinical innovations becomes essential in the practice of psychiatry.

REFERENCES

1. *Diagnostic and Statistical Manual of Mental Disorders,* ed 3 revised. Washington, DC, American Psychiatric Association, 1987.

2. Cummings JL, Benson DF: *Dementia: A Clinical Approach.* Boston, Butterworths, 1983.
3. Cummings JL: Treatable Dementias. *Adv Neurol* 38:165–183, 1983.
3a. Reisberg B, Ferris SH, DeLeon MJ, et al: The Global Deterioration Scale (GDS): An instrument for the assessment of primary degenerative dementia (PPD). *Am J Psychiatry* 139:1136–1139, 1982.
4. Fauci AS, Masur H, Gelmann EP, et al: The acquired immunodeficiency syndrome: An update. *Ann Intern Med* 102:800–813, 1985.
5. Sande MA, Volberding PA: *The Medical Management of AIDS.* Philadelphia, WB Saunders Co., 1988.
6. Navia BA, Jordan BD, Price RW: The AIDS dementia complex. I. Clinical features. *Ann Neurol* 19:517–524, 1986.
7. Gabuzda DH, Hirsch MS: Neurologic manifestations of infection with human immunodeficiency virus: Clinical features and pathogenesis. *Ann Intern Med* 107:383–391, 1987.
8. Navia BA, Price RW: The acquired immunodeficiency syndrome dementia complex as the presenting or sole manifestation of human immunodeficiency virus infection. *Arch Neurol* 44:65–69, 1987.
9. McArthur JC: Neurologic manifestations of AIDS. *Medicine* (Baltimore) 66:407–437, 1987.
10. Tross S, Price RW, Navia B, et al: Neuropsychological characterization of the AIDS dementia complex: A preliminary report. *AIDS* 2:81–88, 1988.
11. Price RW, Brew B, Sidtis J, et al: The brain in AIDS: Central nervous system HIV-1 infection and AIDS dementia complex. *Science* 239:586–592, 1988.
12. Perry SW, Tross S: Psychiatric problems of AIDS inpatients in the New York Hospital: Preliminary report. *Public Health Rep* 99:200–205, 1984.
12a. Bredesen DE, Levy RM, Rosenblum ML: The neurology of human immunodeficiency virus infection. *Quart J Med* 68:665–667, 1988.
13. Grant I, Atkinson JH, Hesselink JR, et al: Evidence for early central nervous system involvement in the acquired immunodeficiency syndrome (AIDS) and other human immunodeficiency virus (HIV) infections: Studies with neuropsychologic testing and magnetic resonance imaging. *Ann Intern Med* 107:828–836, 1987.
14. Janssen RS, Saykin AJ, Kaplan JE, et al: Neurological complications of human immunodeficiency virus infection in patients with lymphadenopathy syndrome. *Ann Neurol* 23:49–55, 1988.
14a. Brew BJ, Sidtis JJ, Petito CK, Price RW: The neurologic complications of AIDS and human immunodeficiency virus infection, in Plum F (ed), *Advances in Contemporary Neurology*. Philadelphia, F.A. Davis Company, 1988, pp. 1–49.
15. Catalan J: Psychosocial and neuropsychiatric aspects of HIV infection: review of their extent and implications for psychiatry. *Psychosom Res* 32:237–248, 1988.
16. Navia BA, Cho ES, Petito CK, et al: The AIDS dementia complex. II. Neuropathology. *Ann Neurol* 19:525–535, 1986.
17. Hill JM, Farrar WL, Pert CB: Localization of the T4 antigen–monkey and rat brain: Prominence in cortical regions. *Psychopharm Bull* 22:689–694, 1986.
18. Pumarola-Sune T, Navia BA, Cordon-Cado C, et al; HIV antigen in the brains of patients with the AIDS dementia complex. *Ann Neurol* 21:490–496, 1987.
19. Rotterberg DA, Moeller JR, Strother SC, et al: The metabolic pathology of the AIDS dementia complex. *Ann Neurol* 22:700–706, 1987.
20. Parisi A, Di Perri G, Strosselli M, et al: Testing for neurological involvement in HIV infection. *Lancet* 2:1531–1532, 1987.
21. Parisi A, Di Perri G, Strosselli M, et al: Usefulness of computerized electroencephalography in diagnosing, staging and monitoring AIDS-dementia complex. *AIDS* 3:209–213, 1989.
22. Yarchoan R, Brouwers P, Spitzer AR, et al: Response of human immunodeficiency virus associated neurological disease to 3′-azido-3′-deoxythymidine. *Lancet* 1:132–135, 1987.
23. Brunetti A, Berg G, Di Chiro G, et al: Reversal of brain metabolic abnormalities following treatment of AIDS dementia complex with 3′-azido-2′,3′-dideoxythymidine (AZT, zidovudine): A PET–FDG study. *J Nucl Med* 30:581–590, 1989.
23a. Fernandez F, Levy JK, Pirozzolo FJ: Neuropsychological and immunological abnormalities in advanced HIV infection, *Abstracts of the WHO Fifth International Conference on AIDS,* Montreal, Quebec, Canada, International Development Research Center, 1989.
24. McArthur JC, Sipos E, Chupp M, et al: Immunocytochemical straining of blood and cerebrospinal fluid mononuclear cells in AIDS-spectrum disorders. *Neurology (NY)* 37:319, 1987 (abst).

25. Brew BJ, Bhalla RB, Fleischer M, et al: Cerebrospinal fluid β-2 microglobulin in patients infected with human immunodeficiency virus. *Neurology (NY)* 39:830–834, 1989.
26. Albert ML: Subcortical dementia, in Katzman R, Terry RD, Bick KL (eds): *Alzheimer's Disease: Senile Dementia and Related Disorders.* New York, Raven Press, 1978, pp. 173–180.
27. Van Gorp WG, Mitrushina M, Cummings JL, et al: Normal aging and the subcortical encephalopathy of AIDS. *Neuropsychiatry Neuropsychol Behav Neurol* 2:5–20, 1989.
27a. Fernandez F: Anxiety and the neuropsychiatry of AIDS. *J. Clin Psychiatry* 50(11, suppl):9–14, 1989.
28. Fernandez F, Levy JK, Mansell PWA: Management of delirium in terminally ill AIDS patients. *Int J Psychiatr Med* 19:165–172, 1989.
29. Fernandez F: Pharmacotherapy of HIV related dementia, in *American Psychiatric Association's AIDS Primer.* Washington, DC, American Psychiatric Association, 1987, pp. 5–27.
30. Cassem NH: Critical care psychiatry. in Shoemaker WC, Thompson WL, Holbrook PR (eds): *Textbook of Critical Care.* Philadelphia, WB Sanders, 1984, pp 981–989.
31. Adams F, Fernandez F, Anderson B: Emergency pharmacotherapy of delirium in the critically ill cancer patient: Intravenous combination drug approach. *Psychosomatics* 27(suppl):33–38, 1986.
32. Adams F: Delirium: An optimal treatment approach. *Hosp Ther* January:29–42, 1987.
33. Fernandez F, Adams F, Levy JK, et al: Cognitive impairment in AIDS related complex and its response to psychostimulants. *Psychosomatics* 29:38–46, 1988.
34. Fernandez F, Levy JK, Galizzi H: Response of HIV related depression to psychostimulants: Case reports. *Hosp Community Psychol* 39:628–631, 1988.
35. Holmes VF, Fernandez F, Levy JK: Psychostimulant response in ARC/AIDS patients. *J Clin Psychol* 50:5–8, 1989.
36. Fernandez F, Adams F, Levy JK, et al: Depression and cancer: An update. *Texas Med* 82:46–49, 1986.
37. Woods AM, Niederehe G and Fruge E: Dementia: A family systems perspective, in Zarit SH (ed): *Generations: Quarterly of the American Society on Aging.* San Francisco, 1985.
38. Fernandez F, Levy JK, Holmes VF, et al: Critical care issues in HIV spectrum disorders, in Wise MG (eds): *Problems in Critical Care.* Philadelphia, JB Lippincott, 1988, pp 159–170.
39. Folstein MF, Folstein SE, McHugh PR: "Mini-Mental State": A practical method for grading the cognitive state of patients for the clinician. *J Psychiatr Res* 12:189–198, 1975.
40. Levin HS: Learning and memory, in Hannay HJ (ed): *Experimental Techniques in Human Neuropsychology.* New York, Oxford University Press, 1986.
41. Benton AL: *Revised Visual Retention Test,* ed 4. New York: The Psychological Corporation, 1974.
42. Lezak MD: *Neuropsychological Assessment,* ed 2. New York, Oxford University Press, 1983.
43. Benton AL, des Hamsher K: *Multilingual Aphasia Examination.* Iowa City, The University of Iowa, 1983.
44. Pfeiffer E: A short portable mental status questionnaire for the assessment of organic brain deficit in elderly patients. *J Am Geriatr Soc* 23:433, 1975.
45. Benton AL, des Hamsher K, Varney NR, Spreen O: *Contributions to Neuropsychological Assessment: A Clinical Manual.* New York, Oxford University Press, 1983.
46. Lacks P: *Bender Gestalt Screening for Brain Dysfunction.* New York, John Wiley & Sons–Interscience, 1984.
47. Raven JC, Court JH, Raven J: *Manual for Raven's Progressive Matrices and Vocabulary Scales.* Section 3: *Standard Progressive Matrices.* London, H.K. Lewis & Co., Ltd., 1983.
48. Golden CJ: *WAIS—R Manual.* New York, The Psychological Corporation, 1981.
49. Golden CJ, Osmon DC, Moses JA Jr, et al: *Interpretation of the Halstead–Reitan Neuropsychological Test Battery: A Casebook Approach.* New York, Grune & Stratton, 1981.
50. Pirozzolo FJ, Christensen KJ, Ogle KM, et al: Simple and choice reaction time in dementia: Clinical implications. *Neurobiol Aging* 2:113, 1981.
51. Golden CJ: *Stroop Color and Word Test: A Manual for Clinical and Experimental Uses.* Chicago: Stoelting Company, 1978.

13

HIV Disease

Brain–Behavior Relationships

IGOR GRANT, JOHN R. HESSELINK, CAROLINE J. KENNEDY, and J. HAMPTON ATKINSON III

INTRODUCTION

The earliest reports in the literature of the syndrome we now term acquired immune deficiency syndrome (AIDS) date to 1981.[1,2] Although the initial focus was, and continues to be, the consequences of deficiency of cell-mediated immunity in terms of multiple opportunistic infections, and susceptibility to neoplasia such as Kaposi's sarcoma and lymphomas, reports of neuropsychiatric complications began appearing as early as 1982. Horowitz et al.[3] described nine patients with retinopathy, seven of whom had neurological involvement, which included mental status changes and seizures. These investigators commented that cerebral atrophy and focal lesions were seen on some of the computed tomography (CT) scans and that pathological findings in the three cases that went on to autopsy included acute necrotizing encephalitis with vasculitis due to cytomegalovirus (CMV), multifocal necrotizing toxoplasmosis, and multifocal cerebritis. Britton et al.[4] described four homosexual men with neurological complications. Three of these patients had organic psychosis with paranoid delusions, hostility, and agitation. One of these three also had quadriparesis, resting tremor, rigidity, and dystonia. All three patients had generalized seizures. Autopsy in three of these cases showed changes consistent with encephalitis, and it was suggested that CMV was implicated. A fourth case presented with progressive multifocal leukoencephalopathy (PML) with papovavirus being documented at biopsy.

An autopsy series of 50 brains revealed neuropathology in 18.[5] The most common finding was an encephalitis, which Snider et al.[5] termed *subacute encephalitis*. Clinical manifestations before death included subtle cognitive deficits, disturbances in affect, motivation, and social activity. With mounting clinical experience, the features of *subacute encephalitis* have become defined more clearly. The term AIDS dementia complex (ADC) is now used to describe this neuropsychiatric syndrome.

IGOR GRANT and J. HAMPTON ATKINSON III • Psychiatry Service, San Diego Veterans Administration Medical Center, San Diego, California 92161; Department of Psychiatry, University of California, San Diego, School of Medicine, La Jolla, California 92093. JOHN R. HESSELINK • Psychiatry Service, San Diego Veterans Administration Medical Center, San Diego, California 92161; Department of Radiology, University of California, San Diego, School of Medicine, La Jolla, California 92093. CAROLINE J. KENNEDY • Psychiatry Service, San Diego Veterans Administration Medical Center, San Diego, California 92161; Department of Medicine, University of California, San Diego, School of Medicine, La Jolla, California 92093.

AIDS DEMENTIA COMPLEX, OR AIDS-ASSOCIATED ORGANIC MENTAL DISORDER

The term AIDS dementia complex was proposed by Price and associates.[6] Although we will use the term ADC in deference to the pioneering work of the Memorial Sloan–Kettering investigators in this area, we find this designation problematic. It connotes a severity of disturbance and inexorability of prognosis which may not be justified in many instances. We simply do not know the natural history of neuropsychiatric involvement in AIDS well enough to speculate whether decline into profound dementia is inevitable, or whether alternative outcomes are possible, e.g., mild stable cognitive deficit; or even reversibility of deficit with effective antiviral treatment. A term such as "AIDS-associated organic mental disorder," while more cumbersome, may actually be more precise. Within such a designation, it is then possible to talk about acute, subacute, and chronic progressive clinical courses.

EARLY FINDINGS IN ADC/AAOMD

Navia and Price[6] suggested that general mental and motor slowing may be the most common early sign of neuropsychiatric involvement of AIDS. There may be subjective slowness of thinking, impaired concentration, and apathy. Patients may also notice difficulties in learning new material and in recalling old information, as well as experiencing some unsteadiness in gait, leg weakness, incoordination, and tremor.

On mental status and neurological examination, the patient may have difficulty performing tasks such as serial sevens and may appear to be motorically slowed. Specific neurological examination may reveal impairment in the performance of rapid alternating movements, gait ataxia, hyperreflexia, tremor, dysarthria, and impaired smooth pursuit eye movements. Patients can have mild abnormalities on neurological examination with no apparent mental status findings and vice versa. Indeed, even if the patient has subjective complaints of cognitive inefficiency, the usual "bedside" mental status examination (MSE) may be entirely normal.

LATER SIGNS OF ADC/AAOMD

Those who enter a progressive phase of neuropsychiatric deterioration may evidence psychomotor and mental retardation, a vacant stare, poverty of ideation, severe distractibility, and marked language difficulties, including problems in word finding and comprehension. There may be profound disinhibition and lack of awareness of the illness. A psychotic state, with auditory and visual hallucinations and delusions of suspiciousness or grandiosity can sometimes be found.

Clinical examination may reveal either an apathetic or severely agitated individual whose orientation may be impaired. Patients may have loose associations, perseveration, flight of ideas, varying forms of aphasia, and mutism. Some patients have extreme circumstantiality. Psychotic individuals may evidence any one of a number of delusions as well as hallucinations in any sensory sphere, including auditory. Some patients appear to be profoundly depressed, reminiscent of depressive or catatonic stupor. Others can become severely regressed and incontinent. Neurological findings include spasticity, hyperreflexia, extensor plantar responses, myoclonus, and muscle weakness, greater in the lower extremities. Some patients will show a positive glabella tap; others will have seizures.

The natural history of the progression of neuropsychiatric change is not well understood at this time. At our own center, we have seen cases exhibiting the deteriorating course described by Navia and Price.[6] We have also followed patients with mild neuropsychological deficits for a year or more with no evidence of progression. Still other patients have shown improvement, in some cases related to successful treatment of secondary infections (e.g., toxoplasmosis).

ADC/AAOMD PRESENTING AS A PRIMARY PSYCHIATRIC DISORDER

Whereas depression, anxiety, and other psychiatric symptoms can accompany the diagnosis of AIDS, much as occurs with other debilitating and life-threatening medical diseases,[7] severe psychopathology can also be a presenting feature of ADC/AAOMD. The psychiatric presentation can include profound depression, with lethargy and retardation, paranoia with hallucinations, and, more uncommonly, mania. Of the dozen case reports available at the time of this writing,[8–15] psychiatric symptoms appeared before major changes in cognitive function in seven.[11–15] Despite unremarkable findings on initial clinical assessment of sensorium, all seven cases ultimately progressed to dementia.

A case that we recorded previously serves as an illustrative example.[16] The patient was a 32-year-old bisexual male brought to the emergency room because of a 9-month history of increasing apathy, social withdrawal, and bizarre behavior. On mental status, he was agitated and distracted. His thinking was impoverished and his associations were loose. His affect was inappropriate, and he had delusions of thought control and appeared to be responding to auditory hallucinations. He was oriented to time, place, and person, and, although he had difficulty concentrating, had no problems with simple memory tests. After being admitted to psychiatry, he was found to have lymphadenopathy and skin lesions consistent with Kaposi's sarcoma. Over a period of a few days, he remained psychotic, but formal neuropsychological testing revealed defects in abstracting ability, concentration, information processing speed, and memory. CT scan revealed mild ventricular enlargement, but the magnetic resonance imaging (MRI) scan was interpreted as normal.

The patient's behavior was ultimately brought under control by haloperidol, 2–4 mg/da. This allowed him to be discharged to the care of relatives. He had to be rehospitalized four additional times, however, during the remaining 6 months of his life either to control new infections or exacerbations of his behavioral problems. After the patient's death secondary to pulmonary complications of AIDS, an autopsy was performed. Inspection of the brain revealed meningoencephalitis, ependymitis, and subependymal gliosis. Intracytoplasmic inclusions suggesting CMV were noted in astrocytes. This case, and others in the literature, indicate the importance of careful neuropsychological, neuroradiological, and neurological assessment of patients who are at-risk groups for AIDS, and who present with major psychopathology for the first time.

THE NEUROPSYCHOLOGY OF ADC/AAOMD

Whenever there are clinical grounds for suspecting that a disease is associated with organic mental disorder, it is desirable to confirm the presence of such cognitive deficit by means of neuropsychological testing. Neuropsychology provides a validated and reliable approach to defining the qualitative and quantitative features of neurocognitive disorder.[17]

The Memorial Sloan-Kettering Group presented results of neuropsychological testing of 43 newly diagnosed AIDS patients.[18,19] Only 14% of these patients had no neuropsychological impairment, 16% were impaired on at least one of nine tests administered, 28% on two to four tests, 23% on five to nine tests, and 19% were classified as having "severe" impairment. This group of investigators has speculated that the neuropsychological findings are consistent with "subcortical" dementia, with prominent features including psychomotor and mental slowing, reduction in spontaneity, and reduced flexibility. The same group of investigators has also been examining AIDS and ARC patients who do not have overt neurological symptoms.[20] They have found that AIDS patients had significant impairment in tests of motor speed, concentration, and visual–spatial performance.

Joffe et al.[21] and Rubinow et al.[22] compared neuropsychological impairment of AIDS patients who did not have any evidence of opportunistic infections with that of a matched set of controls. AIDS patients showed impairments on the Category test, on Trail Making part B, and on an attentional measure (cancellation procedure). These patients performed well on a constructional task involving copy of the complex Rey diagram.

Several groups, including our own, have been exploring the neuropsychological correlates not only of confirmed AIDS and ARC, but also of other HIV-infected groups who are asymptomatic or relatively less symptomatic. For example, Janssen et al.[23–25] examined homosexual men diagnosed as having lymphadenopathy syndrome (LAS). The mean duration since onset was approximately four years. They found that one half of LAS patients had some neuropsychological impairment. A limitation of this study was that the controls were considerably better educated (16 years versus 19 years).

Ayers et al.[26] employed the Luria–Nebraska neuropsychological battery (LNNB) to examine subjects in four groups: (1) those who had AIDS for 1 year or more ($N = 15$); (2) those with early AIDS (duration less than 3 months, $N = 13$); (3) ARC ($N = 15$); and (4) seronegative homosexuals ($N = 15$). Whereas the rate of impairment (defined as two or more LNNB scales in the impaired range) was 7% for the seronegatives, it was 40% for ARC, 54% for early AIDS, and 40% for established AIDS. Patients in the AIDS groups performed worse than the others on motor tasks, tactile sensation, receptive speech, reading, and memory. Interestingly, only two of the 21 MRI scans of AIDS patients reported by Ayers et al. showed any abnormality.

Our own group in San Diego has been involved in several neuropsychiatric studies of patients with AIDS, ARC, and other HIV-infected groups. Our initial pilot study[41] showed that 87% of 15 AIDS patients, 54% of 13 ARC patients, and 9% of immune normal seronegative homosexual men were impaired on a battery of tests that included measures of abstracting ability, learning and memory, flexibility, and information-processing speed. The AIDS group had the most pronounced neuropsychological findings, despite having no overt neurological signs at time of initial neuropsychological testing. Tests that significantly differentiated the AIDS group from the controls included performance on Halstead's Category test, story learning from the Wechsler Memory Scale, and paced auditory serial addition (PASAT).

Recently, we were able to perform more detailed neuropsychological assessments of 23 patients with AIDS and ARC as part of a randomized placebo-controlled clinical trial of azidothymidine (AZT). The neuropsychological results were rated in accordance with the method we have described previously.[27–30] On the basis of on these clinical ratings, 17% of AIDS and ARC patients were classified as definitely normal, 35% as atypical but not clearly impaired, and 48% as definitely impaired. In the impaired group, nine (39%) were thought to have mild deficits, whereas two (9%) had moderately substantial impairment.

BRAIN IMAGING IN ADC/AAOMD

There is a substantial literature on cranial CT in AIDS, and there are a growing number of reports using MRI as well. As is the situation with neuropsychology, the precise incidence and prevalence of changes measurable by brain imaging at various stages of HIV infection remain unknown. Most of the reports concerning CT and MRI have involved patients referred for neuroradiological study because neurological involvement was suspected on clinical grounds. The vast majority of such patients have evidence of brain atrophy—dilated ventricles and enlarged sulci—on CT.[5,31–33] One of the largest series of CT studies has emerged from the University of Miami/Jackson Memorial Hospital group.[34] Of 51 patients evaluated for intracranial symptoms, and in whom a neurological diagnosis was confirmed by nonradiological means, 76% had an abnormal CT. The most common abnormalities were the ring-enhancing lesions characteristic of *Toxoplasma gondii* encephalitis. A handful of patients had parenchymal lesions attributed to other causes. These included lesions that enhanced with contrast material and that were attributed to lymphoma, as well as hypodense lesions secondary to PML, CMV, and hemorrhage. There was evidence of brain atrophy in 28 of the 51 cases, all of whom had diffuse cortical sulcal enlargement and 14 of whom had ventricular dilatation.

The CT findings in the cases of pediatric AIDS have been even more dramatic, particularly in those with congenital AIDS. Cerebral atrophy is commonly reported,[35–37] and calcifications in the basal ganglia are observed frequently.[36,37] Some cases have been noted to have hypodense lesions in the centrum semiovale as well as mass lesions and infarctions.[36]

The MRI is coming to the forefront as an important tool for clinicians and investigators concerned with the neuropsychiatry of AIDS and HIV infection. Post et al.[38] demonstrated that the MRI is more sensitive to the presence of lesions than high-resolution-enhanced CT, although it may, on occasion, be less specific in sorting out edema from underlying pathology. The superior sensitivity of MRI has been confirmed by other investigators.[39,40]

The UCSD AIDS Study Group has been documenting patterns of brain involvement in AIDS and ARC using the MRI. The patterns observed in our initial study[41] can be summarized as follows:

1. Multiple small areas of high signal intensity, principally in subcortical white matter: These lesions resemble those seen in patchy viral encephalitis, and could represent HIV or CMV infection. In this study 9 of 13 AIDS patients and 5 of 10 ARC patients presented with such abnormalities (see Fig. 10 and 11 for examples).

2. Larger confluent areas of high signal, involving white matter principally (see Fig. 1). Between a quarter and one-third of AIDS/ARC patients' MRIs had such lesions, which might represent progression of the infective process represented by the type 1 pattern.
3. Ventricular dilation and sulcal enlargement: approximately one half of AIDS/ARC patients showed evidence of "brain shrinkage." (Fig. 11 and 13 illustrate mild cortical atrophy for a 39-year-old man).
4. Solitary focal abnormalities: 3 of 23 AIDS/ARC patients had single lesions including two that might have represented small strokes, and one with focal atrophy in the region of the temporal horn of the lateral ventricle.

It is unclear whether these solitary lesions are related to the AIDS process. In addition, approximately one half of AIDS/ARC patients with abnormal MRI had both a parenchymal lesion and evidence of cerebral atrophy.

NP, MRI, AND CLINICAL PRESENTATION: CASE STUDIES

The following cases, which we reported previously,[42] are presented to illustrate the types of neuropsychological and neuroradiological findings which can be associated with HIV infection.

Case A: Rapidly Progressive Neuropsychiatric Syndrome

Case A was 41 when he presented to the UCSD AIDS Group with symptoms of pneumonia which was determined to be due to *Pneumocystis carinii*. The diagnosis of AIDS was made in January. His medical condition stabilized for a period of 2 months. During February neuropsychological testing and MRI scanning were performed. A list of NP tests used in our studies, the area of cognitive function they are thought to assess, and cutoff scores for probable and definite impairment are displayed in Table 1.

Test results for case A are presented in Table 2. It can be seen that this patient was markedly impaired in most areas of higher cortical functioning despite scoring well on measures of verbal intelligence (WAIS-R vocabulary = 11) and simple attention (WAIS-R Digit Span = 12). The impairments included defects in abstract reasoning, speeded information processing, and memory.

The MRI scan is shown in Fig. 1. There are multiple areas of increased signal intensity within the white matter of both cerebral hemispheres. The right hemisphere is involved more than the left. The lesions have poorly defined margins and are confluent in many areas, particularly the right hemisphere. The pattern of abnormality is most consistent with a white matter encephalitis secondary to HIV or CMV.

Over the next 4 months Case A underwent progressive deterioration of cognitive function, which was readily apparent on clinical examination. Decline in episodic memory (i.e., learning and recalling new information) was complicated by disturbance in semantic memory, as judged by decline in fluency to letters. He also developed a painful, bilateral sensorimotor neuropathy. In the last months of his life Case A became so somnolent that he was unable to stay awake during neurological examination. The final neurologic exam with which he could cooperate to some degree revealed a man oriented to

TABLE 1. Neuropsychological Tests, Areas of Function They Are Thought to Reflect, and Criteria for Impaired Performance[a]

	Probable	Definite	
Vocabulary (scaled score)	6–7	0–5	Verbal intelligence
Digit span (scaled score)	6–7	0–5	Simple attention
Digit symbol (scaled score)	6–7	0–5	Speeded information
Category errors	50–60	>60	Abstraction
Trails B (time, sec)	85–99	>99	Speed and flexibility of thinking
Tactual performance test (total time)	15–18	>18	Perceptual motor speed, spacial learning
Finger oscillation (dominant) (taps in 10 sec)[b]	42–47	<42	Motor speed
Story learning (no. of trials to reach criterion)[c]	3	4,5	Verbal learning
Story recall (% loss after 1 hr)	25–30	>30	Verbal recall (forgetting)
Figure learning (no. of trials to reach criterion)[c]	3	4,5	Visual learning
Figure recall (% loss after 1 hr)	25–30	>30	Visual recall
Selective reminding (best score out of 6 trials)	7–8	<7	Verbal learning
Symbol digit paired associate learning (SDPAL) (correct, 4 trials)	16–21	<16	Associative learning
Paced auditory serial addition task (PASAT) (no. correct, trial 1)	25–35	<25	Speeded information processing
FAS	20–25	<20	Verbal fluency

[a]The criteria for "probable" and "definite" abnormality on these tests assume a young or mid-years (age ≤50) adult with a high school education.
[b]Criteria for men; subtract 5 for women.
[c]The criterion (minimum acceptable) score is 15 memories for the story "Anna Thompson" taken from the Wechsler Memory Scale (WMS) and 15 memories for the WMS figures, scored according to the method of Heaton, et al. A maximum of 5 trials is given.

year and month, but not place. His affect was flat, and he had difficulty following single commands. His speech was dysarthric. He displayed slow saccadic eye movements. Reflexes were generally hyporeflexic and a snout reflex was present. He had painful polyneuropathy of both lower extremities.

In the final weeks he developed urinary and fecal incontinence and became completely unable to care for himself. As a terminal event he developed pyelonephritis which responded poorly to treatment. Case A died 6 months after initial diagnosis.

Case B: Subclinical Organic Mental Disorder: Neuropsychological Abnormality Precedes MRI Findings

Case B is a 35-year-old accountant who was diagnosed as having AIDS in November, following a bout of pneumocystis pneumonia, from which he recovered uneventfully after treatment with Septra. His neuropsychometry and MRI were performed in March, the following year, at which time he was medically and neurologically asymptomatic. The NP testing and MRI were repeated 6 months later (he was in the placebo arm of an AZT trial during this period). His follow-up physical assessment, including a structured neurologic exam were unremarkable.

TABLE 2. Neuropsychological Test Results of Cases Presented

Test	Case A	Case B		Case B		Case B	
		Initial	Follow-up	Initial	Follow-up	Initial	Follow-up
WAIS–R							
Vocabulary	11	14	15	10	10	15	16
Digit Span	12	12	12	10	11	15	19
Digit Symbol	6	8	7	9	13	10	12
Category Test	104	79	91	80	60	9	5
Trail Making B	300	84	74	139	62	50	37
Tactual Performance Test (total time)	—	10.4	10.6	11.5	9.4	11.6	10.0
Tapping Test[a]	(78) 52	54	(66) 44	(67) 45	(77) 52	(67) 45	(70) 47
Story Learning (no. of trials)	>5	2	2	2	>5	1	2
Story Recall (% loss)	100	0	0	25	29	4	5
Figure Learning	>5	1	1	1	1	1	1
Figure Recall (% loss)	36	5	0	0	0	0	0
Selective Reminding—best of 6 trials	5	12	8	10	9	11	12
Symbol Digit PAL	2	28	28	16	18	28	28
PASAT (no. of correct—trial 1)	13	30	40	26	46	—	49
FAS	19	45	37	30	37	34	40

[a] In the AZT trial a nonstandard time of 15 sec was used. The values in parentheses are the actual taps in 15 sec; the other values are the estimated scores for a 10-sec (standard) trial, obtained by multiplying the 15-sec value by 0.67.

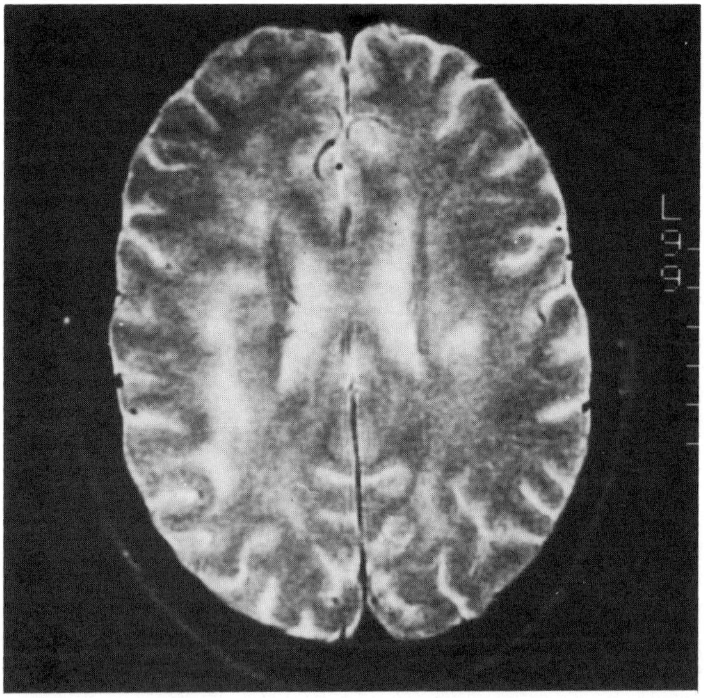

FIGURE 1. Case A shows multiple areas of increased signal intensity within white matter of both cerebral hemispheres.

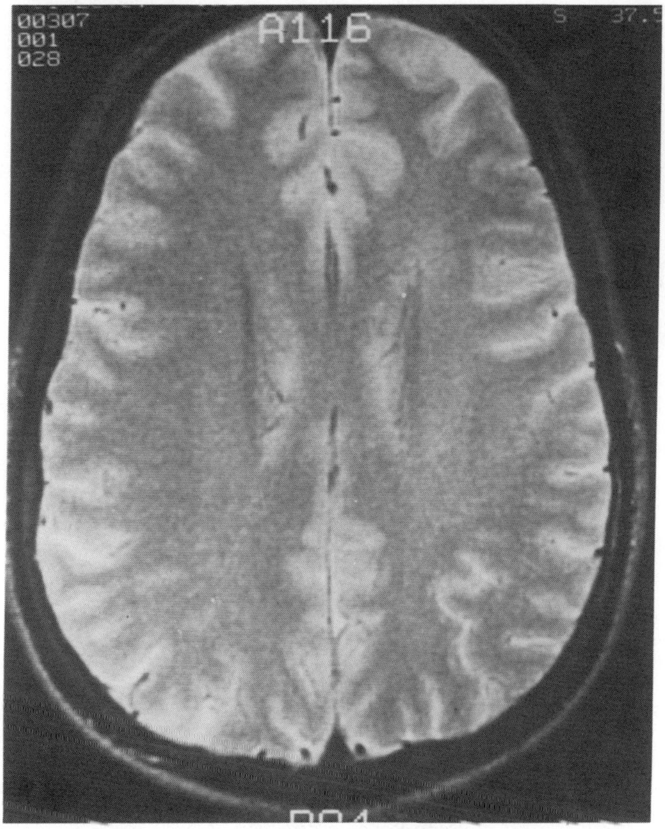

FIGURE 2. Case B shows normal magnetic resonance imaging scan initially.

Table 2 shows that case B had mild neuropsychological impairment at initial testing. Specifically, he was somewhat slowed in speeded information processing (PASAT, Digit Symbol) and made an unexpectedly large number of errors on the Category Test, a measure of abstraction. Despite these mild abnormalities, MR scans of the brain appeared normal in March (Figs. 2 and 3).

Six months later, although there was little change in general clinical symptomatology case B showed some further neuropsychological decline, particularly in measures related to abstraction, memory, and motor speed (Table 2). Concurrent MRI scanning revealed diffuse patchy regions of high signal intensity throughout the white matter of both cerebral hemispheres, which developed in the interval (Figs. 4 and 5). The lesions have poorly defined margins and are confluent in some areas. Inferior extension of the abnormality was noted in the internal capsules bilaterally. Once again, the MR findings appeared to be most consistent with white matter encephalitis, such as HIV or CMV encephalitis. At physical examination one year after initial testing, case B was still medically asymptomatic but at approximately 18 months he developed clinical signs of dementia as well as pneumocystis pneumonia. He was markedly demented at time of death, 20 months after initial assessment.

This case illustrates that the neuropathic process associated with AIDS can exist in a

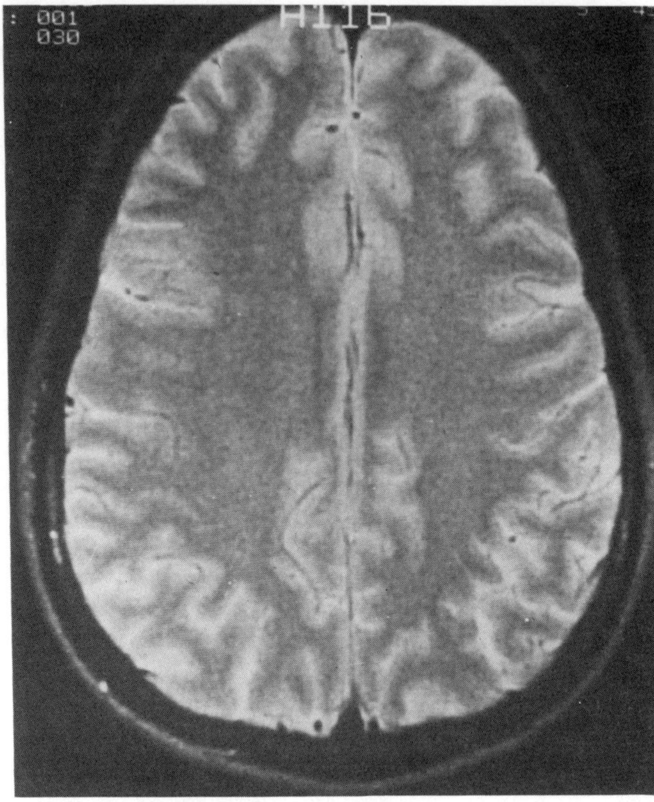

FIGURE 3. Case B, another section from initial scan.

subacute form, and can remain subclinical despite evidence of slowly progressive neuropsychological deficit. The appearance of MRI changes at a later stage suggests that the disease process might manifest itself first in subtle disturbance in brain function which can be detected by comprehensive neuropsychological testing, but which remains occult on the basis of MRI. With respect to case B, it seems possible that during the 6 months between first and second NP and MRI studies there was a progression of brain involvement by HIV with changes reaching a threshold which allowed visualization by MRI at second evaluation. Despite NP and MRI confirmation of brain disease, it is important to note that case B continued to be unremarkable on general physical and neurological exam, and remained employed as an accountant for over a year, before entering an accelerated phase of his illness.

Case C: Partial Reversal of CNS Findings Concurrent with a 6-Month Course of AZT

Case C was a 39-year-old fiscal clerk who was diagnosed as having AIDS in December. At the time he had marked lymphadenopathy and recurrent urinary tract infections. Mental status examination was abnormal, with reduced attention span and fluency. Neurologic exam was remarkable only for slowness of saccadic eye movements.

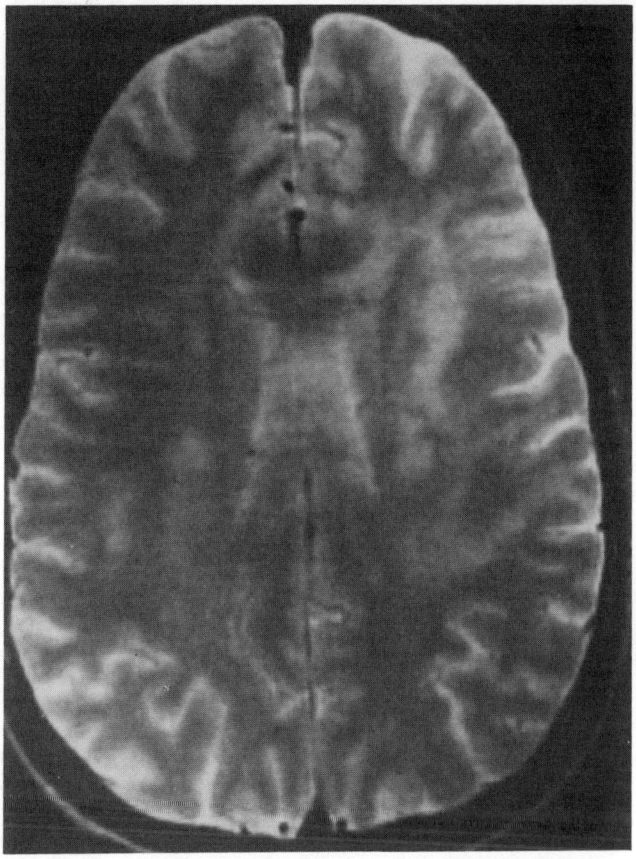

FIGURE 4. Case B shows new white matter lesions 6 months later.

The following February, prior to randomization as participant in a clinical trial of AZT, Case C received neuropsychological testing and MRI. The former revealed mild impairment of a broad range of cognitive functions, including difficulty with abstraction, memory, and speeded information processing (Table 2).

Images from the MRI showed areas of increased signal intensity within the basal ganglia and internal capsule, bilaterally (arrows, Fig. 6). The abnormality extends to the left inferiorly to involve the middle cerebral peduncle on the left side (arrowheads, Fig. 7). The lesions are fairly well defined and have a homogeneous internal texture. While these findings are non-specific and could represent toxoplasmosis or lymphoma, as well as HIV infection, the clinical course of this patient, as described below, renders the first two possibilities highly unlikely.

Case C was re-examined neuropsychometrically and by means of MRI after 6 months of treatment with AZT. The neuropsychological testing showed improvement on some tests, e.g. Trail Making B, Digit Symbol and PASAT, but deficits in abstraction and memory were still evident (Table 2).

By contrast, the 6 month follow-up MRI scan revealed complete resolution of abnor-

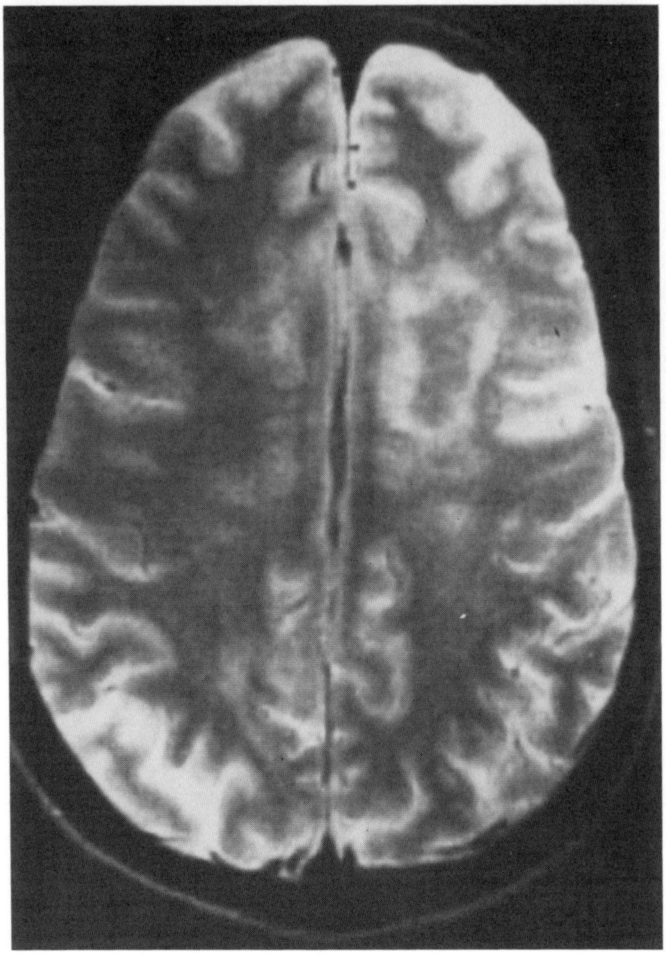

FIGURE 5. Another section from 6-month follow-up scan from case B showing white matter involvement especially in left hemisphere.

malities (Figs. 8, 9). Indeed, these scans were rated as normal for this individual's age.

On clinical examination during the interim Case C developed transiently a positive glabella tap and snout reflexes. At the most recent physical available (1 year later), case C had no remarkable neurological signs, and was deemed stable on continuing treatment with AZT. Case C died 23 months after first assessment without any gross signs of dementia.

Experience with case C suggests that AZT treatment might, in selected cases, be accompanied by resolution of brain lesions visualized by MRI. More troublesome are the neuropsychological findings which, while showing some improvement, also indicate persisting impairment. It has yet to be determined whether neurobehavioral abnormalities take longer to clear than do the sorts of neuroanatomic lesions seen on MRI. If so, then such slow normalization of cognitive function might be akin to the slowly reversible

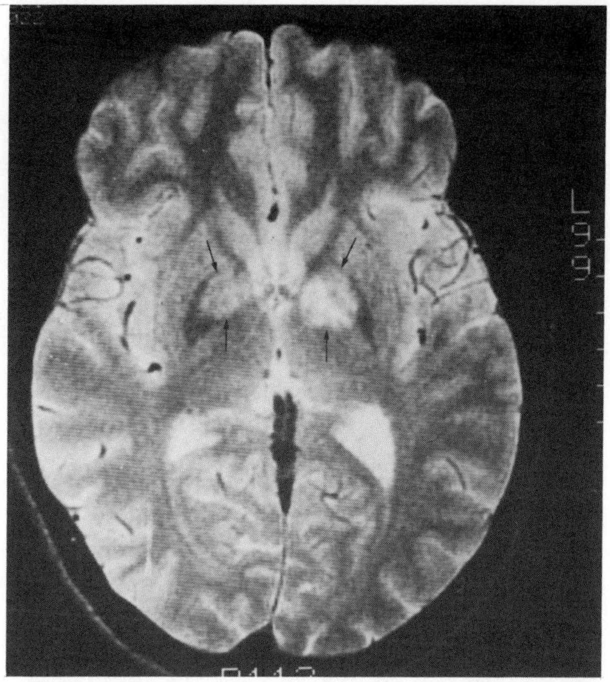

FIGURE 6. Initial scan from case C shows bilateral basal ganglia lesions (arrows).

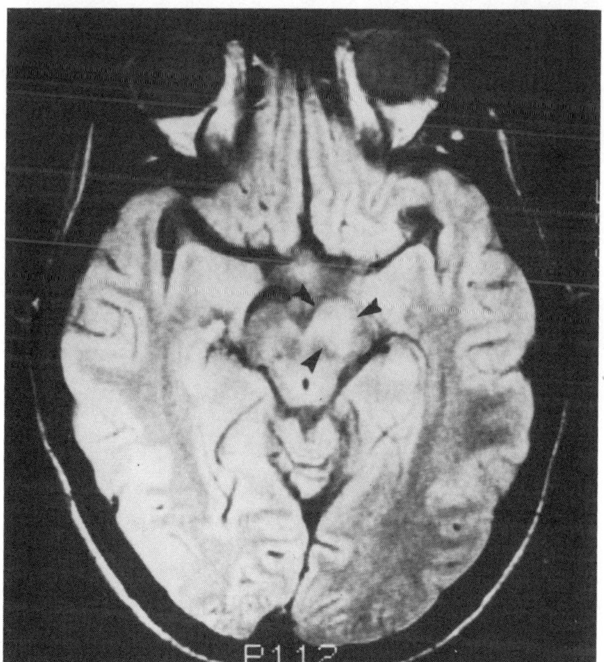

FIGURE 7. A more inferior section from the initial scanning of case C shows involvement of the left cerebral peduncle. (Note: left and right are reversed on this scan.)

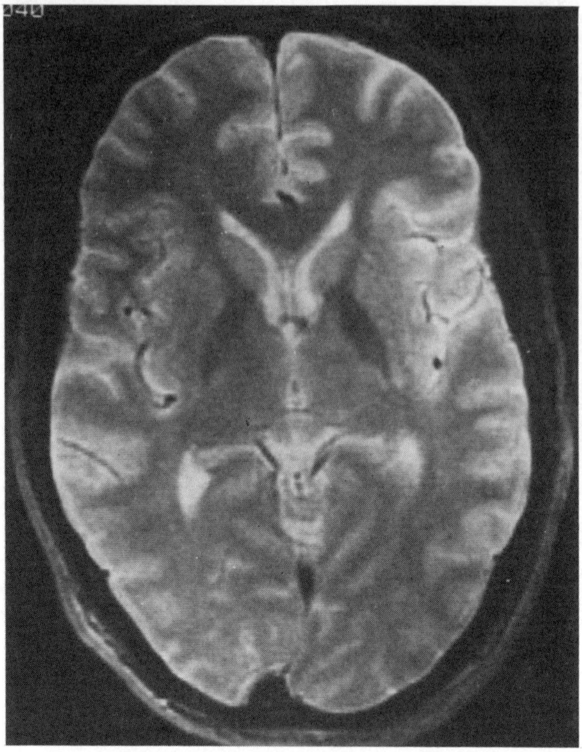

FIGURE 8. After 6 months, the magnetic resonance scan for case C is normal. This patient received AZT in the interim.

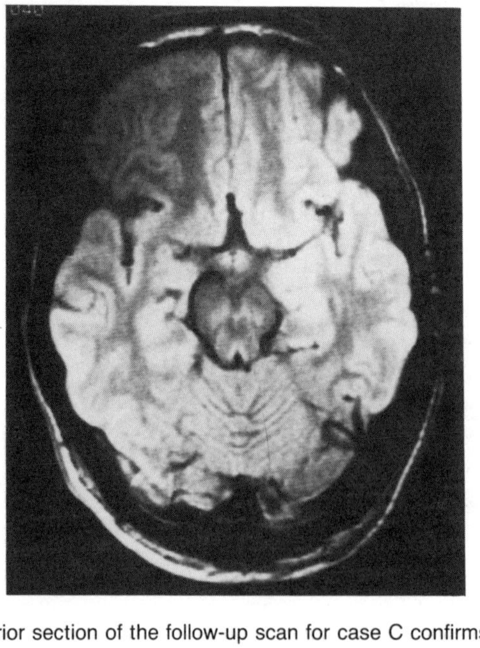

FIGURE 9. A more inferior section of the follow-up scan for case C confirms resolution of lesions.

intermediate duration organic mental disorders described among recovering alcoholics[43,44] or patients with head injuries.[45]

Alternatively, persisting neuropsychological deficit might reflect permanent injury, a residuum of the acute infective process, or continuing disease sputtering at a low level without provoking the marked edema or inflammatory response which would tend to be visualized by MRI.

Case D: Neuropsychological, MRI, and Clinical Neurological Signs Can Have Differing Natural Histories

Case D was a 39-year-old computer programmer who was diagnosed as having AIDS in February. He presented with CMV retinopathy and herpes simplex virus (HSV) related diarrhea. In April he was randomized into the active treatment arm of a 6-month clinical trial of AZT.

His prerandomization clinical exam revealed CMV retinopathy with cotton wool spots, present glabella sign and snout reflex, and slightly asymmetry of deep tendon reflexes. His mental status was unremarkable. The initial neuropsychological test results, obtained in April, are shown in Table 2. Beyond slight motor slowness, the neuropsychological evaluation was entirely normal.

In contrast, the initial MR scan taken a week later showed small focal punctate lesions (arrows, Figs. 10 and 11) within the white matter of the frontal lobes. There was also some cortical atrophy.

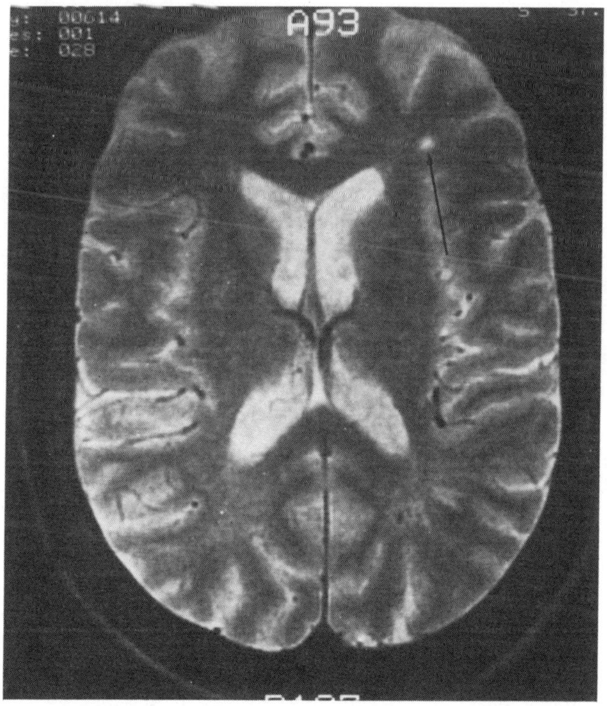

FIGURE 10. Case D shows small white matter lesions (arrow).

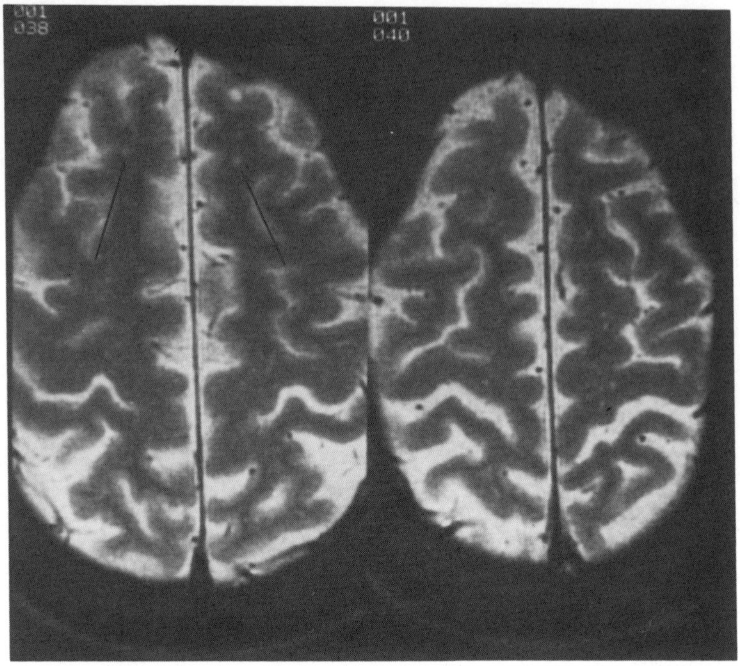

FIGURE 11. Another section from case D shows more punctate lesions and mild cortical atrophy.

Clinical examination of 6-month follow-up revealed clearing of the retinopathy, but evidence of peripheral neuropathy. Mental status was unremarkable but glabella sign and snout reflex persisted. Neuropsychological testing performed in October remained normal (Table 2). MRI scans obtained at the same time showed resolution of the two white matter abnormalities noted initially (Figs. 12 and 13). There was no change in degree of cortical atrophy. Approximately one year after initial assessment his peripheral neuropathy had worsened markedly. AZT was stopped because of leukopenia. Neuropsychological testing showed no decline in cognitive functioning. Case D died at 16 months with no evidence of CNS involvement.

This case illustrates that changes in peripheral neurological, cognitive, and neuroradiological indicators of HIV-associated CNS diseases need not parallel each other. Case D had definite but small parenchymal lesions in the frontal lobes. Evidently, for their location these lesions were not sufficiently large or active to be reflected in neuropsychological performance, even though tests sensitive to frontal lobe injury were administered. The lesions resolved after 6 months, during which time case D received AZT. Whether treatment was actually responsible for MR improvement remains speculative, although one report from a large multicenter series suggests psychometric improvement associated with AZT.[46] At the same time that MRI seemed to improve and NP stayed normal, case D developed peripheral neuropathy. This underscores that, in common with other diseases such as Wernicke–Korsakoff syndrome and vitamin B_{12} deficiency, central and peripheral signs need not coexist, and progression of neuropathy can be unrelated to neuropsychiatric symptomatology, and vice versa. It remains to be seen whether central and peripheral symptoms respond differently to various treatments.

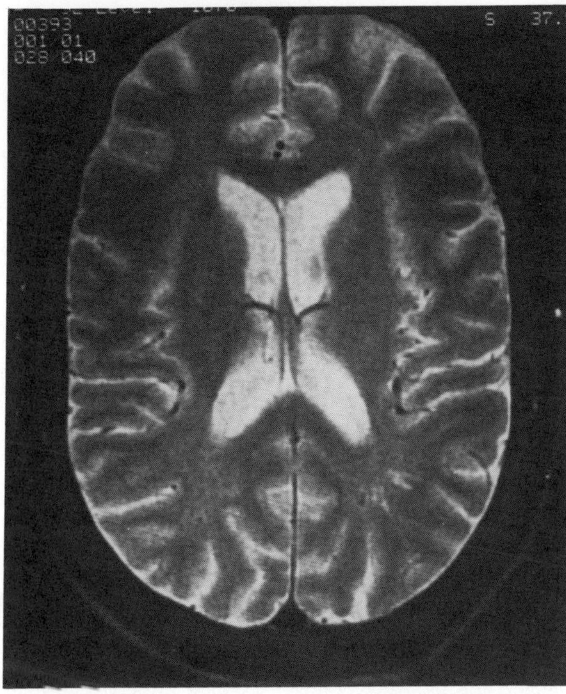

FIGURE 12. A 6-month follow-up of case D shows resolution of lesion noted earlier in Fig. 10.

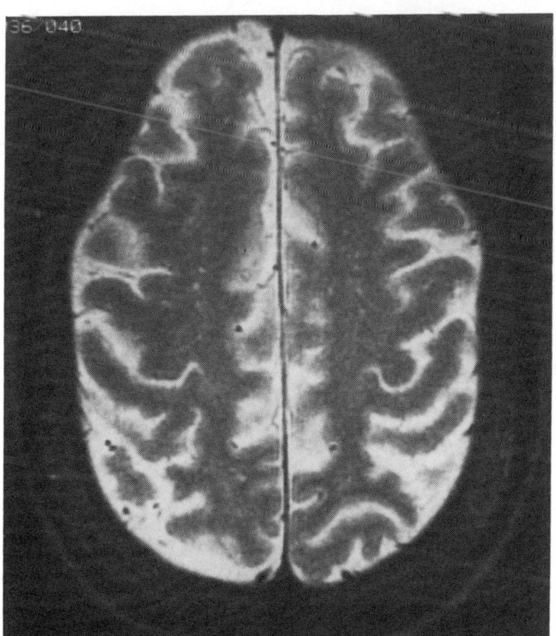

FIGURE 13. A more superior section from the 6-month follow-up scan for case D shows disappearance of previously noted frontal lesions (see Fig. 11). The patient received AZT in the interim.

SUMMARY

AIDS and related HIV syndromes are neuropsychiatric diseases even as they are infectious and immunological diseases. In the early days of AIDS research and treatment, psychiatrists, behavioral neurologists, and behavioral scientists came on the scene as an afterthought—to provide support or understanding to victims of a catastrophic illness, or to manage the occasional neurologic or neuropsychiatric complication. The data we have reviewed here, and information contained elsewhere in this book indicate that neuropsychiatric symptoms and signs are regular concomitants of HIV infection. Indeed, our preliminary results suggest that subtle cognitive changes can occur even in otherwise asymptomatic HIV seropositive homosexual men,[41] although some other investigators have not confirmed this.[20,47] Furthermore, retrovirus has been visualized in brain, and cultured from neural tissue and CSF.[48,49] Although the precise pathogenesis of HIV infection of the brain remains unclear, there is little doubt that many HIV seropositive individuals are at risk of developing an organic mental disorder. While the late stage of this disorder—AIDS-associated organic mental disorder (AAOMD)—is well recognized, we do not know the natural history of AAOMD. In what proportion of seroconverting persons does HIV enter the CNS? Which cells are infected? What is the mechanism of neural injury? How quickly do early cognitive signs develop? Is progression to dementia inevitable, or do some cases stabilize? What is the effect of antiviral treatments? It is possible that the brain disease can continue to progress despite improvement in immunodeficiency? What are the neuropsychiatric adverse effects of prospective treatments? From the data presented and the questions raised it is evident that neuroscientists and behavioral scientists will need to work closely with colleagues in virology and immunology to map the pathogenesis and natural history of AAOMD.

While the neuropsychological and MRI findings reviewed here indicate a higher prevalence of subclinical organicity than had heretofore been suspected, it would be imprudent to conclude that all HIV-infected persons are bound for dementia. Even among those with definitive AIDS, a proportion, perhaps as many as one third,[50] never develop neuropsychiatric symptoms. Through prospective studies of recent seroconvertors it should be possible, in the next several years, to estimate more accurately the incidence of brain involvement in the earlier stages of HIV-infection. Such research will need to combine psychiatric, neuropsychological, neurological, and radiological assessments, coupled with virologic study capable of documenting presence of HIV in cerebrospinal fluid, while excluding other organisms as causes of neuropathology. In the same vein, clinical trails must be sure to include comprehensive neuropsychiatric assessment to assure that potential treatments protect and heal the brain as well as the immune system.

ACKNOWLEDGMENTS. This work was supported in part by award SA 325 from the Medical Research Service of the Veterans Administration, by the University of California Universitywide AIDS Task Force, and by NIMH grant 1 RO1 MH43298-01. Some of the data presented in this review chapter have been reported previously in Grant et al., *Annals of Internal Medicine* 107:828–836, 1987 and in Grant et al., *J. Royal College of Physicians of London* 22:149–157, 1988.

REFERENCES

1. Gottlieb MS, Schroff R, Schanker HM, et al: *Pneumocystis carinii* pneumonia and mucosal candidiasis in previously healthy homosexual men: Evidence of a new acquired cellular immunodeficiency. *N Engl J Med* 305:1425–1431, 1981.
2. Masur H, Michelis MA, Green JB et al: An outbreak of community acquired *Pneumocystis carinii* pneumonia: Initial manifestation of cellular immune dysfunction. *N Engl J Med* 305:1431–1438, 1981.
3. Horowitz SL, Benson DF, Gottleib MS, et al: Neurological complications of gay-related immunodeficiency disorder. *Ann Neurol* 12:80, 1982 (abst).
4. Britton CB, Marquardt MD, Koppel B, et al: Neurological complications of the gay immunosuppressed syndrome: Clinical and pathological features. *Ann Neurol* 12:80, 1982 (abst).
5. Snider WD, Simpson DM, Nielsen S, et al: Neurological complication of acquired immune deficiency syndrome: Analysis of 50 patients. *Ann Neurol* 14:403–418, 1983.
6. Navia BA, Jordan BD, Price RW: The AIDS dementia complex. I. clinical features. *Ann Neurol* 19:517–524, 1986.
7. Faulstich ME: Psychiatric aspects of AIDS. *Am J. Psychiatry* 144:551–556, 1987.
8. Nurnberg HG, Prudic J, Firoi M, et al: Psychopathology complicating acquired immune deficiency syndrome (AIDS). *Am J Psychiatry* 141:95–96, 1985.
9. Hoffman RS: Neuropsychiatric complications of AIDS. *Psychosomatics* 25:393–400, 1984.
10. Kermani EJ, Drob S, Alpert M: Organic brain syndrome in three cases of acquired immune deficiency syndrome. *Compr Psychiatry* 25:294–297, 1984.
11. Kermani EJ, Borod JC, Brown PH, et al: New psychopathologic findings in AIDS: Case report. *J Clin Psychiatry* 46:240–241, 1985.
12. Price WA, Forejt JF: Neuropsychiatric aspects of AIDS: A case report. *Gen Hosp Psychiatry* 8:7–10, 1986.
13. Beresford TP, Blow FC, Hall RCW: AIDS encephalitis mimicking alcohol dementia and depression. *Biol Psychiatry* 21:394–397, 1986.
14. Thomas CS, Toone BK, El Komy A, et al: HTLV-III and psychiatric disturbance. *Lancet* 2:395–396, 1985.
15. Perry S, Jacobsen P: Neuropsychiatric manifestations of AIDS-spectrum disorders. *Hosp Community Psychiatry* 37:135–142, 1986.
16. Cummings MA, Cummings KL, Rapaport MH, et al: Acquired immune deficiency syndrome (AIDS) presenting as schizophrenia. *West J Med* 146:615–618, 1987.
17. Grant I, Adams KM: *Neuropsychological Assessment of Neuropsychiatric Disorders*. New York, Oxford University Press, 1986.
18. Sidtis JJ, Tross S, Navia BA, et al: Neuropsychological characterization of the AIDS dementia complex, in *International Conference on AIDS, Paris, June 23–25, 1986*, p 160 (communication 207).
19. Tross S: Neuropsychological complications of AIDS, in *NIMH/NIDA Conference, AIDS: Challenge to Neuroscience, Psychology, and Drug Abuse Research, Washington, DC. May 30, 1986.*
20. Tross S, Price RW, Navia B, et al: Neuropsychological characterizations of the AIDS dementia complex. A preliminary report. *AIDS* 2:81–88, 1988.
21. Joffe RT, Rubinow DR, Squillace BS, et al: Neuropsychiatric aspects of AIDS. *Psychopharmacol Bull* 22:684–688, 1986.
22. Joffe RT, Rubinow DR, Squillace BS, et al: Neuropsychiatric aspects of AIDS. *Psychopharmacol Bull* 22:684–688, 1986.
23. Janssen RS, Saykin AJ, Kaplan JE, et al: Neurological manifestations of lymphadenopathy syndrome, in *International Conference on AIDS, Paris, June 23, 1986*, p 45 (poster 70).
24. Janssen RS, Saykin A, Kaplan J, et al: Neurologic and neuropsychologic complications of lymphadenopathy syndrome, in *International Conference on AIDS, Washington, DC, June 2, 1987*, p 55 (communications T.5.2).
25. Janssen RS, Saykin AJ, Kaplan JE, et al: Neurological symptoms and neuropsychological abnormalities in lymphadenopathy syndrome. *Ann Neurol* 23(suppl):S17, 1988.
26. Ayers M, Newell T, Beardslee D, et al: Neuropsychological deficits associated with AIDS retrovirus infection, in *International Conference on AIDS, Paris, June 23, 1986*, p 161 (poster 219).
27. Grant I, Adams KM, Carlin AS, et al: The collaborative neuropsychological study of polydrug users. *Arch Gen Psychiatry* 35:1063–1074, 1978.

28. Heaton RK, Grant I, Anthony WZ, et al: A comparison of clinical and automated interpretation of the Halstead–Reitan Battery. *J Clin Neuropsychol* 3:121–141, 1981.
29. Heaton RK, Grant I, McSweeney AJ, et al: Neuropsychological findings in hypoxemic chronic obstructive pulmonary disease. *Arch Intern Med* 142:1470–1476, 1982.
30. Grant I, Heaton RK, McSweeney AJ, et al: Psychological effects of continuous and nocturnal oxygen therapy in hypoxemic chronic obstructive pulmonary disease. *Arch Intern Med* 143:1941–1947, 1983.
31. Bursztyn EM, Lee BCP, Bauman J: CT of acquired immunodeficiency syndrome. *AJNR* 5:711–714, 1983.
32. Koppel BS, Wormster Gp, Tuchman AJ, et al: Central nervous system involvement in patients with acquired immune deficiency syndrome (AIDS). *Acta Neurol Scand* 71:337–353, 1985.
33. Jordan BD, Navia BA, Petito C, et al: Neurologic syndromes complicating AIDS. *Front Radiat Ther Oncol* 19:82–87, 1985.
34. Post MJD, Kursonoglu SJ, Hensley GT, et al: Cranial CT in acquired immunodeficiency syndrome: Spectrum of diseases and optimal contrast enhancement technique. *AJR* 145:929–940, 1985.
35. Dei Cas A, Michelone G, Azzini M, et al: AIDS, ARC observation of eight pediatric cases, in *International Conference on AIDS, Paris, June 23, 1986,* p 47 (poster 79).
36. Belman AL, Horoupian D, Ultmann M, et al: Pediatric AIDS: Central nervous system involvement, in *International Conference on AIDS, Paris, June 23, 1986,* p 50 (poster 276).
37. Kairam R, Kaul A, Bhalani K, et al: Pediatric AIDS—variability of clinical disease, in *International Conference on AIDS, Paris, June 23, 1986,* p 47 (poster 78).
38. Post MJD, Sheldon JJ, Hensley GT, et al: Central nervous system disease in acquired immunodeficiency syndrome: Prospective correlation using CT, MR imaging, and pathologic studies. *Radiology* 158:141–148, 1986.
39. Delapaz R, Floris R, Brand-Zawadzki M: Magnetic resonance imaging of central nervous system complications of AIDS, in *Annual Meeting of the Society of Magnetic Resonance in Medicine, London, August, 1985.*
40. Levy RM, Bredesen, DE, Moore S, et al: Cranial magnetic resonance imaging in AIDS: Superiority to computed tomography, in *Annual Meeting of the Society of Magnetic Resonance in Medicine, London, August, 1985.*
41. Grant I, Atkinson JH, Hesselink JR, et al: Evidence for early central nervous system involvement in the acquired immunodeficiency syndrome (AIDS) and other human immunodeficiency virus (HIV) infections. Studies with neuropsychologic testing and magnetic resonance imaging. *Ann Intern Med* 107:828–836, 1987.
42. Grant I, Atkinson JH, Hesselink JR, et al: Human immunodeficiency virus-associated neurobehavioural disorder. *J R Coll Physicians Lond* 22:149–157, 1988.
43. Grant I, Reed R, Adams K: Diagnosis of intermediate-duration and subacute organic mental disorders in abstinent alcoholics. *J Clin Psychiatry* 48:319–323, 1987.
44. Grant I, Adams KM, Reed R: Intermediate-duration (subacute) organic mental disorder of alcoholism, in Grant I (ed): *Neuropsychiatric Correlates of Alcoholism.* Washington, DC, American Psychiatric Press, 1986, pp 37–60.
45. Bond MR: The psychiatry of closed head injury, in Brooks, DN (ed): *Closed Head Injury: Psychological, Social and Family Consequences.* Oxford, Oxford University Press, 1984, pp 148–178.
46. Schmitt FA, Louge PE, et al, and AZT Collaborative Working Group: Short-term longitudinal change in AIDS and ARC patients: Neuropsychological effects on AZT. *J Clin Exp Neuropsychol* 10:77, 1988 (abst).
47. Selnes OA, Miller EN, Becker JT, et al: Normal neuropsychological performance in healthy HIV-1 infected homosexual men. The multicenter AIDS cohort study (MACS), in *The Fourth International Conference on AIDS, Stockholm,* 1988.
48. Gabuzda DH, Hirsch MS: Neurologic manifestations of infection with human immunodeficiency virus. Clinical features and pathogenesis. *Ann Intern Med* 107:383–391, 1987.
49. Price RW, Brew B, Sidtis J, et al: The brain in AIDS: Central nervous system HIV-1 infection and AIDS dementia complex. *Science* 239:586–592, 1988.
50. Price RW, Brew BJ. The AIDS dementia complex. *J Infect Dis* 158:1079–1083, 1988.

14

Somatic Treatment of Psychiatric Symptoms in HIV Disease

KATIE A. BUSCH and SARZ MAXWELL

INTRODUCTION

In June 1981, the *Morbidity and Mortality Weekly Report* published an account of five homosexual men infected with *Pneumocystis carinii* pneumonia (PCP).[1] As case reports mounted of PCP, of previously rare Kaposi's sarcoma (KS), and of other opportunistic infections,[2] the symptom cluster was given the name acquired immune deficiency syndrome (AIDS). In 1983, a retrovirus was isolated that is currently believed to be etiologic in AIDS, which now carries the official name human immunodeficiency virus (HIV). After a brief introduction on HIV illness in general, we review the literature to date on its neuropsychiatric aspects, with a major focus on the complicated diagnostic and treatment issues at this interface. Psychosocial issues[3,4] so essential in treatment, are described elsewhere in this volume and are beyond the scope of this chapter

Since 1981, the number of cases has increased drastically. The Centers for Disease Control (CDC) has projected 270,000 cases by 1991, more than one half of whom will have died from this illness. Seroprevalence is difficult to assess accurately, but it is known to be highest in urban areas, particularly New York, California, Florida, New Jersey, and Texas. Hispanics and blacks have a seroprevalence many times higher than whites for most risk groups.[5,6] As this epidemic spreads so silently, it is essential to focus more on "risky behavior" rather than on membership in a "risk group" as a means of transmission control.

The CDC classifies HIV infection into four mutually exclusive groups,[7] which define the continuum of AIDS-spectrum illness. Full-blown AIDS is defined only by group IV. Group I describes the acute infection associated with exposure to the virus. These patients are described as usually being asymptomatic or as having an acute, limited glandular fever type of illness. Group II is asymptomatic infection with the serum being positive for HIV antibody. Group III is persistent generalized lymphadenopathy (PGL) with enlarged lymph nodes, but no opportunistic infection or persistent constitutional symptoms. An increasing proportion of group III progresses to the full-blown AIDS syndrome with increasing length of follow-up. Group IV includes those with constitutional neurologic, or

---

KATIE A. BUSCH and SARZ MAXWELL • Department of Psychiatry, Rush–Presbyterian–St. Luke's Medical Center, Chicago, Illinois 60612.

TABLE 1. CDC Classification

Group/subgroup	Description
Group I	Acute infection (aka Seroconversion)
	May occur up to 12 weeks after contact
	Usually asymptomatic, but may have acute reversible glandular feverlike illness, encephalopathy, and/or myelopathy
Group II	Asymptomatic infection (aka seropositive, HIV+)
	Serum positive for HIV
Group III	Persistent generalized lymphadenopathy (PGL)
	Nodes at least 1 cm in diameter in two or more noncontiguous extrainguinal sites for at least 3 months
	No history of opportunistic infections or persistent constitutional symptoms
Group IV	Constitutional, neurologic, secondary, or other conditions (subgroups are not mutually exclusive)
Subgroup A:	Constitutional disease (aka AIDS-related complex-ARC)
	Fever, weight loss, fatigue, night sweats
Subgroup B:	Neurologic disease
	Dementia, encephalitis, meningitis, peripheral neuropathy
Subgroup C:	Secondary infectious disease
Subgroup D:	Secondary cancers
Subgroup E:	Other conditions

secondary infectious diseases or with various "other" conditions, including AIDS wasting syndrome[7] (Table 1).

NEUROPSYCHIATRIC SYMPTOMS AND SYNDROMES

As the rapidly increasing numbers of persons with AIDS (PWAs) are studied, significant neuropsychiatric effects of this virus have become manifest.[7–12] Information about these various neuropsychiatric symptoms comes from clinical reports of single cases or small groups. There are currently few published controlled studies either of these symptoms of AIDS-spectrum illness or of treatment effects, so the following information must be evaluated with awareness of the limitations this places on the validity of the data.

It is clear that, in addition to the opportunistic infections and neoplasms that affect central nervous system (CNS) structure and function in AIDS-spectrum illness, HIV itself has a predilection for invasion of nervous tissues. There are various hypotheses about how HIV may enter the CNS, with more recent hypotheses focusing on the newly discovered receptor sites for T lymphocytes at the blood–brain barrier (BBB) or on macrophage carriers. However the virus enters the brain, CNS manifestations of this infection are so prevalent that the Centers for Disease Control (CDC), in August 1987, included AIDS encephalopathy among official criteria for diagnosis of group IV.[7] (Table 2). This AIDS dementia complex (ADC)[13] has become one of the most prominent features of this illness and is discussed in more detail elsewhere in this volume. Clinically, the picture is that of a subcortical dementia more similar to multi-infarct problems than to Alzheimer's disease (Table 3). With subcortical dementias, there are more problems with alertness and inatten-

TABLE 2. CDC Definition of HIV Encephalopathy

Disabling cognitive/or motor dysfunction
Interfering with occupation or activities of daily living (ADL) or loss of behavioral milestones (pediatric)
Progressing over weeks to months
In absence of concurrent condition that explains findings
Methods to rule out concurrent condition must include
  CSF examination
  Either brain imaging (CT/MRI) or autopsy

TABLE 3. Clinical Symptoms of AIDS Dementia Complex

Cognitive impairments
  Short-term memory deficit; ''forgetfulness'' rather than amnesia
  Concentration and attention
  Confusion and disorientation
  Overall intellectual ability generally well preserved until late
  Visuospatial—serious deficits

Personality/behavior changes
  Apathy, decreased interest
  Impaired judgment, erratic behavior
  Social withdrawal
  Rigidity of thought
  Language-slow, dysarthria, hypophonia; no impaired comprehension

Psychotic symptoms
  Hallucinations
  Suspiciousness/delusions
  Agitation and inappropriate behavior

Motor symptoms
  Ataxia/loss of coordination/weakness
  Tremors

Generalized/systemic symptoms
  Fatigue, sleep changes (hypersomnia)
  Anorexia/decreased weight
  Eneuresis
  Increased sensitivity to medications and alcohol

Advanced dementia—cognitive symptoms
  Global cognitive impairment
  Rudimentary social functioning
  Disorientation
  Psychomotor retardation, decreased spontaneity
  Agitation, sundowning
  Mutism, vacant stare
  Coma

Advanced dementia—motor symptoms
  Ataxia
  Spastic weakness
  Paraplegia, quadraparesis
  Hyperreflexia, myoclonus, seizures
  Bladder and bowel incontinence

tion, but these patients are often aware of, and can acknowledge, their deficits. The dementia seen often coexists with various psychiatric symptoms, particularly depression, but also with anxiety or psychotic symptoms. The course of the neuropsychiatric symptoms in HIV illness is not clear cut: severe dementia is often seen in terminal stages, but 10–20% of patients may present with a wide range of neuropsychiatric symptoms up to and including a severe dementia, even up to 2 years before any symptoms of immune deficiency.[14,15]

The recognized incidence of neuropsychiatric symptoms in PWAs, particularly dementia, has been increasing yearly. Current reports of these neuropsychiatric symptoms range from 40 to 70%[13,16] to "almost all."[3] Most current speculations on this rise in the incidence of dementia focus on the rapidly increasing effectiveness of treatment of the opportunistic illnesses. Most current medications used in HIV-infected patients with the possible exception of zidovudine, do not cross the BBB and therefore have no effect on the CNS. The differential diagnosis of HIV dementia is presented in Table 4. In early January 1988, our AIDS care team evaluated 13 inpatients, all of whom were moderately to severely demented as measured on the Mini-Mental State Exam[17] (scores of below 20) or general mental status testing, behaviorally, and on the Trail making subtests of the Halstead–Reitan neuropsychological battery.[18,19] Five of these patients also showed symptoms of depression, and one other showed severe anxiety. The difficulty of diagnosing these psychiatric syndromes, particularly regarding etiology, within the context of severe medical and/or CNS illness will be discussed below.

On CNS evaluation, in general, with primary HIV infection, the literature describes a cortical atrophy visible on computed tomography (CT) scan or magnetic resonance imag-

TABLE 4. Differential Diagnosis of Dementia in HIV Illness

Etiology	Insidious course	Acute symptoms	Diagnostic findings
HIV	Weeks–months Dementia may be only symptom		CT—cortical atrophy EEG—generalized slowing CSF—may be HIV-Ab reactive
Cryptococcus	Weeks	Headache	CT—may show thickened meninges
	Nonspecific constitutional symptoms		CSF—India ink or culture
Toxoplasmosis	1–2 weeks	Headache	CT—usually ring-enhancing lesion
	Confusion, lethargy	Focal deficits	CSF—serology may be negative
Lymphoma	Weeks Personality change Confusion	Headache Focal deficits	CT—may be normal May need brain biopsy
Progressive multifocal leukoencephalopathy	Weeks–months Dementia may be only symptom		CT—usually nonenhancing MRI—may see white matter lesion
Major depression	Weeks–months Mood, social, vegetative, and psychotic symptoms usually more severe than cognitive	Suicidality	Stimulant challenge may make diagnosis; may coexist with any other etiologies

TABLE 5. Psychiatric and Neurological Side Effects of Medication Used in Treating HIV Illness[a]

Pneumocystis	
Trimethoprim/Sulfa (Bactrim)	Psychosis, mutism, bizarre mannerisms, depression, loss of appetite, insomnia, apathy, headache, neuritis
TB and *Mycobacterium avium*—intracellulare	
Isoniazid	Depression, agitation, auditory, and visual hallucinations, paranoia, peripheral neuropathy, memory impairment
Ethambutol	Headache, dizziness, confusion, visual disturbances
Rifampin	Headache, fatigue, loss of appetite, visual disturbances
Cycloserine	Anxiety, depression, confusion, disorientation, hallucinations, paranoia, loss of appetite, fatigue
Ethionamide	Depression, hallucinations, neuritis, diplopia, headache, drowsiness
Candida, Cryptococcus	
Ketoconazole	Headache, dizziness, photosensitivity
Amphotericin B	Delirium, peripheral neuropathy, blurred vision, diplopia, weight loss, loss of appetite, headache
5-Flucytosine	Confusion, headache, sedation
Toxoplasmosis	
Sulfonamides	Headache, neuritis, insomnia, loss of appetite, photosensitivity
Strongyloids stercoralis	
Thiabendazole	Hallucinations, olfactory disturbance
Herpes simplex/zoster	
Acyclovir	Depression, agitation, auditory and visual hallucinations, depersonalization, tearfulness, confusion, hyperaesthesia, hyperacusis, insomnia, thought insertion, headache
Kaposi's sarcoma	
Vincristine	Hallucinations, headache, neuritis, ataxia, sensory loss
Vinblastine	Depression, loss of appetite, headache, neuritis
Etoposide (VP 16)	Neuropathy, loss of appetite
α-Interferon	Depression, weakness
Lymphomas	
Methotrexate	Headaches, blurred vision, fatigue, photosensitivity, encephalopathy in high doses
Procarbazine	Mania, loss of appetite, headaches, insomnia, nightmares, confusion, malaise
Anti-HIV	
Azidothymidine (AZT)	Headache, restlessness, severe agitation, insomnia, mania
Suramin	Malaise, paresthesis
Ribavirin	?

[a] Adapted from Strain.[28a]

ing (MRI).[9,20,21] With cerebral toxoplasmosis,[22] a ring-enhancing mass effect may be seen. The electroencephalogram (EEG) may show a diffuse bilateral slowing, and cerebrospinal fluid (CSF) results are nonspecific other than identifying specific infectious agents. At autopsy, the literature reports that 75–90% of PWAs have some brain pathology.[23–26] This is described in detail elsewhere in this volume.

In addition to the cognitive and behavioral problems of dementia in PWAs, the full range of psychiatric symptoms and syndromes is seen.[27,28] These are described more fully by Miller (Chapter 10, this volume) but may be the first clinical presentation of AIDS-spectrum illness. In our experience, neurologic deficits and psychiatric symptoms usually coexist.

Many of the symptoms have treatable causes, and impairment in cognitive or behavioral capacity has major management implications, making the differential diagnosis of all neuropsychiatric changes essential. Most, if not all, of the medications used for the treatment of opportunistic disease in PWAs have neuropsychiatric side effects (Table 5). Fluctuating medical status, especially the decreased PO_2 level seen in pneumonia, and the electrolyte imbalance seen with the severe diarrhea, worsens the cognitive status in a patient with a compromised CNS. In addition, as described in detail below, the sedative and anticholinergic side effects of psychiatric medications often cause increased difficulties in patients with dementia.

DIAGNOSIS OF PSYCHIATRIC SYMPTOMS

The differential diagnosis of depressive and anxiety syndromes in the severely medically ill or CNS-compromised patient is extremely difficult. This is primarily attributable to the fact that all somatic symptoms used for psychiatric diagnosis are also caused by medical/CNS impairment and may therefore not be used reliably for psychiatric diagnosis. (As in any psychiatric evaluation, personal or family psychiatric history is useful in establishing diagnoses.) For clinical purposes, however, as various psychopharmacologic

TABLE 6. Symptoms of Major Depressive Syndrome[a,b]

Somatic symptoms[c]
Significant weight loss or weight gain when not dieting (e.g., more than 5% of body weight in a month), or decrease or increase in appetite nearly every day (in children, consider failure to make expected weight gains).
Insomnia or hypersomnia nearly every day.
Psychomotor agitattion or retardation nearly every day (observable by others, not merely subjective feelings or restlessness or being slowed down).
Fatigue or loss of energy nearly every day.
Diminished ability to think or concentrate, or indecisiveness, nearly every day (either by subjective account or as observed by others).
Markedly diminished interest or pleasure in all, or almost all, activities most of the day, nearly every day (as indicated either by subjective account or observation by others of apathy most of the time)[d]
Affective symptoms
Depressed mood (or can be irritable mood in children and adolescents) most of the day, nearly every day, as indicated either by subjective account or observation by others.
Feelings of worthlessness or excessive or inappropriate guilt (which may be delusional) nearly every day (not merely self-reproach or guilt about being sick).
Recurrent thoughts of death (not just fear of dying), recurrent suicidal ideation without a specific plan, or a suicide attempt or a specific plan for committing suicide.

[a]From ref. 29.
[b]As defined by DSM-III-R, 1987, Criterion A; at least 5 of the symptoms must be present to meet criteria for criterion "A".
[c]All of the somatic symptoms are also caused by organic illness.
[d]Apathy is often observed in dementia.

TABLE 7. Symptoms of Anxiety[a,b]

Generalized anxiety disorder, Criterion "D"[c]
Motor Tension
Trembling, twitching, or feeling shaky[d]
Muscle tension, aches, or soreness[d]
Restlessness[d]
Easy fatigability[d]
Autonomic hyperactivity
Shortness of breath or smothering sensations[d]
Palpitations or accelerated heart rate (tachycardia)[d]
Sweating or cold clammy hands[d]
Dry mouth[d]
Dizziness or light headedness[d]
Nausea, diarrhea, or other abdominal distress[d]
Flushes (hot flashes) or chills[d]
Frequent urination[d]
Trouble swallowing or "lump in throat"[d]
Vigilance and scanning
Feeling keyed up or on edge
Exaggerated startle response
Difficulty concentrating or "mind going blank" because of anxiety[d]
Trouble falling or staying asleep[d]
Irritability[d]
Panic disorder, Criterion "C"[e]
Shortness of breath (dyspnea) or smothering sensations[d]
Dizziness, unsteady feelings, or faintness[d]
Palpitations or accelerated heart rate (tachycardia)[d]
Trembling or shaking[d]
Sweating[d]
Choking[d]
Nausea or abdominal distress[d]
Depersonalization or derealization[d]
Numbness or tingling sensations (paresthesias)[d]
Flushes (hot flashes) or chills[d]
Chest pain or discomfort[d]
Fear of dying
Fear of going crazy or of doing something uncontrolled

[a] From ref. 29.
[b] For either diagnosis to be made, it cannot be established that an organic factor initiated and maintained the disturbance.
[c] At least six symptoms must be present.
[d] Symptom may commonly be due to an organic illness.
[e] At least four symptoms must be present.

treatment modalities are very effective for symptom relief, it may be advisable to be inclusive in the use of symptoms to diagnose syndromes presumptively, rather than delay treatment.

Table 6 lists somatic symptoms used for the diagnosis of Major Depression in DSM-III-R,[29] all of which may be attributable to other causes. What then remains for diagnostic use is an evaluation of mood, interest or pleasure, and feelings of worthlessness or guilt.

Anhedonia, usually considered a particularly psychologic symptom, is easily confused with the apathy commonly seen in dementia. As depressive symptoms in PWAs may exist for years, there may often be little information to differentiate between Adjustment Disorder with Depressed Mood (DSM-III-R #309), Dysthymic Disorder (DSM-III-R #300) or Major Depression (DSM-III-R #296).

There is some evidence that certain items on the Beck Depression Inventory may be particularly helpful in differentiating depression from symptoms of medical or CNS etiology.[30] These items relate to symptoms of suicidal ideation, sense of failure, sense of punishment, loss of social interest, indecision, and dissatisfaction and may represent criteria of depressive severity that are not confounded by the presence of physical illness. We are currently developing an instrument for more accurate assessment of both anxiety and depression in the context of severe medical illness and/or CNS compromise.

Table 7 lists the somatic symptoms used in the diagnosis of Generalized Anxiety Disorder and Panic Disorder.[29] As in PWAs with depression, this can all be due to causes other than anxiety, again making diagnosis difficult. In terms of the differential diagnosis of the more psychotic symptomatology, distinction of etiology is important to be able to direct specific treatment toward causes. However, as antipsychotic medications are effective for psychotic symptoms of "organic" as well as "functional" etiology,[31] differential diagnoses for purposes of treatment of psychotic symptoms is less crucial.

TREATMENT

Treatment of the psychiatric states in PWAs, for the reasons described above, has often depended more on identification of target symptoms and assessment of symptom severity than on DSM-III-R diagnoses. Because of the CNS compromise, these patients are often extremely sensitive to the side effects of psychiatric medication. The choice of somatic psychiatric treatment, when necessary because of symptom severity, depends on the interplay of target symptoms, CNS compromise, and the severity of the current medical condition. Patients with AIDS-related complex (ARC) may be as severely CNS compromised as patients with full-blown AIDS.[11,14] In general, if there is minimal or no CNS compromise on clinical evaluation, standard somatic treatments for psychiatric symptoms may be effective. Comparable to the geropsychiatric population, PWAs may only be able to tolerate dosages significantly small than usual, with slower titration upward.

TABLE 8. Short-Intermediate Antianxiety Medications

Medication	"t-1/2" (hr)[a]
Alprazolam (Xanax)	12–15
Lorazepam (Ativan)	12–18
Oxazepam (Serax)	5.7–10.9

[a]From ref. 32.

TABLE 9. Opiate-Dosage Equivalencies Compared to Morphine[a]

	IM(mg)	PO(mg)	Duration of action (hr)
Morphine	1.0	6.0	4–5
Hydromorphone (Dilaudid)	0.15	0.75	4
Levorphanol (Levodromoran)	0.2	0.4	6–8
Codeine	12.0	20.0	4–6
Methadone	1.0	2.0	3–5[b]
Meperidine (Demerol)	7.5	30.0	2–4
Propoxyphene (Darvon)	N/A	40.0	3–4

[a]From ref. 33.
[b]On repeated administration, active metabolites result in significantly increased duration of action.

ANXIETY

Somatic treatment of anxiety in PWAs is particularly limited by the CNS intolerance of the sedating side effects of anxiolytic medications. In the less severely medically or patients with little or no CNS compromise, small doses of the short to intermediate acting benzodiazepines have been effective and frequently well tolerated[32] (Table 8). Those who are more severely medically ill or clinically demented, however, cannot tolerate the sedation. In these patients, we have found that very small dosages of opiates are very effective in lysing the anxiety, with few or no side effects[33] (Table 9). Opiates have the added benefits of also treating pain, subjective difficulty breathing, and the raging diarrhea often seen in PWAs. Our use of opiates has primarily been intermittent dosing on a PRN basis, titrating anxiolytic effect with sedation. We have treated only a small series of inpatients partially due to the fact that, as the dementia increases, the severity and incidence of anxiety appears to decrease.

DEPRESSION

Comparable to the situation with anxiety, somatic treatment of depressive symptoms in PWAs depends on medical and CNS status. There have been single case or small group reports in the literature of positive responses to tricyclic antidepressants.[28,34] These patients are highly sensitive to anticholinergic side effects of medication; we have seen two cases of an atropine psychosis in a PWA, presumptively due to a scopolamine patch prescribed for nausea. In the medically stable PWA with little or no CNS compromise, it seems reasonable to prescribe a standard antidepressant, starting in the lowest dosage possible. It is advisable to start treatment with those agents with fewer anticholinergic side effects, whose metabolites are for the most part, pharmacologically inactive, such as nortriptyline or desipramine.[35] We have also used low-dose fluoxetine (Prozac) in one severely demented PWA (who lost his response to methylphenidate) with improvement in general alertness and decrease in subjective symptoms of depression after 14 days. Fluoxetine is a pure presynaptic serotonin reuptake blocker with little or no anticholinergic activity and minimal sedative properties but which may result in agitation. Whichever antidepressant is used, upward titration of dosage should proceed very slowly. There are no reports in the literature regarding the use of monoamine oxidase inhibitors in AIDS patients.

In the severely CNS-compromised PWA, treatment of depressive symptoms is more problematic. The use of psychostimulants has been extremely effective in these clinical situations, with little or no side effects seen. Both dextroamphetamine[11,12] and methylphenidate are reported to be effective. There is nothing in the literature to date regarding the use of pemoline in this context. For those concerned about psychostimulant addiction, it is reasonable to try pemoline, as it is reported to result in less drug craving. In our usage of methylphenidate, we have had two patients continue on this as outpatients, both at 5 mg/day p.o. for 3 months, with apparent relief of depressive symptomatology, and no indication of drug tolerance. Patients with symptoms of severe depression in the context of moderate to severe dementia were tried on 5–20 mg of methylphenidate p.o., daily with rapid (within hours) relief of depressive symptomatology.

There is evidence from Dr. Fernandez et al.[11] that amphetamines may specifically improve general neuropsychiatric functioning as well as help relieve depressive symptoms. In some patients, the apparent antidepressant response may, at least partially, be due to an improvement in alertness and attention, but the improvement on neuropsychological testing in this study was dramatic.

PSYCHOSIS

In our experience, psychiatric symptoms of psychotic severity have occurred primarily during an acute medical episode or as a side effect of medication. In terms of the treatment of psychotic symptomatology in patients with HIV illness, it does not appear to be quite as essential to separate the medically/CNS-compromised patient from those patients who are more stable except regarding dosages. Very low doses of the high potency neuroleptic medications have been extremely helpful in controlling psychotic symptoms, especially the severe agitation although case reports suggest that there may be an increased incidence of extrapyramidal or parkinsonian side effects in this group[36] (Table 10). Slow titration of dosage upwards has been necessary although we have not needed to use more than the equivalent of 10 mg/day of haloperidol in the patients we have treated. Patients whose medical and CNS status is more stable may tolerate somewhat larger doses.

TABLE 10. Antipsychotic Medications (High Potency, Low Anticholinergic)

Medication	Recommended starting dosages
Haloperidol (Haldol)	0.5–1 mg up to QID
Fluphenazine (Prolixin)	1 mg up to QID
Trifluoperazine (Stelazine)	1–2 mg up to BID
Thiothixene (Navane)	1–2 mg up to BID

ROUTES OF ADMINISTRATION

Owing to the AIDS wasting syndrome, and the often very severe diarrhea seen in PWAs, route of administration often becomes problematic; nothing p.o. is absorbed and there is little muscle mass available for injections. Although there is preliminary data on various treatments to increase muscle mass (Von Roenn J: personal communication) and to control the diarrhea, our repertoire of effective medications available by sublingual and subcutaneous routes needs to be expanded. (For those medications effective sublingually, but which taste terribly, we have found it effective to place the pill in the center of a Lifesaver®).

CONCLUSION

Knowledge of the neuropsychiatric aspects of HIV illnesses is increasing rapidly. This includes data both regarding the complicated differential diagnosis of psychiatric symptomatology and regarding safe and effective treatments. Research is in process to more clearly delineate diagnostic criteria and course of illness, in order to make treatment more specific. Currently, treatment of psychiatric symptoms in the context of HIV-related organic brain disease is based on very pragmatic considerations. Nevertheless, this treatment can be very rewarding, both in terms of relief of suffering and increased ability to cooperate with the complicated management necessary in this devastating condition.

REFERENCES

1. Centers for Disease Control: *Pneumocystis pneumonia*—Los Angeles. *MMWR* 30:250–252, 1981.
2. Centers for Disease Control: Kaposi's sarcoma and Pneumocystis pneumonia among homosexual men—New York City and California. *MMWR* 30:305–307, 1981.
3. Holland JC, Tross S: The psychosocial and neuropsychiatric sequelae of the acquired immunodeficiency syndrome and related disorders. *Ann Intern Med* 103:760–764, 1985.
4. Nichols SE: Psychosocial reactions of persons with the acquired immunodeficiency syndrome. *Ann Intern Med* 103:765–767, 1985.
5. Centers for Disease Control: Weekly Surveillance Report 1/11/88, *AIDS Rec* 2(3):6, 1988.
6. Di Clemente RJ, Boyer CB, Morales ES: Minority and AIDS: *Am J Public Health* 78:55–57, 1988.
7. Centers for Disease Control: Revision of the CDC surveillance case definition for acquired immunodeficiency syndrome. *MMWR* 36(suppl):15, 1987.
8. Price RW, Navia BA, Cho E-S: AIDS encephalopathy. *Neurol Clin* 4:285–303, 1986.
9. Faulstich ME: Acquired immune deficiency syndrome: An overview of the central nervous system complications and neuropsychological sequelae. *Int J Neurosci* 30:249–254, 1986.
10. Snider WD, Simpson DM, Nielson S, et al: Neurological complications of acquired immune deficiency syndrome: Analysis of 50 patients. *Ann Neurol* 14:403–418, 1983.
11. Fernandez F, Adams F, Levy JK, et al: Cognitive impairment due to AIDS-related complex and its response to psychostimulants. *Psychosomatics* 29:38–46, 1988.
12. Perry S, Jacobsen P: Neuropsychiatric manifestations of AIDS-spectrum disorders. *Hosp Community Psychiatry* 37:135–142, 1986.
13. Navia BA, Jordan BD, Price RW: The AIDS dementia complex. I. Clinical Features. *Ann Neurol* 19:517–524, 1986.
14. Navia BA, Price RW: The acquired immunodeficiency syndrome dementia complex as the presenting or sole manifestation of human immunodeficiency virus infection. *Arch Neurol* 44:65–66, 1987.

15. Beckett A, Summergrad P, Manschreck T, et al: Symptomatic HIV infection of the CNS in a patient without clinical evidence of immune deficiency. *Am J Psychiatry* 144:1342–1344, 1987.
16. Detmer WM, Lu FG: Neuropsychiatric complications of AIDS: A literature review. *Int J Psychiatry Med* 16:21–29, 1986–1987.
17. Folstein MF, Folstein SE, McHugh PR: "Mini-Mental State." *J Psychiatr Res* 12:189–198, 1975.
18. Reitan RM: The relation of the Trail-making test to organic brain damage. *J Consult Psychol* 19:393–394, 1955.
19. Davies ADM: The influence of age on Trail-making test performance. *J Clin Psychol* 24:96–98, 1968.
20. Shaw GM, Harper ME, Hahn BH, et al: HTLV-III infection in brains of children and adults with AIDS encephalopathy. *Science* 227:177–181, 1985.
21. Belman AL, Ultmann MH, Horoupian D, et al: Neurological complications in infants and children with acquired immune deficiency syndrome. *Ann Neurol* 18:560–566, 1985.
22. Navia BA, Petito CK, Gold JWM, et al: Cerebral toxoplasmosis complicating the acquired immune deficiency syndrome: Clinical and neuropathological findings in 27 patients. *Ann Neurol* 19:224–238, 1986.
23. Navia BA, Cho E-S, Petito CK, Price RW: The AIDS dementia complex. II. *Neuropathology Ann Neurol* 19:525–535, 1986.
24. Nielson SL, Petito CK, Urmacher CD, et al: Subacute encephalitis in the acquired immune deficiency syndrome: A postmortem study. *Am J Clin Pathol* 82:678–682, 1984.
25. Epstein LG, Sharer LR, Joshi VV, et al: Progressive encephalopathy in children with acquired immune deficiency syndrome. *Arch Neurol* 17:488–496, 1985.
26. Stoler MH, Eskin TA, Benn S, et al: Human T-cell lymphotropic virus type III infection of the central nervous system. A preliminary in situ analysis. *JAMA* 256:2360–2364, 1986.
27. Perry SW, Tross S: Psychiatric problems of AIDS inpatients at the New York Hospital: Preliminary report. *Public Health Rep* 99:200–205, 1984.
28. Rundell JR, Wise MG, Ursano RJ: Three cases of AIDS-related psychiatric disorders. *Am J Psychiatry* 143:777–778, 1986.
28a. Strain J: Paper presented at the May 1987 American Psychiatric Association Meeting, New York, May, 1987.
29. American Psychiatric Association: *Diagnostic and Statistical Manual of Mental Disorders,* ed 3, revised. Washington, DC, American Psychiatric Association, 1987.
30. Clark DC, Cavanaugh SVA, Gibbons RD: The core symptoms of depression in medical and psychiatric patients. *J Nerv Ment Dis* 171:705–713, 1983.
31. Cummings JL: Organic psychosis. *Psychosomatics* 29:16–26, 1988.
32. *Physicians' Desk Reference,* ed 42. Oradell, New Jersey, Medical Economics Company, 1988.
33. Schnoll SH: Pain. in Buchwald C, Cohen S, Katz D, Solomon J (eds): *Frequently Prescribed and Abused Drugs.* State University of New York, 1980.
34. Perry SW, Markowitz J: Psychiatric interventions of AIDS-spectrum disorders. *Hosp Community Psychiatry* 37:1001–1006, 1986.
35. Reynolds CF, Maren RS, Spiker D: Clinical considerations in prescribing antidepressants for geriatric patients. *Geriatr Med Today* 2:45–55, 1983.
36. Baer JW, Hall JM, Holm K, et al: Challenges in developing an outpatient psychiatric program for patients with AIDS and ARC. *Hosp Community Psychiatry* 38:1299–1303, 1987.

15

Adjuvant Treatment of HIV Dementia with Psychostimulants

FRANCISCO FERNANDEZ and JOEL K. LEVY

INTRODUCTION: NEUROPSYCHIATRIC IMPAIRMENT IN HIV DISEASE

Individuals infected with the human immunodeficiency virus (HIV) manifest signs and symptoms of the disease ranging from asymptomatic infection to full-blown AIDS.[1] The virus preys upon T cells, thus destroying immune function and eventually leaving the body open to overwhelming opportunistic infections or cancer. HIV is now believed to be neurotropic as well, and may attack the central nervous system (CNS) at any point during the infection.[2] The results are indeed protean, and this infection has been compared to other neurodegenerative pathogens, including syphilis.[3]

Patients who are seropositive for HIV often exhibit a range of psychological and psychiatric disturbances that run the spectrum from stress/distress-related symptomatology to organic mental disorders.[4] The exact nature of how HIV gains entry into the brain is unknown, but it has been speculated that it does so through endothelial gaps in the capillary vascular bed.[5] From there it may bind to glial and perhaps neural cells which contain the T4 receptor whereby it may enter the cells and replicate.[6–8] A cellular reaction occurs, with inflammation and degeneration of myelin causing the white matter changes which often take place with HIV–CNS involvement.

The most frequent neurological impairment that occurs with HIV disease is the progressive dementia which affects as many as 90% of individuals with AIDS.[9] HIV-related cognitive and neuropsychiatric disturbances have also appeared before any signs of immune compromise have arisen.[10] The exact incidence of cognitive impairment and dementia in pre-AIDS conditions, such as lymphadenopathy syndrome (LAS) and AIDS-related complex (ARC), and in asymptomatic individuals is presently unknown. However, the recognition of these syndromes caused by HIV–CNS involvement is important given the frequency of subjective complaints and objective clinical findings of neuropsychiatric disturbances in HIV-spectrum disorders.

FRANCISCO FERNANDEZ • St. Luke's Episcopal Hospital, Houston, Texas 77030; Department of Psychiatry and Behavioral Sciences, Baylor College of Medicine, Houston, Texas 77030. JOEL K. LEVY • Department of Psychiatry and Behavioral Sciences, Baylor College of Medicine, Houston, Texas 77030.

Unfortunately, no effective treatment for HIV-related cognitive impairment and dementia is yet known. Conceivably, psychopharmacological strategies could be formulated to palliate HIV-related cognitive dysfunction, with resultant qualitative and quantitative improvement in cognition. The use of adjuvant psychopharmacotherapy in these disorders is underused.[4] As with other medically ill patients, physicians tend to avoid psychotropic agents because of the adverse side effects generally, but often erroneously, ascribed to psychotropic agents. Moreover, a historical bias exists against medical intervention for psychological symptoms ("psychopharmacologic calvinism").[11] Nevertheless, optimal care of patients who suffer from HIV infection and secondary neuropsychiatric disturbances should include rapid recognition and management of these syndromes in order to provide improved functioning for the patients and avoid exacerbation, possibly, to the point of delirium. In this chapter, we will address the treatment of HIV-related cognitive impairment and dementia with psychostimulants.

THE ROLE OF STIMULANTS IN MEDICINE AND HIV DISEASE

Since their formal introduction into general medical practice more than 50 years ago, controversy has surrounded the therapeutic role of amphetamines in psychiatry.[12] Several states have legislation banning amphetamine production altogether and have limited their therapeutic use even for FDA-approved conditions. These actions were prompted to a large degree by the dramatic rise in illicit amphetamine use in the 1960s and the often indiscriminate prescription of amphetamines for varying conditions. Because anyone can become addicted to these agents, it is still a commonly held notion that universal restriction is the safest means of controlling stimulant abuse. However, continued clinical and investigative experience with these psychostimulants has demonstrated them to be both safe and useful when prescribed appropriately.

Current FDA approval is limited to narcolepsy, attention deficit disorder with hyperactivity, and obesity. Clinical reports have found them useful in nocturnal enuresis, postencephalitic parkinsonism, analgesic adjuvants, neurasthenia fatigue syndromes, hiccups, and some forms of seizures.[12] In cases of "secondary" depressive syndromes in medically ill patients, the general experience is that psychostimulants are useful for apathetic and withdrawn states in the elderly and major depression.[13–15] The clinical response is highlighted by quick remission of depression and cognitive dysfunction without treatment-related side effects. Thus, the psychostimulants can be considered to be an effective therapeutic strategy for depression in medically ill patients and, in particular, for HIV patients with or without cognitive impairment.[16]

RECOGNIZING NEUROPSYCHIATRIC DISTURBANCE IN HIV INFECTION

As more and more individuals have developed HIV infection and AIDS, it has become clear that significant CNS involvement was present.[2–4,9,10,16,17] AIDS patients have presented with organic cognitive impairment, language disorders, movement disorders, delirium, and dementia. Therefore, having a working knowledge of HIV-related psychiatric disease is important in order to provide optimal and timely assessment and intervention for each individual. This implies that in any case in which HIV infection may be possible, a shift in theoretical approach is required. Any psychiatric symptom occurring in conjunction with HIV infection must be considered to be organic first and foremost until proven otherwise. Given that the onslaught of this disease complex upon a patient's mental health is multifactorial, it is important to evaluate systematically the possible neuropsychiatric basis of any psychological disturbance before ruling in, as the sole source of the patient's problem, any of the possible psychological and psychosocial complications attributable to HIV disease. This also assures that prompt medical intervention for any of these medical complications will be rendered.

Most cognitively impaired HIV individuals can be diagnosed using the Diagnostic and Statistical Manual 3rd Edition-Revised (DSM-III-R) criteria.[18] However, given recent reports of cognitive impairment as an early and presenting feature of HIV–CNS involvement, finer distinctions in observed cognitive function are required. In our own studies, the Mini-Mental State Examination[19] did not seem to discriminate degrees of cognitive impairment in HIV-infected patients as opposed to those who are asymptomatic with either LAS, ARC, or AIDS.[16,20] However, when an observational scale like Reisberg's Global Deterioration Scale (GDS)[21] (Table 1) for primary degenerative dementia of the Alzheimer type was applied, finer distinctions in observed cognitive function could be made.[20] Our results indicate that the most severe impairment occurred in ARC and AIDS patients and that there were no significant differences between the distributions of ARC, AIDS, or AIDS complicated with Kaposi's sarcoma. However, levels of cognitive functioning for the PGL patients were significantly different from that of the other groups, suggesting that once systemic effects of HIV infection appear, with or without opportunistic infection, serious cognitive impairment is more likely to be present. One must not overlook the fact, however, that this virus appears to be opportunistic itself in its access to and degenerative effects upon the brain. Studies have shown that even in the early stages of HIV symptomatic infection in PGL, as many as 40% show measurable cognitive dysfunction.[22] And, when rated with the GDS, 21% of our PGL sample showed early confusional to early dementia characteristics. It seems unlikely that these impairments arose acutely and neuropathological studies have demonstrated that HIV subacute encephalitis may have an indolent, demyelinating course.[23] While this process is possible, the

TABLE 1. Global Deterioration Scale[a,b]

GDS stage	PGL	ARC	AIDS	AIDS/KS
1. Normal	11	6	1	1
2. Forgetfulness	4	10	12	5
3. Early confusional	2	7	8	2
4. Late confusional	1	3	2	1
5. Early dementia	1	2	2	4
6. Middle dementia	0	4	1	3
7. Late dementia	0	5	4	1

[a] Adapted from Fernandez et al.[20]
[b] Chi square ($N = 103$): PGL vs. ARC vs. AIDS vs. AIDS/KS, $p < 0.05$; PGL vs. ARC vs. AIDS + AIDS/KS, $p < 0.05$; ARC vs. AIDS + AIDS/KS, n.s.; ARC vs. AIDS, n.s.; AIDS vs. AIDS/KS, n.s.

clinician should be alert to subtly progressive cognitive changes as time postinfection passes.

NEUROBEHAVIORAL ASSESSMENT

In view of the potential for HIV to undermine an individual's cognitive function, early evaluation of the patient with sensitive neuropsychological tests is mandatory. Not only will issues of organic versus functional diagnoses be clarified, but test results will help to understand the patient's abilities to comprehend and comply with his or her treatment. The ability of the patient to understand is salient, as shown by recent reports that verbal memory problems and psychomotor slowing are early but persistent features of HIV-related cognitive disturbance.[24] At the other end of the HIV spectrum disorders (the end-stage associated with AIDS), neurocognitive assessment may be restricted to behavioral observations because of the severity of the illness. As with other medically ill patients, the range of cognitive dysfunction is quite wide and the selection of neuropsychological evaluative instruments will have to be based on the patient's stamina and ability to respond.

TABLE 2. HIV Neuropsychological Screening Battery[a]

General
Mini-Mental State Examination[19]
Memory
Verbal Selective Reminding Test[33]
Benton Visual Retention Test[34]
Rey-Osterrieth Complex Figure[26]
Language/speech
Controlled Oral Word Association (from Benton Multilingual Aphasia Examination)[35]
Visual Naming Test (from Benton Multilingual Aphasia Examination)[35]
Orientation
Pfeiffer Short Portable Mental Status Questionnaire[36]
Benton Temporal Orientation Test[37]
Visuospatial
Bender–Gestalt Test[38]
Raven Progressive Matrices[39]
Intellectual/executive/psychomotor
Digit Span, Arithmetic, Digit Symbol from the WAIS or WAIS-R[40]
Trail Making Test, Parts A and B[41]
Wisconsin Card Sorting[26]
Finger Oscillation Test[41]
Grooved Pegboard[26]
Reaction Time–Simple Auditory, Simple Visual, and Four-Choice Visual[40]
Shipley Institute of Living Scale [42]
Stroop Color Word Test[44]

[a]Suggested battery for evaluating the CNS effects of HIV infection and neurotoxic effects from antiviral and chemotherapeutic agents.

HIV-related cognitive disorder was initially characterized as a "subcortical"[25] dementing process. This suggests that neuropsychological instruments that test memory (registration, storage and retrieval), psychomotor speed, and rate of information processing are essential in the evaluation for this syndrome. Table 2 lists a suggested battery for evaluating not only the effects of HIV infection, but also the effects of any neurotoxicity from antiviral and chemotherapeutic agents. As the patient's stamina and ability to respond permit, elements of this battery may be added or omitted. Many of these tests have age-related norms whereby the patient's performance can be compared with normal functioning persons of his or her same age. For a patient who is affected by HIV primary dementia, this battery, although comprehensive, would be too time-consuming and cumbersome. Nevertheless, elements can be adapted for the assessment of grossly demented patients. For those who are unable to respond other than with a "yes/no" pattern of response, observations may be limited to only gross disturbances of behavior. However, comprehension can still be tested with the Illinois Test of Psycholinguistic Abilities Auditory Reception Subtest.[24] It is a series of yes/no questions graded according to difficulty to permit establishment of a cognitive age. The test also permits a determination of whether the patient is responding in a random or chance manner through analysis of response pattern. This test is useful to assess comprehension for any HIV demented patient with a limited response repertoire. Thus, neuropsychological testing can answer a number of important questions including those of competency, organic versus functional diagnosis, and progression of cognitive decline. Finally, these tests also help determine the type of clinical management and the selection of pharmacotherapy in HIV disease.

PSYCHOSTIMULANT TREATMENT OF COGNITIVE IMPAIRMENT, DEMENTIA, AND OTHER ORGANIC MENTAL DISORDERS IN HIV DISEASE

In their report regarding HIV and psychosis, Maccario and Scharre attributed to Hollander a hypothesis about dopamine dysregulation in HIV-CNS infection.[28] They speculated that HIV affects dopaminergic or catecholaminergic systems preferentially, although it can attack cell lines anywhere from the CNS to the periphery. Evidence for this hypothesis has gained support from several clinical observations. One is that there have been scattered cases of reported schizophreniform psychosis presenting in HIV-infected patients who do not have AIDS or prior histories of thought disorders. The reported episodes responded to haloperidol, however, parkinsonian symptoms then developed. When treated with anticholinergics, the parkinsonian symptoms resolved but hallucinations resumed. In other patients, parkinsonism developed first on metoclopramide, prochlorperazine, or chlorpromazine, suggesting sensitivity to these compounds, or an instability of the dopaminergic systems in HIV-infected patients. Another individual became floridly psychotic with anticholinergics. Nath et al. reported several cases of dystonia, tremor and dyskinesia, implicating basal ganglia involvement.[29] Anatomically, support for the hypothesis has come from Price and colleagues, who have found HIV viral protein in white matter and basal ganglia[30] that parallels the clinical findings. All patients with those neuroanatomical findings have had the AIDS dementia complex. Hill, Farrar and Pert have also demonstrated a localization of the T4 antigen/HIV receptor in primate amygdala, cingulate, and medial temporal cortex and caudate nucleus, among others.[31]

We were aware of evidence implicating catecholaminergic dysfunction that correlated with the findings of cognitive slowing and verbal forgetfulness in the presence of intact higher level abstract reasoning (indicative of a subcortical process). In view of this evidence and due to the fact that many of these patients also complain of fatigue and dysphoria, we tried our population on a regimen of the stimulant methylphenidate (Ritalin).[16] ARC and AIDS patients both showed statistically significant improvement in speed of cognitive tracking and long-term verbal memory function after psychostimulant treatment. AIDS patients had higher performance variability and thus only demonstrated statistically significant improvement on Trail Making Test Part B. Patients who had affective or other psychiatric complaints also tended to show improvement when treated with the psychostimulant. Subjects who did not show a clinical response to methylphenidate when crossed over to dextroamphetamine (Dexedrine) demonstrated a significant improvement. Methylphenidate and dextroamphetamine have also been used in patients with the AIDS dementia complex, organic personality disorders, amnestic syndromes, and organic mood disorders with marked improvements in both affective and cognitive impairments.[16,32] Even in cases of severely demented patients when cognition may not improve, patients will become less negative, more interested in their environment, and family members will frequently report dramatic qualitative improvement in the patient's mood and outlook on life. It must be noted that such improvements were made without precipitating a psychosis in our patients. A few patients developed abnormal involuntary dyskinetic movements which occurred exclusively with the use of dextroamphetamine in excess of 20 mg. Thus, dextroamphetamine should be used cautiously and at lower doses to avoid precipitating a dyskinesia which may not be reversible, even with drug discontinuation.

CONCLUSIONS

There have now been several studies demonstrating the usefulness and the important role of stimulants in the treatment of HIV-related depression and cognitive impairment. The responsiveness of HIV-related behavioral and cognitive deficits to psychostimulant therapy is remarkable for both qualitative and quantitative improvement in higher cortical functions, self-esteem, self-sufficiency and for the absence of treatment-related side effects. When used appropriately, these drugs are both safe and effective, as convincingly demonstrated by their long-term success in the treatment of other disorders such as narcolepsy or childhood hyperkinesis. Side effects are trivial and their occurrences uncommon, even in debilitated HIV patients with multisystem disease.

Psychostimulants, like other potentially addicting agents, must be prescribed with caution to carefully selected HIV patients. However, instances of abuse have not been reported when prescribed for depression, even in HIV-infected populations. Thus, the place of psychostimulants and other pharmacotherapies in the treatment of HIV-related psychiatric disorders will need continuing study to firmly establish their role in the management of depression and cognitively impaired patients with HIV disease. Until then, stimulants should be used to provide a measure of relief not only from the psychological morbidity associated with this disease but also from the infection's pathological effect on neurocognitive production.

REFERENCES

1. Fauci AS, Masur H, Gelmann EP, et al: The acquired immunodeficiency syndrome: An update. *Ann Intern Med* 102:800–813, 1985.
2. Price RW, Brew B, Sidtis J, et al: The brain in AIDS: Central nervous system HIV-1 infection and AIDS dementia complex. *Science* 239:586–592, 1988.
3. Felgenhauer K: Another venereal disease with frequent nervous system involvement: neuro-AIDS. *J Neurol* 234:65–66, 1987.
4. Fernandez F: Psychiatric complications in HIV-related illnesses, in *American Psychiatric Association's AIDS Primer*. Washington, DC, American Psychiatric Association, 1989, pp. 5-1–5-7.
5. Gyorkey F, Melnick JL, Gyorkey P: Human immunodeficiency virus in brain biopsies of patients with AIDS and progressive encephalopathy. *J Infect Dis* 155:870–876, 1987.
6. Vazeux R, Brousse N, Jarry A, et al: AIDS subacute encephalitis: Identification of HIV-infected cells. *Am J Pathol* 126:403–410, 1987.
7. Wiley CA, Schrier RD, Nelson JA, et al: Cellular localization of human immunodeficiency virus infection within the brains of acquired immunodeficiency syndrome patients. *Proc Natl Acad Sci USA* 83:7089–7093, 1986.
8. Funke I, Hahn A, Rieber EP, et al: The cellular receptor (CD4) of the human immunodeficiency virus is expressed on neurons and glial cells in the human brain. *J Exp Med* 165:1230–1235, 1987.
9. Grant I, Atkinson H, Hesselink JR, et al: Evidence for early central nervous system involvement in the acquired immunodeficiency syndrome (AIDS) and other human immunodeficiency virus (HIV) infections: Studies with neuropsychological testing and magnetic resonance imaging. *Ann Intern Med* 107:828–836, 1987.
10. Navia BA, Price RW: The acquired immunodeficiency syndrome dementia complex as the presenting or sole manifestation of human immunodeficiency virus infection. *Arch Neurol* 44:65–69, 1987
11. Klerman GL: Psychotropic hedonism versus pharmacological Calvinism. *Hastings Center Rep* 2(4):1–3, 1971.
12. Tesar GE: The role of stimulants in general medicine. *Drug Ther* July:186–196, 1982.
13. Woods SW, Tesar GE, Murray GB, et al: Psychostimulant treatment for depressive disorders secondary to medical illness. *J Clin Psychiatry* 47:12–15, 1986.
14. Jenicke MA: Assessment and treatment of affective illness in the elderly. *J Geriatr Psychiatry Neurol* 1(2):91–107, 1988.
15. Fernandez F, Adams F, Holmes VF, et al: Methylphenidate for depressive disorders in cancer patients. *Psychosomatics* 28:455–461, 1987.
16. Fernandez F, Adams F, Levy JK, et al: Cognitive impairment due to AIDS-related complex and its response to psychostimulants. *Psychosomatics* 29:38–46, 1988.
17. McArthur JD: Neurologic manifestations of AIDS. *Medicine (Baltimore)* 66:407–437, 1987.
18. American Psychiatric Association: *Diagnostic and Statistical Manual of Mental Disorders,* ed 3, revised. Washington, DC, American Psychiatric Press, 1987.
19. Folstein MF, Folstein SE, McHugh PR: "Mini-Mental State": a practical method for grading the cognitive state of patients for the clinician. *J Psychiatr Res* 12:189–198, 1975.
20. Fernandez F. Levy JK, Salmeron G: The incidence of dementia and other organic mental disorders (OMDs) associated with human immunodeficiency virus (HIV) infection. *Current Concepts in Psycho-Oncology and AIDS*. Syllabus of the Postgraduate Course. New York, Memorial Sloan-Kettering Cancer Center, September 17–19, 1987, p. 399.
21. Reisberg B, Ferris SH, de Leon MJ, et al: The global deterioration scale (GDS): An instrument for the assessment of primary degenerative dementia (PDD). *Am J Psychiatry* 139:1136–1139, 1982.
22. Janssen RS, Saykin AJ, Kaplan JE, et al: Neurological complications of human immunodeficiency virus infection in patients with lymphadenopathy syndrome. *Ann Neurol* 23:49–55, 1988.

23. Navia BA, Cho E-S, Petito CK, et al: The AIDS dementia complex. II. Neuropathology. *Ann Neurol* 19:525–535, 1986.
24. Levy JK, Fernandez F, Pirozzolo FJ: Patterns of cognitive impairment in HIV infection: A preliminary report. *J Clin Exp Neuropsychol* 10:77, 1988.
25. Whitehouse P: The concept of subcortical and cortical dementia: Another look. *Ann Neurol* 19:1–7, 1986.
26. Lezak MD: *Neuropsychological Assessment,* ed 2. New York, Oxford University Press, 1983.
27. Levy JK, Fernandez F: Neuropsychiatric care for critically ill AIDS patients. *J Crit Illness* 4:33–42, 1989.
28. Maccario M, Scharre DW: HIV and acute onset of psychosis. *Lancet* 2:342, 1987.
29. Nath A, Jankovic J, Pettigrew LC: Movement disorders and AIDS. *Neurology (NY)* 37:37–41, 1987.
30. Pumarola-Sune, T, Navia BA, Cordon-Cardo C, et al: HIV antigen in the brains of patients with AIDS dementia complex. *Ann Neurol* 21:490–496, 1987.
31. Hill JM, Farrar WL, Pert CB: Localization of the T4 antigen/AIDS virus receptor in monkey and rat brains: Prominence in cortical regions. *Psychopharm Bull* 22:689–694, 1986.
32. Fernandez F, Levy JK, Galizzi H: Response to HIV-related depression to psychostimulants: Case reports. *Hosp Comm Psychiatry* 39:628–631, 1988.
33. Levin HS: Learning and memory, in Hannay HJ (ed): *Experimental Techniques in Human Neuropsychology.* New York, Oxford University Press, 1986, pp. 309–362.
34. Benton AL: *Revised Visual Retention Test,* ed 4. New York, The Psychological Corporation, 1974.
35. Benton AL, deS Hamsher K: *Multilingual Aphasia Examination.* Iowa City, The University of Iowa, 1983.
36. Pfeiffer E: A short portable mental status questionnaire for the assessment of organic brain deficit in elderly patients. *J Am Geriatr Soc* 23:433, 1975.
37. Benton AL, deS Hamsher K, Varney NR, Spreen O: *Contributions to Neuropsychological Assessment: A clinical Manual.* New York, Oxford University Press, 1983.
38. Lacks P: *Bender Gestalt Screening for Brain Dysfunction.* New York, John Wiley—Interscience, 1984.
39. Raven JC, Court JH, Raven J: *Manual for Raven's Progressive Matrices and Vocabulary Scales: Section 3: Standard Progressive Matrices.* London, H.K. Lewis & Co., Ltd., 1983.
40. Wechsler D: *WAIS-R Manual.* New York, The Psychological Corporation, 1981.
41. Golden CJ, Osmon DC, Moses JA Jr, et al: *Interpretation of the Halstead—Reitan Neuropsychological Test Battery: A Case book Approach.* New York: Grune & Stratton, 1981.
42. Pirozzolo FJ, Christensen KJ, Ogle KM, et al: Simple and choice reaction time in dementia: clinical implications. *Neurobiol Aging* 2:113, 1981.
43. Zachary RA: *Shipley Institute of Living Scale Revised Manual.* Los Angeles, Western Psychological Services, 1987.
44. Golden CJ: *Stroop Color and Word Test: A Manual for Clinical and Experimental Uses.* Chicago, Stoelting Company, 1978.

IV

Health Care Delivery Issues

16

Consultation/Liaison Psychiatry and AIDS

JAMES W. DILLEY and JAY BAER

INTRODUCTION

Consultation/liaison psychiatry is the subspecialty of psychiatry which focuses on the evaluation, treatment, and management of medical and surgical patients with emotional and cognitive problems. Psychiatrists active in this area of expertise are usually based in a hospital setting, or work closely with the patients of internists, family practitioners, surgeons or obstetricians/gynecologists. The psychiatric consultant must possess a firm grounding in general psychiatry as well as a familiarity with common medical/surgical problems and their treatments, the use of psychopharmacologic agents in the medically ill, and the usual structure and functioning of hospitals.[1–3] He/she brings knowledge of the complex interactions among the biological, psychological, and social factors that are always at play at any given moment in a person's life and is expert in assessing the impact of these factors on a person's current condition. Consultation/liaison psychiatry, then, stands as the bridge between the specialties of psychiatry and medicine, bringing the expertise of the psychiatrist to bear on the physically ill patient who demonstrates disorders of mood or cognition.

The primary focus of this chapter is on the application of the consultation process to patients with the acquired immune deficiency syndrome (AIDS) and those infected with the human immunodeficiency virus (HIV). The increasing numbers of patients with AIDS underscore the need for a discussion of consultation issues in a disease which is not always well understood by either the general medical practitioner[4] or the consultation psychiatrist. In particular, there are aspects of this disease which raise especially vexing problems for the psychiatric consultant and the entire treatment team.[5]

This chapter focuses on the consultation process with this group of patients and will highlight information about the spectrum of disease associated with HIV infection. Comparisons with the general practice of consultation/liaison psychiatry is made where the comparison seems pertinent or especially illustrative of a particular point. Emphasis is placed on a description of the variety of psychiatric consultations commonly requested for

JAMES W. DILLEY • Department of Psychiatry, University of California, San Francisco, California 94105; University of California, San Francisco–AIDS Health Project, San Francisco, California 94143–0884. JAY BAER • Department of Psychiatry, Tufts University School of Medicine, Boston, Massachusetts 02111.

people with AIDS or HIV infection as well as the commonly encountered spectrum of psychological reactions seen across the progression of clinical disease. A discussion of psychotropic medication is also included. Finally, a brief discussion of common ethical issues raised by these patients and the role of the psychiatric consultant in working with these issues is presented.

PROCESS OF PSYCHIATRIC CONSULTATION

Whether the psychiatric consultant is asked to evaluate a person with AIDS or any other medical/surgical patient, the process of consultation is similar. During the course of caring for a patient in the hospital, the primary care provider may become concerned about his/her patient's psychological reaction to illness or may feel uncomfortable in managing an underlying major psychiatric disorder. In either case, consultation may be requested by calling the consultant or by submitting a written request. Usually, but not always, the patient is made aware that the consultation has been requested.

Once the consultation has been requested, the psychiatric consultant will try to ascertain as clearly as possible the concerns of the primary provider. Sometimes this is obvious, as when a patient is hospitalized following a suicidal gesture and an evaluation of the patient's current suicidal intent and recommendations for ongoing treatment are needed. At other times, the focus of the consult request may not be as clear: for example, consult requests are sometimes received when the primary provider feels there is something unusual about the way a patient is behaving or reacting to his or her illness. In either case, a brief discussion between the consultant and the primary provider is helpful to clarify the concern of the primary care provider and to ensure that the consultant addresses the specific consultation question.

Once the focus of the consultation is determined, the consultant reviews the medical chart to understand the course of treatment, paying close attention to the kinds and quantities of medication the patient is taking. In addition, the consultant will often confer with the nursing staff and with the patient's family to gather pertinent information about the patient's social history and present functioning.

The consultant then interviews the patient asking about present and past social and psychiatric history, medical problems, and current medications. Mental status examination is performed and the consultant is then usually prepared to make an assessment of the questions raised in the consultation request. A differential diagnosis is formulated and discussed with the primary provider. The nursing staff and the family are also apprised of the evaluation results and the recommendations for treatment. For example, a depressed patient with suicidal ideation should be discussed at length with the staff so they better understand the context of the patient's depression and the specific precautions that need to be taken.

The consultant then summarizes his findings and recommendations in a consultation note in the medical chart. Follow-up examinations by the consultant are an essential part of the consultation process and allow for ongoing support of the patient and treatment team as well as an evaluation of the effectiveness of the recommended treatment plan.

PSYCHIATRIC CONSULTATION IN HIV-SPECTRUM PATIENTS

General Considerations

Much has been written about the psychological and social impact of the AIDS epidemic.[6–8] By now, those issues which most contribute to the unique psychosocial nature of AIDS and infection with HIV are well known: AIDS is a new, essentially untreatable illness that is transmissible and that markedly reduces life-expectancy; it is primarily contracted through sexual contact or through the sharing of unsterilized intravenous needles; it has mostly affected young, previously healthy gay or bisexual men or those with a history of intravenous drug use; and it is a worldwide pandemic with cases reported in the majority of countries throughout the world. For these reasons, a variety of strong responses are encountered in those most affected by the disease—those who are patients, their families and significant others, and those who care for them.[9–11]

For the psychiatric consultant, the two most salient psychological responses engendered by AIDS are fear and the veil of moral judgements that surround the disease and those who are most commonly affected. Examples of the consequences of public fear are common. Perhaps the most dramatic example was the burning of the Reye family home in Arcadia, Florida, by unknown arsonists because the family's three hemophiliac sons were known by the community to be seropositive. Examples of the moral judgements are usually less blatant, but are nonetheless common not only among the general public but within the medical community as well. An editorial about AIDS in the *Southern Medical Journal* is a case in point: "Might we be witnessing, in fact, in the form of a modern communicable disorder, a fulfillment of St. Paul's pronouncement: 'the due penalty of error.' "[12] These underlying issues run throughout the care of people with AIDS, and the psychiatric consultant asked to intervene must have some appreciation for the multiple, complex issues which both the consultant and the person with AIDS must face.

In addition to an appreciation for the unique constellation of social and psychological factors that confront the person with AIDS, so too, must the consultant have an awareness of basic facts about the medical complications of HIV disease and the general prognostic implications of each. The consultant needs to know, for example, that the length of expected survival post-AIDS-diagnosis is correlated with the particular disease state that initially resulted in diagnosis. For example, individuals first diagnosed with Kaposi's sarcoma may be essentially healthy from a subjective point of view and may remain so for several years. Based on the cumulative survival in a cohort of 5833 patients with AIDS diagnosed in New York City between 1981 and December, 1985, a homosexual man whose AIDS diagnosis was on the basis of Kaposi's sarcoma alone, had the most favorable survival pattern, with a cumulative probability of survival of 72.1% at 1 year and 30.9% at 5 years.[13] The patient whose AIDS diagnosis is first made by the appearance of cryptococcal meningitis on the other hand, faces a life expectancy of less than six months.[14] By far most people with AIDS survive their first year post-diagnosis and many live several years beyond. However, quality of life is most often progressively difficult as the numbers and degree of medical complications require coping with multiple hospitalizations, a variety of medication regimens and their side effects, and the psychosocial stress of living with chronic disease and the spectre of a premature death.

TABLE 1. Neurological Complications in AIDS Spectrum Patients

CNS disease	Percent	Known medical treatment
Viral syndromes		
Atypical aseptic meningitis	7	None
Herpes simplex encephalitis	3	Ara-a or Acyclovir
Progressive multifocal leukoencephalopathy	2	Possibly Ara-a
CMV retinitis	?	Ganciclovir, foscarnet
AIDS dementia	?	None
Nonviral syndromes	51	
Toxoplasma gondii	32	Pyrimethamine and sulfadiazine
Cryptococcus neoformans	13	Amphotericin B and fluconazole
Candida albicans	2	Amphotericin B and fluconazole
Atypical mycobacteria	2	INH, ethambutol and rifampin
Other	2	
Neoplasms	10	
Primary CNS lymphoma	5	Radiation therapy
CNS and systemic lymphoma	4	Radiation therapy and chemotherapy
Kaposi's sarcoma	1	Radiation therapy and chemotherapy
Cerebrovascular accidents	3	Treat etiology
Endocarditis		
Herpes zoster arteritis		
Idiopathic thrombocytopenia		
Neuropathies, myopathy	?	
Distal symmetrical neuropathy		Amitriptyline
Chemic inflammatory polyneuropathy		Consider plasma pheresis
Vacuolar myelopathy		
Metabolic and systemic changes	?	Treat etiology
Hypoxia secondary to PCP		
Electrolyte imbalance		
Nutritional deficiencies		

Adapted from Levy et al.[13]

Neuropsychiatric Complications

It is now well recognized that clinically apparent central nervous system (CNS) and/or peripheral nervous system disease occurs in at least 30–40% of AIDS patients. The most common causes of neurological disease in AIDS patients include infection with HIV itself, other viral and non-viral infections, neoplasms and cerebrovascular disease (Table 1).

Because of the neurotropism of HIV, autopsy studies of AIDS patients indicate that 70–90% of the brains of these patients will show gross and/or microscopic evidence of CNS disease. In fact, several reports have shown that subclinical cognitive impairment due to HIV infection may precede the diagnosis of AIDS in 10–25% of patients. Some degree of the AIDS dementia complex[15] may be present in as many as two thirds of AIDS patients prior to death. It is clear, then, that neurological disease in HIV-infected individuals is a major source of medical and psychiatric morbidity and psychiatric consultant must be familiar with signs and symptoms commonly encountered in these patients.

AIDS Dementia Complex

The presence of a chronic, debilitating encephalitis in people with AIDS has been reported from early in the experience of caring for these patients. Subsequently, a good deal of evidence has converged to enable researchers to document a distinct clinical and neuropathological syndrome now referred to as AIDS dementia complex (ADC). Clinically, the ADC is characterized by a triad of cognitive, behavioral, and motor symptoms.[16] The absolute incidence of the ADC in AIDS patients prior to death is unknown, although clinical experience would suggest that it is a common sequelae of the disease, particularly in the later stages of the illness. In one study, evidence of the ADC was shown in about 70% of autopsied AIDS patients in whom all focal neurological disease or confounding metabolic encephalopathy had been excluded.[15] Typically, the dementia has an insidious onset and progression although sudden accelerations may also occur. At times, the dementia has an acute onset and may be accompanied by an acute organic psychosis.

Table 2 details the specific clinical symptoms and signs found in patients with the ADC at both early and later stages of the disorder. The presence, timing and onset, and

TABLE 2. Manifestations of AIDS Dementia

- Symptoms—early
  - Cognitive
    - Memory loss (names, historical details, appointments)
    - Impaired concentration (lose track of conversation or reading)
    - Mental slowing ("not as quick," less verbal, loss of spontaneity)
    - Confusion (time or person)
  - Behavioral
    - Apathy, withdrawal, "depression"
    - Agitation, confusion, hallucinations
  - Motor
    - Unsteady gait
    - Bilateral lag weakness
    - Loss of coordination, impaired handwriting
    - Tremor
- Symptoms—late
  - Cognitive
    - Global dementia
    - Confusion
    - Distractibility
    - Delayed verbal responses
  - Behavioral
    - Vacant stare
    - Restlessness
    - Disinhibition
    - Organic psychosis
  - Motor
    - Slowing, truncal ataxia
    - Weakness: legs > arms
    - Pyramidal track signs: spasticity, hyperreflexia, tremor

relative severity of cognitive, motor, and behavioral symptoms/signs in patients suffering from a psychological depression: the presence of symptoms such as apathy/social withdrawal and dysphoric mood can be seen in both diagnostic entities. The following case examples will highlight these concerns.

Marie is a 39-year-old female intravenous drug user with a 2-year history of symptomatic HIV disease admitted for fevers, severe diarrhea and wasting. The nurses report that she is usually withdrawn, often cannot or will not comply with simple directions and wanders about the hospital at night. She is occasionally incontinent of urine. Her physician feels that she needs a lumbar puncture but is unsure of Marie's ability to give consent. Psychiatric consultation is requested to "assess altered mental status and make recommendations for management."

As mentioned above, the differential diagnosis of cognitive compromise is complex and requires a detailed workup. The requesting physician is aware of this and usually has the workup under way at the time of consultation, but at times must be encouraged to proceed with brain imaging, toxicology screening, trimming excess medications and reviewing or correcting possible metabolic abnormalities. Formal neuropsychological evaluation is often a helpful adjunct to the psychiatric assessment and can help differentiate early HIV dementia from other clinical entities.

The diagnosis of ADC largely depends on the documentation of typical cognitive, behavioral, and motor abnormalities in individuals with AIDS, and on performing those neurodiagnostic tests necessary to rule out the other possible CNS disease states common in this population (see Table 1). The psychiatric consultant can be helpful in those cases in which a diagnosis is made by educating the staff about management strategies for the cognitively compromised patient. Helping the staff to understand the importance of orienting cues, the use of clocks and calendars to help manage poor short-term memory, and the importance of using short, simple sentences in communicating with the patient are helpful helping interventions. Recommendations for the use of medication for control of agitation and to reverse altered sleep/wakefulness cycles are also important (see under Psychopharmacology section). Lastly, understanding and controlling these potentially difficult behavioral problems is extremely important to social workers and discharge planners in arranging for the most appropriate placement for cognitively impaired patients.

Depression

John is a 32-year-old gay white male hospitalized for his first bout of *Pneumocystis carinii* pneumonia. It is the ninth day of his hospitalization and John is being successfully treated with the antibiotic Septra. John's pulmonary status is slowly but steadily improving, but his doctor and nurses have noticed that he appears unusually fatigued, is doing little to care for himself, suffers from insomnia and poor appetite, and withdraws from most attempts to engage him in conversation. Psychiatric consultation for evaluation of depression is requested.

Evaluation for depression may well be the most common psychiatric consultation request in people hospitalized with AIDS. The differential diagnosis of apparent depression is large and includes a number of organic etiologies such as early ADC, metabolic disorder, medication side effects (e.g., nausea and appetite suppression from Septra), as well as recurrent depressive illness and/or reaction to the severe current stress of receiving a AIDS diagnosis. The emotional needs of patients differ somewhat based on their physical condition and their place on the trajectory of AIDS complications (Table 3).

TABLE 3. Common Psychological Issues in the AIDS Patient as a Function of Physical State

New diagnosis
Affective numbing vs. affective discharge; denial
Need for emotional, financial, and social support; possibly impaired self-esteem
Fear of contamination, treatment issues
Fear of rejection by family and friends
Feelings of guilt and self-blame over previous lifestyle—illness as retribution
Is there sex after diagnosis? Other lifestyle changes
Mid-stage
Loss of hope, emotional exhaustion
More detailed grief worrk—anticipating and mourning loss of important people and objects
Extent of treatment, pain control
Unfinished business—life review; putting one's affairs in order
Terminal care
Adequate pain control, personal contact
Work with family and friends
Death and dying, honoring patient's wishes

While it is important to be sensitive to the psychological meanings of the patient's illness and the current psychosocial environment, it is also helpful to remain aware of the potential contribution of organic factors in assessing a patient with AIDS. An absolutely normal CNS may be rare in these patients, especially those with significant psychiatric symptoms. Purely functional disorders, with the exception of adjustment disorders[17] are probably also rare. The likelihood of this "blending" of organic and functional psychiatric disorders complicates the diagnostic picture, as well as the psychopharmacologic and psychotherapeutic management.

Some clinical rules of thumb can be helpful in teasing apart these aspects of a patient's presentation. First, a predominantly functional disorder is more likely in: patients who have more intact immune function, i.e., those more recently diagnosed and those without other opportunistic infections; those patients with a previous personal or family history of major psychiatric disorder; and, those patients for whom a clearly identifiable psychosocial stressor can be identified. Searching for cognitive signs of depression (e.g., hopelessness, guilt, or concerns about being a "bad" person, and suicidal plans) can also be helpful. Again, the use of formal neuropsychological testing is useful in helping to determine the relative proportion of organic versus functional components.

Treatments for patients felt to have major mood disturbances may include brief, supportive psychotherapy and psychopharmacologic and/or social interventions. The use of antidepressant and stimulant medications will be discussed below.

Psychotic Symptoms

Leon is a 42-year-old bisexual white male brought to the emergency room by two of his friends. They report that Leo, who has had a diagnosis of ARC for nearly a year, has undergone a radical personality change in the past few weeks. Formerly a rather shy accountant with no history of psychiatric problems, Leo has become increasingly "speedy," irritable, and promiscuous. His friends became particularly worried when they learned he had not slept for several nights and had spent $12,000 on home appliances he didn't need. The emergency-room physician notes that Leo has markedly pressured speech, admits to auditory hallucinations and voices, and the grandiose delusion that he has become the chief of the United States' Health and Welfare Division and has ordered that its entire budget be utilized for AIDS research. Psychiatric consultation is requested for evaluation of this apparent manic episode and consideration for psychiatric hospitalization.

Psychotic symptoms may arise in many contexts in HIV-spectrum patients, including dementia and delirium. There have been several patients without a history of affective disorder who develop a manic episode and the extent of HIV-related disease progression in these individuals at the time of the episode has varied widely. It appears that over weeks to months the affective symptoms fade away while the patient becomes progressively demented.

In assessing a patient with psychotic symptomatology, the consultant may attempt to elicit a history of psychotic illness including drug and alcohol abuse as well as ADC. He/she must decide if psychiatric hospitalization is indicated and whether or not the patient meets criteria for acute medical and psychiatric treatment (e.g., if Leo had suffered pneumonia in addition to his behavioral problems) and his collaborating physicians must decide which acute hospital service should host his comprehensive treatment.

Treatment for patients with psychotic disorders may include supportive psychotherapy, social interventions, and psychopharmacology. The use of antipsychotic medications will be discussed below.

Family/Support System Conflicts

As mentioned above, one of the psychosocial aspects of AIDS which sets it apart from other life-threatening illnesses is the fact that AIDS is most commonly found among members of socially stigmatized groups. This fact can be a particularly confounding factor in the ability or willingness of the patient's traditional support system to rally to the side of the patient. It should be noted that among gay men who have lived an openly gay lifestyle, it is not uncommon for a nontraditional family to have developed over the years. The patient may have a steady, life-partner relationship that is indistinguishable in tone and form from that of a heterosexual marriage. He may also be single, but have a close circle of friends that substitutes for the biological family. In some cases, the biological family may be aware of their son's homosexuality, though knowledge of the patient's lifestyle does not necessarily imply that the family either condones or approves. There may, in fact, be open conflict that results between the patient's biological family and his nontraditional family of friends. This outcome is particularly likely when the parents have either not known of their son's homosexuality or have known, but have refused to acknowledge it openly or have become emotionally distant because of past conflicts over this issue. These parents are sometimes the most difficult, because they may carry a sense of guilt for having rejected their son and now, with his illness, feel they have to make up for the hard feelings between them over the years. This can lead to difficulty in negotiating with the patient and his current family because the parents may resent or simply cannot accept the legitimacy of the commitment between their son and his male partner, or his friends.

Stephen is a 33-year-old black gay man who had AIDS for 3 years. Initially diagnosed with Kaposi sarcoma, Stephen has felt well for the most part and has continued to work at his job as a computer programmer for a large financial company. Because his homosexuality has never been acceptable to his middle class East Coast parents, it has remained in large part an issue which was known, but never directly discussed. Contact between Stephen and his parents has been minimal, and Stephen decides not to tell his parents about his illness. He is quite open about the fact that he moved to the West Coast some 10 years prior because he needed to feel free to live an openly gay lifestyle, and he "knows" that his parents wouldn't be supportive of his illness. Joseph is Stephen's partner of 8 years. On returning home from a 3-day business trip, Joseph finds Stephen seriously ill, and rushes him to the hospital where Stephen is admitted to the intensive care unit and placed on a respirator. Because of the grave prognosis, Joseph notifies Stephen's family that Stephen is critically ill with "pneumonia" and the parents arrive the next day. After learning that her son has AIDS and may not recover, Stephen's mother, believing that Joseph had "given" AIDS to Stephen, turns on Joseph and demands that he leave the hospital and never return. She insists to the nursing staff that "this man" not be allowed to visit her son and demands to see the hospital administrator. She begins to make plans to have Stephen flown back to the East Coast, where she will "be able to take care of him when he gets out of the hospital." Joseph threatens to sue the hospital if attempts are made to prohibit him from seeing his lover. An immediate psychiatric consultation is requested.

Variations on this basic scenario are common. This case underscores the potential for emotional crisis that exists in working with people with AIDS. The potential for multiple emotional blows for friends and families of those with AIDS is significant. When individuals are forced to confront several difficult issues, including homosexuality, long-term estrangement, and unexpected death simultaneously, the results can be dramatic.

The psychiatric consultant can be extremely helpful by working individually with both parties and initially acknowledging the enormity of conflict and distress each is feeling. The consultant can serve to defuse the immediacy of the situation and eventually help both appreciate the difficult feelings on each side. Acting as an advocate for the patient, the consultant serves both as a crisis intervention specialist and as a mediator to achieve a resolution, or at least, a compromise that is mutually acceptable to both parties. At worst, the consultant can serve as a liaison between the two sides, conveying information and establishing limits which respect the wishes of both sides as much as possible. After the crisis has passed, the consultant can offer psychological assistance or referral to the individuals involved. Frequently, families grieving over loved ones with AIDS must suffer alone, sensing that it is unacceptable for them to bring their concerns home to their communities.

PSYCHOPHARMACOLOGY

General Principles

The consultant working with HIV patients will have become familiar with the sensitivity to medications that the human brain, damaged by HIV, may exhibit. He/she will also need to become familiar with common medications used to treat opportunistic infections in this population and their side effects (Table 4). In our experience, combining commonly used psychotropic medications with these drugs is not contraindicated, nor are there problematic drug interactions.

TABLE 4. Common Opportunistic Infections in HIV-Spectrum Patients, Their Treatments and Neurobehavioral Side Effects

Opportunistic infections	Common medications	Side effects
Pneumocystis carinii pneumonia	Sulfa/trimethoprim	Rash Nausea/vomiting (often leading to Rx with lorazepam or other antiemetics)
	Pentamadine	Hypoglycemia
Cryptococcal meningitis	Amphotericin B	Bone marrow suppression and renal compromise
	Fluconazole	GI upset, nausea, occasional skin rash
Toxoplasma gondii encephalitis	Sulfadiazine Pyramethamine Clindamycin	
Mycobacterium (*M. tuberculosis,* avium intercellulare)	Ethambutol INH Rifampin Dapsone	Hepatitis, bone marrow suppression
Candidiasis		
Oral	Mycelex Nystatin	
Esophageal	Ketoconazole	Hepatitis
CMV retinitis	DHPG (ganciclovir)	Irritability, mild euphoria, increased energy
Prophylaxis	AZT (zidovudine)	Insomnia, irritability, euphoria, increased energy

Antidepressants

Medical practitioners may have a bias against the use of antidepressants in HIV patients. The expectation that it is "normal" to be depressed if one is ill with AIDS or ARC can mistakenly preclude consideration of antidepressant therapy, even when symptoms are of sufficient severity to warrant it. For many patients who evidence signs of depression and dementia, it is incorrect to assume that the presence of the latter absolutely contraindicates treatment for the former. The cognitive symptoms may in part be caused by depression (pseudodementia); even if this is not the case, depressive symptoms are, at least, potentially treatable. Many patients with AIDS have received benefit from antidepressant therapy.

If the patient is acutely medically ill and depressed, it is advisable to wait a few days before instituting drug treatment. This will allow for correction of metabolic abnormalities that may have a profound effect on mood and may make treatment with medication more complex or simply less well tolerated.

As with the use of psychopharmacologic agents in the general population, it is important to choose agents with the most favorable side-effect profile for each individual patient. For HIV patients it is often desirable to minimize sedation, anticholinergic side effects should be minimized because of the potential for exacerbating cognitive deficits and because the drying of mucous membranes may contribute to the growth of candidiasis throughout the alimentary tract. Nortripyline and desipramine are particularly recommended, though many others have been used successfully. Dosing should be modest at first but will often need to be comparable to doses used in the general population. Finally, tricyclics are sometimes helpful in controlling or reducing the pain and discomfort of peripheral neuropathies in these patients.

Stimulants

If tricyclics are refused, ineffective, or contraindicated, the consultant should consider the use of methylphenidate[18] or dextroamphetamine.[19] Methylphenidate has been used with some success in patients with both AIDS and symptomatic HIV disease (Fernandez F: personal communication) and has recently been shown to be a treatment that is well tolerated and results in little abuse in depressed cancer patients.[20] The consultant contemplating the use of psychostimulants should take into account the patient's drug history and be alert for the possibility of drug-induced psychotic reactions.

Antipsychotics

There are several indications for the use of antipsychotics in this patient population. First, they are useful for decreasing psychotic symptoms in those with organic mental disorders. Patients without significant neurological symptoms or cognitive compromise can tolerate dosages comparable to those tolerated by the general population. However, prophylaxis against extrapyramidal side effects is recommended. Secondly, these agents can be used to control agitation in demented patients. Dosing should always begin very modestly as these patients are particularly sensitive to drug side effects and may already have neurological findings that can easily be confused with extrapylaxis for the development of extrapyramidal symptoms. Lastly, antipsychotics in modest dosages can be useful in controlling agitation, dysphoria, and severe anxiety in severely character-disordered patients.

The choice of antipsychotic agent should be dictated by the side-effect profile. Midrange potency agents such as perphenazine and thiothixene may be first drugs of choice, rather than the more commonly used high-potency haloperidol. Haloperidol has been associated with severe extrapyramidal reactions in some patients with AIDS.

Benzodiazepines

These medications are widely and often successfully used to lessen anxiety in HIV-spectrum patients. However, the consultant should be alert for several common mistakes made with their use. Medically hospitalized patients are frequently prescribed multiple psychoactive drugs, including multiple benzodiazepines (e.g., diazepam for anxiety, lorazepam for nausea, temazepam for sleep, etc.). This increases the likelihood of central-nervous-system toxicity. Patients with HIV encephalopathy or other cognitive deficits are at particular risk for such side effects, such as worsening memory deficits or other cognitive performance, disinhibition, visual hallucinations, and excessive sedation. Benzodiazepines can be used successfully to relieve anxiety and agitation in demented patients who have difficulty tolerating antipsychotics, but these drugs must be used cautiously.

Other Treatments

For patients who develop significant agitation in conjunction with a diagnosis of ADC, antipsychotics are the first drug of choice. However, these agents may prove ineffective because of the development of dose-limiting side effects. In these cases, the consultant should consider alternative treatments. Lithium carbonate in usual doses has been successfully used in patients presenting with a manic component to their symptom complex. Carbamazepine and beta-blockers have also been helpful in controlling agitation.

Psychiatric Sequelae of AIDS Treatments

Azidothymidine (AZT), the only commonly prescribed antiviral at this time, has been anecdotally reported to cause anxiety, irritability, racing thoughts, and insomnia shortly after its administration is begun. Cases of mania have been attributed to AZT, but it is currently unclear as to whether the drug played an etiological role in the affective disturbance.

There are also striking case reports of the effectiveness of AZT in the amelioration of the ADC. Patients with significant cognitive deficits have, in individual cases, responded dramatically with marked improvements in their symptoms. Others have shown little or no change. Because AZT is known to cross the blood-brain barrier, there is a theoretical rationale for attempting such treatment. Placebo controlled studies are currently underway to determine the relative effectiveness of AZT on cognitive symptoms.

ETHICAL CONSIDERATIONS

The psychiatric consultant asked to intervene in the care of a person with AIDS must be aware of the difficult ethical dilemmas that may arise. No other disease in recent times has so clearly illuminated the psychological and social implications of medical information and treatment. Because of the interplay among the various unique aspects of AIDS outlined throughout this chapter, ethical considerations are often a part of the consultation requests received by the consultant. The psychiatrist who is well informed about these issues is in a position to promote quality patient care and to provide much appreciated assistance to the treatment team who may be struggling with these issues. What follows is a brief summary of common ethical issues which are raised in the care of people with AIDS and those who are HIV positive. Importantly, most of these issues are equally applicable to members of both groups at highest risk for AIDS (gay and bisexual men and intravenous drug users). For ease of presentation, these issues are presented in a sequence based loosely on the course of the illness.

New Diagnosis

Because of the complex social implications of an AIDS diagnosis or of being told that one is seropositive for antibodies to the AIDS virus, the issue of confidentiality is critical. Because the patient's right to the confidentiality of information concerning his/her medical diagnosis and treatment can sometimes appear to be in conflict with the right of health care providers, actual or potential sexual partners, and household members to have access to this information, the psychiatrist consultant is sometimes called in to help mediate these issues as is illustrated in the following case history.

The HIV Antibody Test

Jim is a 33-year-old married, bisexual architect referred for consultation for depression by his primary care provider. Although Jim does not appear severely clinically depressed, he is certainly anxious and ruminating about a series of events that began 5 months previously. At that time Jim was referred, again by his primary care provider, to a surgeon for elective hernia repair. When the surgeon discovered that Jim was bisexual he informed him that he would be required to undergo the AIDS antibody test and that he would only have access to the operation if he was seronegative. Jim refused these conditions, but was troubled by his discussion with the surgeon, and began to think seriously about whether or not he wanted to take the test. Two months later, he had the test done at an anonymous city-sponsored health center and learned that he was positive. He was greatly upset by this news and has not been able to discuss it with his wife. In addition, he was referred to another surgeon who does not require the test, and plans to have surgery next month.

Receipt of a positive HIV antibody test can have tremendous emotional sequelae for any patient including anxiety, depression, and hypchondriasis. Issues regarding confidentiality and the test can be a significant source of stress for patients and caregivers alike.

As well as dealing with the personal implications of the test result (e.g., Will I become ill? When? Could I have avoided infection?), patients like Jim have to consider the effect of their seropositive status on others in their lives, whom to tell about it, and how to cope with their reactions. Patients may be motivated by a need to protect others and to gain support for themselves but run the risk of losing access to important relationships (e.g., spouse, health care provider). As they struggle with these decisions, patients often require education about the meaning of the antibody test—Do they really understand what their test results mean?—and support through the difficult explorations of their alternatives and fears.

In undertaking these supportive tasks with patients, the psychiatrist may well be faced with ethical dilemmas. If a patient reveals that he/she is seropositive and is unwilling to reveal that fact to the referring physician or to those whom he/she may place at risk via sexual or other activity (e.g., sharing needles), is the consultant obligated more by patient confidentiality or by his duty to warn others at risk? The consultant must carefully scrutinize the extent of the risk posed by his patient's behavior. In the case above, for example, the consultant may decide that the referring physician need not be told because his relationship with the patient is essentially "casual contact," and therefore poses no real risk, although the consultant may be troubled by providing incomplete information in his consultation, including some that is relevant to the patient's ongoing health care. Alternatively, he may simply suggest that hepatitis B precautions should be followed with this patient without stating the exact reason. The question of whether or not to inform the surgeon may be more difficult, if he believes that the surgeon is placing himself at risk by unknowingly operating on a seropositive patient. The greatest difficulty will likely be with the question of whether or not to inform the patient's wife, particularly if the patient indicates that he is continuing to have unprotected intercourse with her. He will need to integrate his beliefs regarding all individuals' responsibility for the prevention of HIV infection—Are all the individuals in these scenarios responsible for protecting themselves or are they "victims" of the patient?—with his wish to prevent illness and, perhaps, his fear of litigation.

Related to confidentiality is the principle of truthful communication between patient and physician. Honest and forthright disclosure by the patient is required for accurate diagnosis and treatment. Similarly, honest and straightforward information from the physician is required if the patient is to be able to make informed and responsible decisions. The ability of the patient to make decisions regarding the type and extent of care desired, the types of medications and procedures he/she wishes, and the ultimate disposition of belongings, depends in large measure on the patient's being fully and honestly informed of the implications of his/her medical status.

Medical personnel are ethically and legally bound to abide by the treatment decisions of mentally competent patients.

Also at this early stage, patients with AIDS should be informed about the potential for developing cognitive impairments that could rob them of their right to participate in treatment decisions. Especially important for gay-identified patients is informing the patient of his right to delegate health care decisions to a Power of Attorney. This legal authorization allows the patient to designate a friend or lover to make decisions relating to medical care if and when the patient is unable to do so. This mechanism is particularly important for gay couples because family members of gay patients have been known to interfere with treatment decisions of the patient and/or his lover. A similar line of reasoning supports the view that these patients are also well advised to be sure to properly execute a will to ensure that their wishes will be honored. The number of patients with AIDS whose wills are contested because of the frequent assumption that patients were affected by the ADC and thus, were unaware of what they were doing appears to be rising. The consultant can often generally relieve a patient's anxiety by helping him understand these issues and develop a plan for addressing them.

Mid-Stage

Suicidal ideation is almost uniformly present among people with AIDS. When asked to intervene with a patient with AIDS who is considered actively suicidal, the consultant may feel a personal conflict between his/her own views about the right of an individual to end his life in the face of a terminal illness, and his/her legal obligation to intervene. Few physicians have qualms about intervening with the physically healthy patient who is suicidal. Clinical experience has shown that after the crisis has passed the majority of suicidal patients are grateful that they were prohibited from harming themselves, even when this has meant involuntary hospitalization or physical restraint. These measures, of course, are justified largely because of the belief in the patients' chances for improvement: despair and hopelessness will lift and he/she will return to a productive life. In the case of terminal diseases, however, medical and legal scholars continue to debate whether suicide is a moral wrong and/or whether intervention by physicians or the police is warranted.[21,22] Thus, there is no clear medical, moral, or legal consensus that suicide is always wrong in this group. Our experience has been that suicidal patients with AIDS who are at an early point in their disease have responded well to traditional psychiatric interventions.[23] Nonetheless, the psychiatric consultant asked to intervene in those instances where the outcome is less certain may find these requests personally difficult.

Terminal Care

While a medical, legal, and ethical consensus has been reached that life-sustaining treatment may be limited when further therapy is medically futile,[24,25] the patient's participation in all other treatment decisions should be solicited. This should, of course, include the right of the patient to refuse treatment or to ask that treatment be stopped. The psychiatrist is almost uniformly asked to evaluate such patients to render an opinion as to the patient's competence. When the opinion of the medical experts is in agreement that the continuation of treatment is not expected to render any benefit and the patient is felt to be competent, his wish should be respected. The psychiatric consultant can sometimes be particularly helpful to the family or lover in accepting this situation. We believe the scope of the physician's responsibility includes a duty to provide care to the significant others identified by the patient as well as the patient himself. Thus, physicians have a duty not to abandon patients or their families during the dying process. Potentially contentious situations can also be avoided or minimized if the patient or his legal surrogate is well informed and encouraged to participate in treatment decisions.

CONCLUSION

We have identified some of the psychiatric and ethical issues raised in the care of patients with AIDS that are frequently encountered by the practicing consultation/liaison psychiatrist. Many of the issues presented here are also potentially present in the care of other chronically or terminally ill patients. However, because of the unique psychosocial ramifications of AIDS, these issues come more to the forefront. We believe this review highlights the importance and contribution of the psychiatric consultant as an active member of the AIDS treatment team.

REFERENCES

1. Lipowski ZJ: Psychiatric Consultation: Concepts and controversies. *Am J Psychiatry* 134:523–528, 1977.
2. Strain JJ: Needs for psychiatry in the general hospital. *Hosp Community Psychiatry* 33:996–999, 1982.
3. Barsky A, Brown H: Psychiatric tracking and consultation in a primary care clinic. *Psychosomatics* 23:9–13, 1982.
4. Lewis CE, Freeman HE, Corey CR: AIDS-related competence of California's primary care physicians. *Am J Pub Health* 77:795–802, 1987.
5. Dilley JW, Shelp E, Batki S: Psychiatric and Ethical issues in the care of patients with AIDS. *Psychosomatics* 27:562–566, 1986.
6. Morin SF, Batchelor WF: Responding to the psychological crisis of AIDS. *Public Health Rep* 99:4–10, 1984.
7. Forstein M: The psychosocial impact of the acquired immunodeficiency syndrome. *Semin Oncol* 11:77–82, 1984.

8. Nichols SE: Psychological reactions of persons with the acquired immunodeficiency syndrome. *Ann Intern Med* 103:765–777, 1985.
9. Wackter RM: The impact of the acquired immunodeficiency syndrome on medical residency training. *N Engl J Med* 314:177–180, 1986.
10. Polon HJ, Hellerstein D, Auchin J: Impact of AIDS-related cases on an inpatient therapeutic milieu. *Hosp Community Psychiatry* 36:173–175, 1985.
11. Cooke M: Learning to care: health care workers respond to AIDS. FOCUS: A Guide to AIDS Research, UCSF AIDS Health Project. 7:1–2, 1987.
12. Fletcher J: Homosexuality: Kick and kickback. (Editorial.) *South Med J* February:47, 1984.
13. Levy R, Bredeson D, Rosenblum M: Neurological manifestations of the acquired immunodeficiency syndrome (AIDS): Experience at UCSF and review of the literature. *J Neurosurg* 62:475–495, 1985.
13. Rothenberg R, Woelfel M, Stoneburner R, et al: Survival with the acquired immunodeficiency syndrome: Experience with 5833 cases in New York City. *N Engl J Med* 317:1297, 1987.
14. Rivin BE, Monroe JM, Hubschuman BP, et al: AIDS outcome: A first follow-up, (Letter.) *N Engl J Med* 311:857, 1987.
15. Rothenberg R, Woelfel M, Stoneburner R, et al: Survival with the acquired immunodeficiency syndrome: Experience with 5833 cases in New York City. *N Engl J Med* 311:857, 1984.
16. Navia BA, Price RW: Dementia complicating AIDS. *Psychiatric Ann* 16:3, 1986.
17. Dilley JW, Ochitill HN, Perl M, et al: Findings in psychiatric consultations with patients with AIDS. *Am J Psych* 142:82, 1985.
18. Woods SW, Tesar GE, Murray GB, et al: Psychostimulant treatment of depressive disorders secondary to medical illness. *J Clin Psychiatry* 47:12, 1986.
19. Kaufmann MW, Murray GB: The use of d-amphetamine in medically ill depressed patients. *J Clin Psychiatry* 43: 463, 1982.
20. Fernandez F, Adams F, Holmes VF, et al: Methylphenidate for depressive disorders in cancer patients. *Psychosomatics* 28:455, 1987.
21. Batlin P: *Ethical Issues in Suicide*. Englewood Cliffs, New Jersey, Prentice-Hall, 1982.
22. Schneidman ES: *Suicide Thoughts and Reflections, 1960–1980*. New York, Human Sciences Press, 1981.
23. Baer JW, Holm K, Lewitter Koehler S: Treatment of AIDS/ARC patients on an inpatient psychiatric unit. FOCUS: A Guide to AIDS Research, UCSF AIDS Health Project. 2:2, 1987.
24. President's Commission For the Study of Ethical Problems in Medicine and Biomedical and Behavioral Research: Deciding to Forego Life-Sustaining Treatment: A Report on the Ethical, Medical and Legal Issues in Treatment Decisions. Washington, DC, Government Printing Office, 1983.
25. Lo B, Steinbrook RL: Deciding whether to resuscitate. *Arch Intern Med* 143:1561–1563, 1983.

17

Mental Health Services Delivery Issues

The HIV Patient

JAMES J. STRAIN and GEORGE FULOP

PSYCHIATRIC MORBIDITY IN THE MEDICAL SETTING

Although it is determined that HIV infection has a physiological etiology, it is a paradigm for illnesses in which both physiological and psychological factors operate. In fact, it is the concomitance of biological and psychological processes that makes HIV infection a prime example of the coexistence of psychiatric and medical morbidity. Since HIV patients are most often treated in the medical setting, the mental health component of their illness will be addressed primarily within the general health sector.

Consequently, there are compelling reasons why the physician needs to know the pathophysiology and psychological concomitants and sequelae of AIDS. Furthermore, significant stresses impact on the patient; on the family, lover, support system; and on the medical/nursing staff. The purpose of this chapter is first to examine the role of the primary care physician in addressing the mental health needs of the patient with HIV illnesses. Second, it will detail the role of psychiatry both directly and indirectly in mental health services delivery for those afflicted with HIV infection.

As the principal gatekeeper for much of the mental health care system, primary care physicians inevitably encounter and, thus, need to assess, triage, diagnose, refer, and treat vast numbers of patients with alcohol, drug abuse, and mental disorders. However, Pincus and Kamerow, in a report to the Administrator of Alcohol, Drug Abuse and Mental Health Administration, not only describe overwhelming evidence of the primary care physician's importance, but also question their effectiveness.[1] The Epidemiological Catchment Area study reports that 19% of American adults in any 6-month period experience anxiety (8.3%), affective disorders (6%), and alcohol (5%) and drug abuse (2%) problems.[2] Alcoholism, drug abuse, and mental disorders result in at least 108,000 deaths per year: 69,000 are alcohol related (up to one half of all motor vehicle crash deaths involve alcohol), 6000 are associated with drug abuse, and 33,000 are mental health related,

JAMES J. STRAIN and GEORGE FULOP • Division of Behavioral Medicine and Consultation Psychiatry, Department of Psychiatry, Mount Sinai School of Medicine, New York, New York 10029.

primarily suicide.[3] The contribution of those patients who have concurrent medical and psychiatric morbidity (e.g., those with HIV infection) to these figures is uncertain.

The cost of these disorders further underscores their importance. In 1983, alcohol, drug abuse, and mental disorders resulted in $50.4 and $250 billion in indirect and direct costs, respectively.[4] The mental health costs of the patients with HIV infection have not been estimated although the anticipated medical costs are staggering.

AIDS ranks near the top of the list of major impairments in terms of average lifetime medical costs: $70,000–$115,000.[5,6] It is estimated that AIDS will account for about 1 percent of total national spending on health and about 3 percent of Medicaid program costs.[7] The Centers for Disease Control (CDC) estimate that over one third of all AIDS cases reported in the United States have been in New York City.[8]

Studies project that the annual costs for treating AIDS patients in New York City will reach $2.9 billion. This reflects only inpatient hospital care, which constitutes the bulk of AIDS-related costs in the City. The AIDS inpatient census could reach 5150 per day by 1991 with 2000 in municipal hospitals: 22% of the actual caseload is in the hospital at any one time with hospital costs, $800 per day (1988), projected to be $1529 by 1991, a large proportion of which falls on Medicaid.[9]

More than one half of all hospitalized patients manifest significant psychologic dysfunction, either as a result of or in conjunction with medical illness, which can interfere with the effectiveness of treatment.[10] Furthermore, between 15% and 50% of all patients encountered in the ambulatory medical setting have psychologic dysfunction that is either primary in nature or secondary to physical illness.[11] No figures are as yet available for those patients with AIDS or AIDS-related complex (ARC). Estimates of neuropsychiatric symptoms have been reported elsewhere in this volume (see Chapter 9). Regier et al. estimate that only 21% of patients with mental disorders in the ambulatory setting receive care from mental health specialists[2]; 62% are seen exclusively in the primary care sector. Although 70% of patients with an alcohol, drug abuse, and mental disorder (in the previous 6 months) made at least one ambulatory health or mental health visit, only 10% saw a mental health specialist.[12] Even though more than half of those received all their care in the general medical sector (usually from a primary care physician), only one fifth stated that they made a visit for mental health purposes.[12]

However, these data do not consider the quality of care patients with alcohol, drug abuse, and mental disorders receive, especially in view of the fact that despite their high prevalence rates they frequently go undetected by the primary care physician. In one study 2.8% were recognized by the physicians as opposed to 27% that were diagnosed by the research team.[13] This extremely low identification rate has added significance because the figure included any indication of recognition, e.g., chart notation or a psychotropic drug prescription. With regard to patients with major depression, between 25% and 50% were identified by primary care physicians.[14,15] Significant undetected cognitive disturbances were observed by Knight and Folstein,[16] as well as by Jacobs et al.[17] Relatively few of the estimated 10% of all adults entering a physician's office who are likely to have a problem with alcohol are detected. The estimates of alcohol and recreational drug use by HIV patients is less well documented than IV drug abuse.

Despite this problem in recognition let alone diagnosis of specific disorders, Unlenhuth et al. found that 70% of tricyclic antidepressants (TCA) and 90% of anxiolytics are administered by primary care physicians.[18] The appropriate use of psychopharmacologic agents in patients with HIV is not known from controlled clinical trials. The employment of antidepressants and neuroleptics for the patient with AIDS needs to be evaluated not only from the perspective of efficacy but tolerance; e.g., TCA for major depressive disorders in the presence of cognitive defects, or with adjustment disorders with depressed moods.

Furthermore, with regard to treatment, surveys show that, despite the high proportion of TCAs used by primary care physicians, there is a low rate of antidepressant and a high rate of antianxiety medications prescribed for their patients with major depression.[18] Admittedly, the tricyclic antidepressants are useful for certain types of depression, but they are commonly prescribed in subtherapeutic doses and for the wrong length of time by primary care physicians.[18] It is necessary to know whether lower doses may be appropriate for those patients seriously ill with HIV disease, and the role of stimulants for depressive disorders. Unfortunately, many physicians recognize neither the depression nor the cognitive deficits in their AIDS patients, and referral rates to a mental health clinician for a recognized mental disorder remain low.[19–21]

There are many barriers to improving the mental health care of HIV patients provided by primary care physicians: the inadequate training and knowledge; the physicians' negative attitude toward the delivery of mental health care[22,23]; the patients' denial of their problems and their negative attitudes about seeking mental health care and/or accepting referral; constraints within the health care systems, e.g., cost, lack of reimbursement for comprehensive interviewing and counseling; availability of psychiatrists; and the impediments between the general health and mental health systems.[24] These barriers overlap and interact to decrease the likelihood of effective mental health care for HIV patients seen in primary care settings.

Investigators report that psychosocial and psychiatric interventions in the general hospital reduce length of hospital stay especially in the elderly and influence discharge placement to home rather than to a health-related facility.[25,26] In addition, Lyons et al. learned that the earlier a hospitalized patient is seen in psychiatric consultation, the earlier the patient with psychiatric and medical comorbidity is discharged (a log linear relationship exists).[27] It is important to investigate whether these observations remain valid for that cohort of patients with HIV who also have psychiatric comorbidity.

DIAGNOSTIC DILEMMAS WITH CONCURRENT MEDICAL AND PSYCHIATRIC COMORBIDITY

Psychiatric diagnosis in the medical setting is problematic for the primary care physician as well as the psychiatrist. It emphasizes one of the most important roles of psychiatry in the collaboration with primary care specialists and the need for future research.[28] With regard to the patient, the psychiatrist may need to deal not only with the potential psychiatric presentation of the illness, but also with the adverse psychological reactions, primary and secondary, of the effect of the HIV virus on the CNS. AIDS may initially present as a cognitive deficit[29]: Patients may seek out their physicians because of a change in memory, problem-solving, or abstracting ability. At times, there may be a frank incipient organic mental disorder, diffuse physiological symptoms suggestive of a somatization phenomena, or acute anxiety and/or depressive disorders.[30] Consequently,

TABLE 1. DSM III and HIV-Illness Examples

Axis	Disorder	ICD-9-CM code
I	Delirium	293.00
	Dementia	294.00
II	Dependent	301.00
III	HIV	042
	Pneumocystis carinii pneumonia	136.3
IV	Psychosocial stressors in last year—severe	(7) (score 1–7)
V	Level of functioning in last year—poor	(25) (score 0–99)

the psychiatrist's skill and competence to render a diagnosis based on biological, psychological, and social parameters is essential to ensure that an organic etiology for psychiatric morbidity is not overlooked. This is further underscored by the fact that psychiatric reactions to medical illness may be superimposed on organically based symptomatology.[29,30]

The *Diagnostic and Statistical Manual* (3rd edition) (DSM-III-R), which describes the criteria for various psychiatric disorders and utilizes a multiaxial approach to diagnosis, ensures that cognizance is taken of state (axis I), trait (axis II), physiology (axis III), stressors (axis IV), and functional level (axis V).[31] It is not expected that the physician will formulate the relationships among the observations on the various axes, e.g., pneumonia (axis III) and delirium (axis I); or that a psychosocial stressor may be a significant contribution to the development or exacerbation of the current mental and/or physical disorder (Table 1).

Emphasis is not placed on axial interrelationships, causality, or etiologic considerations (except on axis III) as would be expected in an integrated biopsychosocial model.[32] The difference between the concepts of a triaxial and the biopsychosocial model is subtle but significant. An interrelationship among biologic, psychologic, and social variables is operative in every disease,[28] whereas in the triaxial conceptual framework, the phenomenologic approach to the various levels of diagnosis supersedes the focus on the dynamics of interaxial effects.

DSM-III-R is a most important step toward making diagnostic efforts more reliable and valid, but it poses problems in the medical setting. Many of the signs and symptoms that would support the diagnosis of a depressive disorder also occur with medical illness. If a symptom is the result of a medical illness, the DSM-III-R decision-making rules dictate that it should not be regarded as supporting a psychiatric diagnosis. For example, dysphoric mood, poor appetite, sleep disturbance, changes in gastrointestinal motility, decreased libido, anhedonia, and so forth, may all accompany a medical illness—AIDS—and be relatively persistent, but they are not necessarily indicative of a major affective disorder. Consequently, one can over- or underdiagnose the depressive disorders in the medically ill as a result of not knowing the etiology of the vegetative symptoms that are present.

Furthermore, psychiatric diagnosis is complicated in the patient with HIV who may be on a variety of drugs for infections (e.g., pneumocystis pneumonia, tuberculosis, candida, toxoplasmosis), Kaposi's sarcoma, lymphomas, or antiviral agents: azi-

TABLE 2. Psychiatric and Neurological Side Effects of Medications Used in Treating AIDS[a]

The following list includes medications for which such side effects have been reported. This list does not include side effects reported for other organ systems and does not include all medications that may be used in the treatment of AIDS-related illnesses.

Medication	Side effects
Pneumocystis	
Trimethoprim/Sulfa (Bactrim)	Psychosis, mutism, bizarre mannerisms, depression, loss of appetite, insomnia, apathy, headache, neuritis
TB and *Mycobacterium avium—intracellulare*	
Isoniazid	Depression, agitation, auditory and visual hallucinations, paranoia, peripheral neuropathy, memory impairment
Ethambutol	Headache, dizziness, confusion, visual disturbances
Rifampin	Headache, fatigue, loss of appetite, visual disturbances
Cycloserine	Anxiety, depression, confusion, disorientation, hallucinations, paranoia, loss of appetite, fatigue
Ethionamide	Depression, hallucinations, neuritis, diplopia, headache, drowsiness
Candida, Cryptococcus	
Ketoconazole	Headache, dizziness, photosensitivity
Amphotericin-B	Delirium, peripheral neuropathy, blurred vision, diplopia, weight loss, loss of appetite, headache
5-Flucytosine	Confusion, headache, sedation
Toxoplasmosis	
Sulfonamides	Headache, neuritis, insomnia, loss of appetite, photosensitivity
Strongyloids stercoralis	
Thiabendazole	Hallucinations, olfactory disturbance
Herpes simplex/zoster	
Acyclovir	Visual halllucinations, depersonalization, tearfulness, confusion, hyperaesthesia, hyperacusis, insomnia, thought insertion, headache
Kaposi's sarcoma	
Vincristine	Hallucinations, headache, neuritis, ataxia, sensory loss
Vinblastine	Depression, loss of appetite, headache, neuritis
Etoposide ((VP16)	Neuropathy, loss of appetite
α-Interferon	Depression, weakness
Lymphomas	
Methotrexate	Headaches, blurred vision, fatigue, photosensitivity, encephalopathy in high doses
Procarbazine	Mania, loss of appetite, headaches, insomnia, nightmares, confusion, malaise
Anti-HIV	
Azidothymidine (AZT)	Headache, restlessness, severe agitation, insomnia
Suramin	Malaise, paresthesias
Ribavirin	?

[a]For further information, readers are referred to the following issues of *The Medical Letter*: Vol 27, Issue 681; Vol 28, Issues 721 and 726.

dothymidine (AZT), suramin, ribavirin. These drugs may precipitate diverse psychiatric symptoms, e.g., depression, agitation, auditory and visual hallucinations, depersonalization, and hyperacusis, which are indistinguishable from similar symptoms that have a psychogenic etiology[33] (Table 2).

At times, specification of the psychiatric diagnosis may defy solution and the clinician is forced to rely on his/her judgment. Depressive and anxiety disorders are not only difficult to assess in the medically ill, but also in the geriatric population. It might be stated that DSM III-R is not only "age unfair",[34] but medically ill unfair. Furthermore, since HIV patients may experience cognitive deficits (dementia), depression, or both, it is necessary for the physician to detect not only an organic mental syndrome, but also the cognitive impairment that frequently accompanies a major affective disorder—pseudodementia. Similarly, since an organic affective disorder may result from the HIV virus affecting the brain, a secondary pseudodepression can be manifestly apparent. These diagnostic difficulties have major implications for psychopharmacological interventions. The clinician should consider an antidepressant medication for a pseudodementia.

Furthermore, the medical illness complicates the employment of standard psychological instruments. The Hamilton Depression Rating Scale has 8 of 20 items that refer to somatic symptoms that commonly accompany medical illness, thereby enhancing the opportunity to overdiagnose depression.[35] And the frequency of cognitive items on the Beck Depression Inventory often forces a score into the depressive range because the patient who is demented or delirious cannot remember all four multiple choices, which forces an overselection of the last option, thereby inflating the score.[36] As mentioned before, many HIV patients experience depression as well as an organic mental disorder which compromises the validity of the results from standard measures. Instruments to assess cognitive deficits, validated in patients with medical illness, may yield a high incidence of false negative and false positive results with HIV illness.

COGNITIVE CAPACITY SCREENING EXAMINATION (CCSE) (APPENDIX I)

The CCSE is a one-page, 30-item questionnaire specifically designed to detect diffuse organic mental disorders, particularly delirium.[37] Administration time is 5 min. Questions relating to orientation, serial sevens, verbal short-term memory, abstraction, digit recall, and arithmetic are included. Since it was believed that a global deficit might influence the patient's ability to shift from one domain to another (rather than his or her ability to perform any single mental operation), the order in which the questions were presented demanded rapid shifts from one mental task to another (e.g., short-term memory to abstraction). Furthermore, questions were formulated that required performance of an interposed task (e.g., "Remember four digits, count 1–10 out loud, recall the four digits"). The test form includes instruction for its use and scoring, and in the event of a score under 20 (which indicates a cognitive deficit), the physician is directed toward possible organic pathology and to review the patient's physiological data.

MINI-MENTAL STATE EXAMINATION (MMS) (APPENDIX II)

The MMS is a one-page, 11-question examination that requires 5–10 min to administer.[38] It is "mini" because it concentrates on only the cognitive aspects of mental functions. The first of its two sections requires vocal responses for orientation, memory, and attention (maximum score: 21). The second section tests the patient's ability to name, follow verbal and written commands, write a sentence spontaneously, and copy intersecting polygons (maximum score: 9). A score of 23 or below suggests an organic mental disorder.

HAND-HELD TACHISTOSCOPE (T-SCOPE)

The T-scope is a 35-mm camera shutter assembly that has the lens aperture set to fully open.[39] The shutter allows exposure times of 1/125, 1/60, 1/30, 1 sec. When the shutter is fully open, a black capital letter—E—from a standard typewriter is visible on a white background. The subject is asked to put on glasses if usually worn and identify the position of the letter E in the open shutter. The first exposure time is 1/125 second, and if the position of the E is identified unsuccessfully after three trials, the exposure is increased stepwise until the patient is correct on two of the trials. That exposure time is recorded as the subject's threshold for the task. Total examination time is three minutes. A score of 1/30 or below on two of three successive correct positional identifications of the letter E is regarded as the cutoff point related to significant cognitive deficits.

A recently reported cognitive screening device with unique psychometric properties may overcome some of the limitations of the measures described above, but it has not been adequately validated in the medically ill.[39]

NEUROBEHAVIORAL COGNITIVE STATUS EXAMINATION (NCSE)

The Neurobehavioral Cognitive Status Examination, a screening examination that assesses cognition in a brief but quantitative fashion, uses independent tests to evaluate functioning within five major cognitive ability areas: language, constructions, memory, calculations, and reasoning.[40] The examination separately assesses level of consciousness, orientation, and attention. This instrument quickly identifies intact areas of functioning, yet provides more detailed assessment in areas of dysfunction. Standardization data are provided for 119 healthy adults (age range, 29–92 years) and for 30 patients receiving neurosurgical care for brain lesions (range, 25–88 years). In the authors' paper, cognitive profiles for several common neuropsychiatric conditions illustrate the usefulness of this examination in clinical practice.[41,42]

PSYCHOSOCIAL DATA COLLECTION METHODS IN THE GENERAL HOSPITAL

Until recently, there was no systematic method for evaluating the consultee's (usually a primary care physician) understanding of a behavioral problem of his/her patients referred for psychiatric consultation in the general hospital, or the outcome of the psychiatrist's recommendations.[43] A computerized data-base schema—MICRO-CARES—for needs assessment, learner appraisal, systems analysis, and fate of the psychiatrist's recommendations has been developed at the Northwestern University and the Mount Sinai School of Medicine by Hammer and Strain.[44–46]

TABLE 3. Reasons for Referral

Rank		Reason for referral stated by consultant HIV (N = 25)	Reason for referral stated by consultant Others (N = 1342)	P	Rank	Assessed by consultee HIV (N = 25)	Assessed by consultee Others (N = 1342)
1.	Coping	8	253	<0.01	1	14	498
2.	Depression	7	376	NS	2	13	483
3.	Suicide Risk	6	299	NS	4	7	299
4.	Behavior management	6	277	NS	5	6	290
5.	Drug	5	77	<0.01	6	6	121
6.	Judgment	5	80	<0.01	7	5	118
7.	Anxiety	4	147	NS	8	5	275
8.	Noncompliance	4	113	NS	9	5	140
9.	Organic brain syndrome	4	145	NS	3	8	315
10.	Alcohol	3	58	NS	10	3	102
11.	Diagnosis	3	229	NS	—	—	—
12.	Terminal illness	3	46	—	—	—	—

Although many investigators describe clinical phenomena and symptoms of the HIV patient in the general hospital, no systematic study has been conducted to date to compare this unique patient group with others seen in the routine psychiatric consultation setting. The MICRO-CARES data-collection system was particularly helpful with regard to characterizing those patients with HIV referred to psychiatry versus "others" on whom a psychiatric consultation had been requested. Examination of 1367 patients in 1982–1986 by the psychiatric consultation staff at the Mount Sinai Hospital of whom 25 had HIV disease revealed that the AIDS patients were significantly younger ($p < 0.01$), more likely to be male ($p = 0.0001$) and from medicine ($p = 0.0001$) in contrast to "other" consult patients.[47] They did not differ with regard to race, education, employment, living situation (alone or with another), urgency of request, or personal help available.

The psychological and behavioral problems "stated" by the consultee and "assessed" by the consulting psychiatrist for the HIV patient versus "Other" referrals are summarized in Table 3. By comparing the problem "stated" by the consultee with the problem "assessed" by the consultant, it is possible to detect the primary care physician's view or "labeling" of the patient's behavior and its etiology.[44] The reasons for referral revealed HIV patients as having significantly greater problems with coping ($p < 0.01$), drug abuse ($p < 0.01$), and judgment ($p < 0.05$). Although nonspecific "behavioral management" and "behavior strange or unexplained" were frequently listed as the problem precipitating the consultation, the underlying etiologic diagnosis for the behavior (e.g., organicity, depression, or anxiety) was often undetected by the referring physician.

Specifically, in 239 of 1065 (22.4%) patients, the consultee did not indicate the presence of an organic mental disorder.[48] It is also possible to note that the incidence of consultee erroneous labeling increases with age, thereby suggesting policy interventions with regard to mandatory screening. Standard organic mental screening devices would be appropriate for those inpatients in the general hospital who are over 65 years of age. Given the frequency of delirium and dementia in HIV patients, it may be important that all AIDS

TABLE 4. DSM-III Psychiatric Diagnoses

Axis	AIDS	Others	χ_2	DF	*p*
Axis I					
Organic mental syndrome					
Degenerative dementia	0 (0%)	87 (6.5%)	1.7	1	0.18
Substance induced	3 (12%)	102 (7.6%)	0.7	1	0.41
Secondary physiologic process	8 (32%)	192 (14.3%)	6.2	1	0.01
Substance use disorder	10 (40%)	173 (12.9%)	15.6	1	0.0001
Adjustment	14 (56%)	343 (25.6%)	11.8	1	0.0006
Affective	0 (0%)	160 (11.9%)	3.4	1	0.07
Schizophrenia/psychoses	0 (0%)	64 (4.8%)	1.3	1	0.26
Anxiety	1 (4%)	46 (3.4%)	0.02	1	0.88
Other	0 (0%)	45 (3.4%)	0.87	1	0.35
Axis II					
Personality	8(32%)	333(24.8%)	0.7	1	0.41
Axis IV					
Psychosocial stressors	5.3 ± 1.4	4.5 ± 1.3	$t = -2.9$	23,1140	0.01
Axis V					
Highest functioning	4.0 ± 1.0	3.7 ± 1.1	$t = -1.6$	23,1171	0.11
Severity of psychiatric illness	4.2 ± 1.2	3.8 ± 1.4	$t = -1.6$	23,1276	0.12

inpatients have a structured cognitive assessment with valid and reliable instruments at admission and discharge from the hospital.

The most common psychiatric diagnoses in HIV versus "Other" consultation patients are described (Table 4). The AIDS patient was more likely to have an organic mental disorder secondary to a physiologic process ($p = 0.01$) and substance abuse disorders ($p = 0.0001$).

Furthermore, in the general hospital it is important to make initial and follow-up psychiatric assessments. For example, Snyder and Strain observed that of 105 patients initially diagnosed as having a major affective disorder (296.30), 22 were no longer evaluated as such at discharge.[49] On the other hand, 38 patients initially not diagnosed as having a major affective disorder were so designated with repeated examination when the consultation was finally terminated. Therefore, within the general hospital setting, it is essential to constantly re-evaluate the working diagnoses: Treatment, especially with chemotherapy (psychotropic medications) for a major depressive disorder, might better be delayed until the early hospital phase has elapsed and until the physician is secure that such a diagnosis persists. In some cases, the physician may want yet a third determination postdischarge to ascertain whether the symptoms for a major affective disorder still exist once the patient is out of the hospital and removed from the environment of an acute medical/surgical illness.

Treatment Issues

From a computerized data-based schema, it is possible to learn which psychotropic drugs and which doses the consultee used before the consultant arrived, thereby gaining

TABLE 5. Psychiatric Treatment/Management

	AIDS	Others	χ^2	p
Unit staff treatment				
Gratify needs	3 (12%)	198 (14.8%)	0.15	0.7
Modify defenses	6 (24%)	171 (12.7%)	2.8	0.10
Set limits	7 (28%)	145 (10.8%)	7.3	0.007
Constant	2 (8%)	92 (6.9%)	0.05	0.8
Consultation needed	2 (8%)	150 (11.1%)	0.25	0.6
Diagnostic tests	4 (16%)	177 (13.2%)	0.17	0.7
Environmental change	2 (8%)	141 (10.5%)	0.17	0.7
Social service	7 (28%)	296 (22%)	0.5	0.5
Consultant treatment				
Psychotherapy	3 (0.2%)	261 (19.5%)	0.9	0.3
Follow-up	20 (80%)	822 (61.3%)		
Psychiatric treatment recommended	2 (8%)	465 (35%)	8.9	0.01
Inpatient psychiatry	0 (0%)	101 (7.5%)	2.0	0.4
Outpatient psychiatry	0 (0%)	178 (13.3%)	3.8	0.15
Against medical advice discharge	2 (8%)	27 (2%)	4.2	0.04
Impaired judgment	2 (8%)	35 (2.6%)	2.7	0.10
Invasive procedure	15 (68%)	217 (25%)	21.2	0.0001

knowledge about the appropriateness of the medication employed and the areas of necessary teaching for the referring physician. Finally, the psychiatrist can discern which of his/her recommendations were followed by the HIV patient's physician. Popkin et al. observed that consultees incorporated recommendations into their assessment and treatment plans for psychopharmacology, consultations, and diagnostic labeling, 71%, 43%, and 39% of the time, respectively.[43]

Patients with HIV had psychiatric in- and outpatient treatment recommended less often ($p = 0.01$), but more limit setting ($p = 0.0007$), follow-up inhospital psychiatric treatment (5.6 ± 9 versus 3.5 ± 5, $p = 0.01$), leaving against medical advice ($p = 0.04$), and death (18% versus 6.7%, $p = 0.05$) (Table 5). The patients with HIV infection were less likely to be seen as having a cognitive deficit by the consultee, who overstated the problem as behavioral management or coping. The consultee often described the HIV patient as depressed and suicidal, while the consultant seldom diagnosed affective disorders or regarded suicide as a major risk. The primary care physician registered disturbances of mood as depressive disorders and any expressions of suicide to be equivalent to a major suicidal risk. In both cases, they "overrated" the mood disturbance and the communication regarding suicidal ideation. In contrast to the fact that psychiatric inpatient and outpatient treatment was seldom recommended, several AIDS patients required intensive psychiatric follow-up while on the medical wards.

Since a number of the HIV patients went on to die during their hospital admission, it was possible, using the MICRO-CARES system to profile those patients (HIV plus "others") referred for a psychiatric consultation who went on to die.[50] A group of 344 inpatients seen by the Mount Sinai Medical Center Behavioral Medicine and Consultation Service in 1984 were evaluated for an inhospital death. Hospital death within 3 months of the consultation was established by examining the Utilization Information Service tape abstracts generated for every hospital admission and discharge. One fifth ($N = 67$) of the consultation population ($N = 344$) (19%) died, whereas the overall hospital death rate was 3.5%. The patients who died were more likely to be living alone ($p = 0.04$); on Medicare/Medicaid ($p = 0.001$); older (mean age 61; $p = 0.0001$); but not characterized as having significantly more substance abuse, adjustment disorders, or personality disorders ($p = 0.01$). The death consultation cohort also had decreased functioning (axis IV, $p = 0.05$).

Demographics, reasons for consultation, and diagnostic data are important variables for identifying patients with medical and psychiatric morbidity who are at risk for death who may require immediate interventions. Earlier detection of organic mental disorders as a consequence of physical illness may heighten awareness for continued physical diagnosis and treatment in an attempt to attenuate mortality in this at-risk population. Therefore, the MICRO-CARES method allows for the identification of clinical situations, including the use of psychopharmacologic agents, that mandate a greater concentration of teaching effort for primary care physicians to become aware, detect, diagnose/refer, and treat some mental disorders, at least for a hospitalized inpatient population. This computerized database system, now being used by a consortium of twenty teaching hospitals, permits multisite investigations of HIV consultation patients across institutions with regard to psychiatric diagnoses, treatment interventions employed, and the fate of recommendations to the consultee.[51]

THE MEDICAL/PSYCHIATRIC HEALTH CARE DELIVERY SYSTEMS

Several medical and psychiatric health care delivery systems are available to treat the patient with HIV disease.

AIDS Cluster Unit

In some hospitals, a scatter bed approach is used to hospitalize HIV patients, while in other AIDS cluster units have been established. However, there are no systematic studies to support the benefits—psychological, social, staff burnout, or economic—of a cluster versus a scatter bed approach to HIV inpatient care. There is no infectious disease reason why HIV patients must be sequestered away from other inpatients. However, the cluster unit does have the advantage over the scatter bed approach in that several therapeutic vehicles can be established to assist the patient, their support system, and the staff.

Medical–psychiatric co-teaching rounds have been found to be a valuable resource to examine. Ombudsmen rounds conducted jointly by a medical attending physician (ombudsman) and a psychiatrist bring the entire staff together weekly.[52] An attempt is made to address both staff and patient needs on the HIV unit. Through group discussions and patient interviews, in which the patient has an opportunity to express his own feelings about this illness and care, the staff becomes aware of the psychosocial issues that are universally evoked by illness and hospitalization. All staff members are also encouraged to relate their reactions to the patient and their interactions with each other. The ombudsmen-rounds concept maximizes the use of the internist and liaison psychiatrist, and makes psychosocial–medical teaching routine on the medical service in a contemporary teaching hospital where the practice of holistic medicine has been so difficult to implement.[52]

In addition, a weekly or biweekly support group for the nursing staff, who have a most difficult job, has been found useful when it addresses the issues of understanding and managing complex neuropsychiatric and psychodynamic behaviors. The nurses' group permits the verbalization and working through of the anxiety and other problems involved in (1) caring for patients with a fatal illness, grieving, bereavement; and (2) understanding and treating mental illness in their seriously medically ill patients. The Communicable Disease Center health care workers study describes the rate of HIV seroconversion in 870 persons exposed percutaneously to HIV-contaminated blood to have been only 4 (less than 1%), and 37% of the exposures could have been preventable, e.g., recapping, penetrated by needle or sharp object, or open wound exposure to contaminated HIV patient blood.[53]

Finally, patients and their support system can be offered group experiences to enhance their coping with serious illness, abnormal mental behavior, and the prospects of dying. In many respects, the HIV Cluster Unit offers the psychosocial advantages and organizational potential encountered in the milieu of an inpatient psychiatric unit.

However, the effects of sequestering AIDS patients together, the stigmatization, isolation from the general hospital population, exposure to fatal illness and death are negative aspects of a centralized unit of care. As said above, carefully controlled studies comparing cluster- and scatter-bed approaches need to be undertaken before one mode versus the other becomes institutionalized in our country. Such health service delivery studies are one of the recommendations of the President's Task Force on HIV Infection.[54] Cluster units are now routine for specific illnesses (e.g., cancer wards, neurology units, coronary care units) and specific problems (e.g., surgical intensive care units). It has been argued that specialty units with specially trained nursing staff, emphasis upon interdisciplinary relationships, and ongoing training, lower morbidity and mortality and enhance the quality of life during hospitalization.

Psych–Med Units

General hospital psychiatric units have been designated and staffed to care for psychiatric patients who are too sick medically to be on a traditional psychiatric inpatient ward, and yet too psychiatrically ill to be on the traditional medical unit.[55] They are units where psychopharmacology can be more carefully monitored in the seriously medically ill and where patients may be cared for who are in danger of hurting themselves. These units also provide a unique opportunity for a biopsychosocial diagnostic assessment by a nursing staff trained to make observations around the clock. The milieu of a psychiatric unit is available for therapeutic interventions: Patient government, group psychotherapy, occupational therapy, rehabilitation, team meetings. It remains to be determined if the medical exigencies of the HIV patient exceed the capacity of these units and whether the psychiatric needs of the patient necessitate the high-level psychiatric skill available in these units.

Med–Psych Units

Medical services in contrast to psychiatric departments have established special units that promote both physical and mental assessment and treatment.[56] Often patients in whom physical dysfunction has resulted in psychological symptomatology (e.g., endocrinopathies, pain) are encouraged to accept placement on these units. Medicine in close collaboration with psychiatry addresses both medical and psychiatric treatment that is often required in patients with HIV illness. It remains to be seen whether HIV patients are better cared for in a Med-Psych Unit (Medicine), Psych-Med Unit (Psychiatry), Cluster Unit, or in a general hospital inpatient scatter bed.

Suicide

Suicidal ideation presents a dilemma in health care for the patient with HIV and the staff. Although suicidal thinking is not unusual for any chronically or fatally ill patient, during the initial phase of the epidemic hope that a medical cure was around the corner stayed the patient's hand. Since 1984, there has been an increase in the rate of documented suicide among HIV patients, bringing into question the use of psychiatric hospitalization, even involuntary admission for those acutely suicidal. At the same time, the issue of "rational" suicide has again surfaced and challenged the position of involuntary admission.[57] In the Netherlands, euthanasia is practiced for those patients in the terminal phase of a terminal illness who are competent to understand the meaning of their request. It is important that the psychiatrist assess such HIV patients requesting assistance to terminate their lives to ensure that they do not suffer from an affective, organic, anxiety, or other psychiatric disorder that could intrude on their judgment and ultimately their legal competence in decision-making. Often the patient who wishes to die fears unbearable pain, abandonment, or out-of-control behavior, as primary concerns to which suicide appears a viable solution. Often when the patient is reassured that his/her pain can be treated and that the physician and support system will stay by his side through a difficult illness the pressure to suicide is diminished.[58]

"Look-Back" Program

The "look-back" program has been established at several blood dispensing institutions to track and council those patients who were originally transfused blood from HIV-negative donors who were found upon a subsequent donation to be positive. In essence, the patient has been given blood that may have been contaminated with HIV. Such patients require medical and psychiatric counseling as they face uncertainty, the need to change their sexual practices, and the prospects of a serious, life-threatening illness.

Similarly, it is essential to provide medical and psychiatric backup to those patients seen in the HIV treatment units which are following randomized therapeutic trials that will hopefully prolong their lives and at the same time enhance our knowledge of how best to treat this illness. Frequently, the standard medical and/or psychiatric clinic is poorly equipped to collaborate on the complex requirements to treat both the medical and psychiatric comorbidity that these patients present.

MENTAL HEALTH SERVICES DELIVERY AND LENGTH OF STAY IN GENERAL HOSPITAL

In this era of cost containment, concurrent medical and psychiatric disorders—psychiatric comorbidity—assume increased importance. Owing to the rapid escalation in medical costs, public policy now emphasizes limiting resource utilization by decreasing the length of stay of hospitalized medical/surgical patients. Coincidentally, there is an increased awareness of the psychosocial concomitants of physical disability and of the potential cost effectiveness of psychosocial interventions for the medically ill. Consequently, it is essential to understand the impact of psychiatric morbidity on HIV patients' length of hospital stay.

As early as 1938 Billings[59] observed that the average length of stay was 28 days among patients with psychiatric comorbidity, but only 15 days among such patients who received rapid diagnosis and subsequent involvement of the psychiatric liaison service when indicated. In a study of discharge abstracts from short-term general hospitals with and without psychiatric units between 1970 and 1977, patients with psychiatric disorders diagnosed according to the hospital adaptation of ICDA (H-ICDA-2)[60] stayed an average of 10.8 days, whereas the mean stay of all patients (including the patients with psychiatric comorbidity) was 7.3 days.[61]

Fulop et al. compared the length of hospital stay of medical and surgical patients with psychiatric comorbidity who were not transferred to a specialized psychiatric unit to the length of stay of patients without psychiatric comorbidity.[62] All medical/surgical patients discharged in 1984 from the Mount Sinai Hospital in New York City (N = 37,370) and Northwestern Memorial Hospital in Chicago (N = 21,889) were examined to assess their length of stay. At both hospitals, the mean ± SD length of stay of the patients with psychiatric comorbidity was significantly longer than that of the other patients: 19.8 ± 33.3 versus 9.2 ± 15.3 days at The Mount Sinai Hospital and 13.7 ± 27.7 versus 8.3 ± 13.2 days at Northwestern Memorial Hospital. This is especially important for patients with HIV disorders, many of whom have psychiatric and medical comorbidity particularly in the more advanced stages of illness. Psychiatric diagnoses and associated length of stay for specific medical disorders are presented (Table 6).

Patients with HIV disease could have any of the psychiatric diagnoses listed. It would be important to learn if earlier detection and psychosocial psychiatric interventions for HIV patients with psychiatric comorbidity influenced the use of hospital resources. The relative insensitivity of diagnostic related groups (DRGs) to issues complicating individual cases (e.g., comorbidity or severity of illness) has been documented by others.[63,64] The current DRG reimbursement mechanism provides incentives for treatment plans that are focused, but not for comprehensive interventions, thereby creating a disincentive for measures aimed at the primary or secondary detection of psychiatric comorbidity in medical illness. Even though many psychiatric disorders experienced during medical hospitalizations are transient, once detected the mental disorders are undertreated and unlikely to receive appropriate psychiatric treatment after hospitalization; it has been reported that only 4–34% receive appropriate treatment.[65–67] HIV patients may have transient delirium and depression that is obscured by their serious medical illness. Furthermore, the lack of detection of psychiatric disorders not only endangers psychiatric aftercare, but threatens compliance with the prescribed medical regimen.[68,69]

If it is discerned that psychiatric detection and intervention for HIV inpatients result in cost savings, let alone enhance medical care and diminish psychiatric morbidity, then strategies for fiscal incentives for the identification and treatment of psychiatric disorders should be undertaken through the DRG system. Perhaps the transfer of select HIV patients with psychiatric comorbidity to psychiatric/medical units not regulated by DRGs would

TABLE 6. Psychiatric Diagnoses and Associated Length of Stay for 2009 Medical/Surgical Inpatients with Psychiatric Comorbidity at Mount Sinai Hospital[a]

Psychiatric disorder[b]	Patients with diagnosis[c]		Length of stay (days)			
	N	Percent	Mean	SD	Range	Geometric mean
Organic mental disorder						
DSM-III section 1						
Dementia	39	1.9	29.7	41.3	1–173	14.8
Substance-induced organic mental disorder	132	6.6	17.3	35.4	1–366	8.5
DSM-III section 2						
Organic mental disorder secondary to physiologic process	483	24.0	23.6	33.4	1–508	14.5
Substance use	561	30.5	13.1	17.3	1–264	7.6
Affective disorder	366	18.2	26.9	33.6	1–273	15.2
Other disorder	193	9.6	18.2	59.5	1–791	7.6
Psychosis	180	9.0	23.3	33.0	1–314	13.5
Anxiety	146	7.3	14.5	15.7	1–88	8.6
Adjustment disorder	75	3.7	27.8	27.7	1–172	17.6
Personality disorder	61	3.0	16.4	23.0	1–150	9.2

[a]*American Journal of Psychiatry* 144:7. Copyright 1987, The American Psychiatric Association. Reprinted by permission.
[b]Determined by *ICD-9*/*DSM-III* codes.
[c]Each patient may have had more than one *DSM-III* category of psychiatric comorbidity had a mean ±SD of 1.2±0.5 psychiatric diagnoses.

promote the treatment of psychiatric disorders discovered on medical units.[70] This would facilitate appropriate psychiatric disposition and protect against the undertreatment of psychiatric morbidity. Premature hospital discharge of patients with psychiatric comorbidity because of the length of stay constraints imposed by DRG fiscal incentives may also be prevented.

However, specialized treatment units, as well as all psychiatric units, may soon lose their prospective payment system exemption, removing this fiscal option. In fact, Fogel et al.[70] reported that under DRGs, specialized medical/psychiatric units (primarily medical) fared worse financially than the DRG-exempt psychiatric/medical units (primarily psychiatric). Unless special considerations for psychiatric comorbidity are included in a new DRG reimbursement formula, treatment of HIV patients with psychiatric comorbidity will likely result in deficits for hospitals.[70] And with the increasing number of AIDS patients, these financial liabilities become an important consideration to even maintain care at its current level.

CONCLUSION

HIV illness with its medical and psychiatric dimensions present new challenges for the primary care physician, the psychiatrist, and the mental health delivery system. Regier has shown that primary care is an important component of the mental health care delivery system—the "de facto mental health service."[71]

Important studies of mental health services delivery are needed for enhancing care of the psychiatric component of HIV disease: (1) prevalence of psychiatric morbidity from studies of HIV populations (denominator) rather than referred cohorts (numerator); (2) enhanced methods of psychiatric assessment and diagnosis, including more reliable and valid instruments; (3) randomized controlled studies of the efficacy of psychotropic medication in the HIV spectrum disorders; (4) controlled investigation of the efficacy of inhospital care units: Psych-Med, Med-Psych, scatter, cluster units; and (5) cost-offset studies of early detection and treatment of the psychiatric component of HIV disease, including impact on length of stay, postdischarge placement, and course of psychiatric morbidity.

Finally, data-based studies of the primary care physician's ability to follow the recommendations of mental health care workers need to be undertaken.[72] Such efforts could give rise to important guidelines to enhance physician adherence to psychiatric interventions in the medical setting.

ACKNOWLEDGMENT. This work was supported in part by the Green Fund. The authors wish to thank Ms. Mirjami Easton for her assistance in the preparation of this manuscript.

APPENDIX 1

Montefiore Hospital and Medical Center Department of Nursing
Mental Capacity Screening Evaluation

Examiner: ______________________ Date: __________

Instructions: Check items answered correctly. Write incorrect or unusual answers in spaces provided. If necessary, urge patient to complete task.

Introduction: "I would like to ask you a few questions. Some you will find very easy and others may be very hard. Just do your best."

1. What day of the week is this? ____
2. What month? ____
3. Day of month? ____
4. Year? ____
5. What place is this? ____
6. Repeat the numbers 8 7 2. ____
7. Say them backwards. ____
8. Repeat these numbers 6 3 7 1 ____
9. Listen to these numbers 6 9 4. Count 1–10 out loud then repeat 6 9 4. (Help if needed. Then use numbers 5 7 3.) ____
10. Listen to these numbers 8 1 4 3, count 1–10 out loud, then repeat 8 1 4 3. ____
11. Beginning with Sunday, say the days of the week backwards. ____
12. 9 + 3 is ____
13. Add 6 (to the previous answer or "to 12.") ____
14. Take away 5 ("from 18.") Repeat these words after me and remember them, I'll ask for them later: hat, car, tree, twenty-six. ____
15. The opposite of fast is slow. The opposite of *up* is ____
16. The opposite of *large* is ____
17. The opposite of *hard* is ____
18. An orange and a banana are both fruits. Red and blue are both ____
19. A penny and a dime are both ____
20. What were those words I asked you to remember? (hat) ____
21. (car) ____
22. (tree) ____
23. (twenty-six) ____
24. Take away 7 from 100, then take away 7 from what's left and keep going: 100 − 7 is ____
25. Minus 7 ____
26. Minus 7 (write down answers ____
27. Minus 7 check correct ____
28. Minus 7 subtraction of 7) ____
29. Minus 7 ____
30. Minus 7 ____

Total correct (maximum score = 30) ____

Patient's occupation (previous, if not employed) ________.
Education ________ Age ______
Estimated intelligence (based on education, occupation, and history, not on test score):
Below average, Average, Above average________.
Patient was: Cooperative ______, Uncooperative ______, Depressed ______, Lethargic ______,
Other ______
Medical Diagnosis: ____.

IF PATIENT SCORE IS LESS THAN 20, THE EXISTENCE OF A DIMISHED MENTAL CAPACITY SHOULD BE SUSPECTED AND THE FOLLOWING INFORMATION SUPPLIED.

Temp.	___	BUN	___	Endocrine dysfunction? ________________
B.P.	___	Glu	___	T3, T4, Ca, P, etc.
Hct	___	PO_2	___	History of previous psychiatric difficulty ________
Na	___	PCO_2	___	Drugs: ________________
K	___			Steroids?, L-Dopa?, Amphetamines?, Tranquil.?, Digitalis?
Cl	___			
CO_2	___			Focal Neurological Signs: ________________
EEG	___			
EKG	___			

APPENDIX 2

Name: ________________
Date: ________________

Mini Mental State
Inpatient Consultation Form

Maximum score	Score	
		Orientation
5	( )	What is the (year) (season) (date) (month)?
5	( )	Where are we: (state) (county) (town) (hospital) (floor)?
		Registration
3	( )	Name 3 objects: 1 second to say each. Then ask the patient all three after you have said them.
		Give 1 point for each correct answer. Then repeat them until he learns all 3. Count trials and record.
		TRIALS: ______
		Attention and Calculation
5	( )	Serial 7s. 1 point for each correct. Stop after 5 answers. Alternatively spell "world" backwards.
		Recall
3	( )	Ask for 3 objects repeated above. (Give 1 point for each correct)
		Language
9	( )	Name a pencil, and watch. (2 points)
		Repeat the following "No if ands or buts." (1 point)
		Follow a 3-stage command: "Take a paper in your right hand, fold it in half, and put it on the floor." (3 points)

Read and obey the following: "Close your eyes." (1 point)
Write a sentence. (1 point)
Copy design. (1 point)

____
Total score

Assess level of consciousness along a continuum. ________________________
(alert drowsy stupor coma)

REFERENCES

1. Jones KP, Vischi TR: Impact of alcohol, drug abuse, and mental health treatment on medical care utilization: A review of the literature. *Med Care* 17(suppl):1–82, 1979.
2. Regier DA, Myers JK, Kramer M, et al: The NIMH Epidemiologic Catchment Area (ECA) Program: Historical context, major objectives, and study population characteristics. *Arch Gen Psychiatry* 41:934–941, 1984.
3. Hoeper EW, Mycz GR, Cleary PD, et al: Estimated prevalence of RDC mental disorder in primary medical care. *Int J Ment Health* 8:6–15, 1979.
4. Health Care Financing Administration 1983 Figures. Quoted in the *Washington Post,* October 17, 1984.
5. Scitovsky A, Rice D, Showstack J, et al: Estimating the direct and indirect economic costs of acquired immune deficiency syndrome, 1985, 1986, and 1990. Final report prepared for the Centers for Disease Control (task order 282-85-0061, no. 2), March 31, 1986.
6. Bloom DE & Carliner G: The economic impact of AIDS in the United States. *Science* 239:604–609, 1988.
7. The costs of treating AIDS under Medicaid: 1986–1991: May 1987 Health Care Financing Administration.
8. AIDS Weekly CDC Surveillance Sheet, US AIDS Program, Center for Infectious Diseases, Centers for Disease Control, August 29, 1988.
9. Projected costs of the treatment of AIDS in NYC, Report No. 11-88.
10. Lipowski ZJ: Review of consultation psychiatry and psychosomatic medicine. I and II. *Psychosom Med* 29:153–171, 201–224, 1967.
11. Lipowski ZJ: Review of consultation psychiatry and psychosomatic medicine. III. Theoretical issues. *Psychosom Med* 30:395–422, 1968.
12. Shapiro S, Skinner EA, Kessler LG, et al: Utilization of health and mental health services: Three epidemiologic catchment area sites. *Arch Gen Psychiatry* 41:971–978, 1984.
13. Hoeper EW, Mycz GR, Cleary PD: The quality of mental health services in an organized primary health care setting. Final report, NIMH Contract No. 278-79-0013 (DB), 1979.
14. Schulberg HC, Saul M, McClelland M, et al: Assessing depression in primary medical and psychiatric practice. *Arch Gen Psychiatry* 42:1164–1170, 1985.
15. Nielson AC, Williams, TA: Depression in ambulatory medical patients: Prevalence by self-report and physicians. *Arch Gen Psychiatry* 37:999–1004, 1980.
16. Knights EB, Folstein MF: Unsuspected emotional–cognitive disturbances in medical patients. *Ann Intern Med* 87:723–728, 1977.
17. Jacobs J, Bernard MR, Delgado A, et al: Screening for organic mental syndrome in the medically ill. *Ann Intern Med* 86:40–46, 1977.
18. Uhlenhuth EH, Balter MB, Mellinger GD, et al: Symptom checklist syndromes in the general population: Correlations with psychotherapeutic drug use. *Arch Gen Psychiatry* 40:1167–1173, 1983.
19. Shepherd M, Cooper B, Brown A: *Psychiatric Illness in General Practice.* London, Oxford University Press, 1966.
20. Thompson TL (II), Stoudemire A, Mitchell WD, et al: Underrecognition of patients' psychosocial distress in a university hospital medical clinic. *Am J Psychiatry* 140:158, 1983.
21. Cohen-Cole SA, Bird J, Freeman A, et al: An oral examination of the psychiatric knowledge of medical house staff: Assessment of needs and evaluation baseline. *Gen Hosp Psychiatry* 4:103, 1982.
22. Weschler H, Levine S, Idelson PK, et al: The physician's role in health promotion: A survey of primary care practitioners. *N Engl J Med* 308:97–100, 1983.
23. Shine D, Demas P: Knowledge of medical students, residents and attending physicians. Final report, NIMH

Contract No. OD-82-0015, 1983.
24. Pincus HA: Linking general health and mental health systems of care: Conceptual models of implementation. *J Psychiatry* 137:315–320, 1980.
25. Lyons JS, Hammer JS, Wise TN, Strain JJ: Consultation-liaison psychiatry and cost-effectiveness research: A review of methods. *Gen Hosp Psychiatry* 7:302–308, 1985.
26. Mumford E, Schlesinger HJ, Glass GV, et al: A new look at evidence about reduced cost of medical utilization following mental health treatment. *Am J Psychiatry* 141:1145–1158, 1984.
27. Lyons JS, Hammer JS, Strain JJ, et al: The timing of psychiatric consultation in the general hospital stay. *Gen Hosp Psychiatry* 8:159–162, 1986.
28. Strain JJ (ed): Diagnostic Dilemmas in the Medical Setting. The Medically Ill Patient. *Psychiatric Clinics of North America.* Philadelphia, WB Saunders Co., 1981.
29. Holland JCB, Tross S: The psychosocial and neuropsychiatric sequelae of the acquired immune deficiency syndrome and related disorders. *Ann Intern Med* 103:760–764, 1985.
30. Strain JJ, Grossman S: *Psychological Care of the Medically Ill: A Primer in Liaison Psychiatry.* New York, Appleton-Century-Crofts, NY, 1975.
31. Diagnostic and Statistical Manual of Mental Disorders (DSM-III-R): Washington, DC, American Psychiatric Association, 1987.
32. Engel GL: The need for a new medical model: a challenge for biomedicine. *Science* 196:129, 1977.
33. Kertzner R: Psychiatric and neurological side effects of medications used in treating AIDS. New York County District Branch Newsletter XI, No. 1, American Psychiatric Association, pp. 7, 14.
34. George L: Personal communication.
35. Hamilton M: Development of a rating scale for primary depressive illness. *Br J Social Clin Psychol* 6:278–296, 1967.
36. Beck A, Ward C, Mendelson M, et al: An inventory for measuring depression. *Arch Gen Psychiatry* 4:561–571, 1961.
37. Jacobs J, Bernhard MR, Delgado A, Strain JJ: Screening for organic mental syndromes in the medically ill. *Ann Intern Med* 86:40–46, 1977.
38. Folstein MF, Folstein SE, McHugh PR: Mini-Mental State. *J Psychiatr Res* 12:189–198, 1975.
39. Pauker NE, Folstein MF, Moran TH: The clinical utility of the hand-held tachistoscope. *J Nerv Ment Dis* 166:126–129, 1978.
40. Kiernan RJ, Mueller J, Langston JW, et al: Neurobehavioral Cognitive Status Examination: A brief but differentiated approach to cognitive assessment. *Ann Intern Med* 107:481–485, 1987.
41. Strain JJ, Fulop G: Screening devices for cognitive capacity. *Ann Intern Med* 107:583–584, 1987.
42. Schwamm LH, Van Dyke C, Kiernan RJ, et al: The Neurobehavioral Cognitive Status Examination: comparison with Cognitive Capacity Screening Examination and the Mini-Mental State Examination. *Ann Intern Med* 107:486–491, 1987.
43. Popkin M, MacKenzie T, Callies A: Consultation-liaison outcome evaluation system. *Arch Gen Psychiatry* 40:215–219, 1983.
44. Taintor Z, Gise L, Spikes J, et al: Recording psychiatric consultations. *Gen Hosp Psychiatry* 1:139–149, 1979.
45. Hammer JS, Lyons J, Strain JJ. Micro-computers and consultation psychiatry in the general hospital. *Gen Hosp Psychiatry* 7:119–127, 1985.
46. Strain JJ, Norvell CM, Strain JJ, et al: CLINFO: A mini-computer approach to consultation/liaison data basing: PEDAGOG ADMINISTRATIVE CLINFO. *Gen Hosp Psychiatry* 7:113–118, 1985.
47. Strain JJ, Fulop G, Strain JW: Misdiagnosis and undertreatment of AIDS referrals. APA Annual Meeting, May 1987 (NY-147), p. 97.
48. Hammond D, Strain JJ, Melonovich T: Detection of organic mental syndromes in the medical setting. (In preparation)
49. Strain JJ, Snyder S: Initial and termination diagnosis. (In preparation)
50. Strain JW, Fulop G, Strain JJ: Establishing predictors for consultation patients. Paper Session 118, p. 246, Amer Psychiatric Assn Annual Meeting, May 1987.
51. Hammer JS, Strain JJ, Lyons JS: Consortium-based consultation/liaison research. *Int J Psychiatry Med* 17(3):237–248, 1987.
52. Strain JJ, Hamerman D: Ombudsmen (medical-psychiatric) rounds. An approach to meeting patient-staff needs. *Ann Intern Med* 88:550–555, 1978.
53. Communicable Disease Center Health Care Workers Study 1987.

54. Watkins JD (Chairman): Presidential Task Force on the Human Immunodeficiency Virus Epidemic, Washington, DC, March 15, 1988.
55. Goodman B, Schwartz M, Kaplan M, et al: The psych-med unit in inpatient psychiatry's future, in *Annual Meeting of American Psychiatric Association, Toronto, May 15–21, 1982.*
56. Stoudemire A, Fogel BS: *Principles of Medical Psychiatry.* New York, Grune & Stratton, 1987.
57. Kertzner R: Rational suicide in the AIDS patient: Questions and answers about AIDS. NY County District Branch Newsletter, American Psychiatric Association, Vol IX, No. 3, Summer/Fall 1986, pp 6–7.
58. Spikes J, Holland JCB: Physician response to death and dying, in Strain JJ, Grossman S (eds): *Psychological Care of the Medically Ill: A Primer in Liaison Psychiatry.* New York, Appleton-Century-Crofts, 1975, pp. 138–150.
59. Billings EG: Value of psychiatry to the general hospital. *Hospitals* 15:305–310, 1941.
60. Hospital Adaptation of ICDA, ed 2 (H-ICDA-2) Ann Arbor, MI, Commission on Professional and Hospital Activities, 1973.
61. Wallen J: Use of short-term general hospitals by patients with psychiatric diagnoses, Hospital and Cost Utilization Project Research Note 8: DHHS Publication PHS 86-3395. Washington, DC, US Government Printing Office, 1985.
62. Fulop G, Strain JJ, Vita J, et al: Impact of psychiatric comorbidity on length of stay for medical/surgical patients: a preliminary report. *Am J Psychiatry* 144:878–882, 1987.
63. Horn SD, Bulkley G, Sharkey PD, et al: Inter-hospital differences in severity of illness: Problems for prospective payment based on diagnosis-related groups (DRG's). *N Engl J Med* 313:20–24, 1985.
64. Berki SE, Ashcraft ML, Newbrander WC: Length-of-stay variations with ICDA's diagnosis-related groups. *Med Care* 22:126–142, 1984.
65. Sensky T: Failure to keep psychiatric follow-up appointments (Letter.) *Gen Hosp Psychiatry* 7:272–273, 1985.
66. Karasu RB, Plutchik R, Steinmuller RI, et al: Patterns of psychiatric consultation in the general hospital. *Hosp Community Psychiatry* 28:291–294, 1977.
67. Burstein A: Psychiatric consultations in a general hospital: Compliance with follow-up. *Gen Hosp Psychiatry* 6:139–141, 1984.
68. Stam M, Strain JJ: Refusal of treatment: The role of psychiatric consultation. *Mt Sinai J Med* 52:4–9, 1985.
69. Strain JJ: *Noncompliance in Psychological Interventions in Medical Practice.* New York, Appleton-Century-Crofts, 1978.
70. Fogel BS, Stoudemire A, Houpt JL: Contrasting models for combined medical and psychiatric inpatient treatment. *Am J Psychiatry* 142:1085–1089, 1985.
71. Regier DA, Goldberg D, Taube CA: De facto U.S. mental health services system. *Arch Gen Psychiatry* 35:685–693, 1978.
72. Huyse F, Strain JJ, Hengeveld M: Interventions in consultation/liaison psychiatry: The development of a model. *Gen Hosp Psychiatry* 10:88–101, 1988.

18

Public Health Policy and Bioethical Issues in AIDS

The Case of HIV-Related Neuropsychiatric Illness

DAVID G. OSTROW, MICHAEL TRAUGOTT, and JEFF STRYKER

BACKGROUND

The ability of HIV to cross the blood–brain barrier is by now well known. In fact, central nervous system (CNS) involvement is a common feature in HIV infection.[1] Organic mental disease is manifested in as many as two thirds of AIDS patients before they die; at autopsy, as many as 90% of AIDS patients show neuropathological changes of HIV encephalopathy.

Grant and colleagues[2] reported the presence of significant early cognitive deficits in HIV-positive individuals who have otherwise not yet developed any symptoms of opportunistic infection. Subtle cognitive changes, including impaired abstract reasoning capabilities, learning difficulties, and slowed speed of information processing, have been demonstrated by batteries of quantitative neuropsychiatric tests. In a high proportion of cases, cognitive deficits were correlated with underlying anatomical abnormalities as demonstrated by magnetic resonance imaging (MRI) (see Chapter 12). The presence of cognitive deficits in some persons with otherwise asymptomatic HIV infection, although not always immediately evident and perhaps "mild" by some standards, raises myriad ethical and public health-related questions (Table 1).

The findings of Grant and colleagues prompted calls for screening programs to remove human immunodeficiency virus (HIV)-seropositive individuals from military and private sector jobs requiring exacting performance and judgment.[3] However, these findings were soon contradicted by other researchers.[4–6] The resolution of questions about the

DAVID G. OSTROW • Midwest AIDS Biobehavioral Research Center, Institute for Social Research, and Department of Psychiatry, University of Michigan School of Medicine, Ann Arbor, Michigan 48109. MICHAEL TRAUGOTT • Center for Political Studies, Institute for Social Research, University of Michigan, Ann Arbor, Michigan 48106. JEFF STRYKER • Department of Public Health Policy and Administration, University of Michigan, School of Public Health, Ann Arbor, Michigan 48109-2029.

TABLE 1. Public Health and Bioethical Issues in AIDS Neuropsychiatric Illness

Drug development and clinical trials
1. What is the role of the physician in monitoring or providing access to unapproved or experimental therapeutics?
2. Should the rules for testing of experimental drugs be changed because of AIDS?

Public health issues
1. Should "recalcitrant" behavior be treated as a psychiatric issue?
   When is evaluation for possible neuropsychiatric etiology warranted?
2. Should mental health facilities be used to isolate persons who pose a threat to others?
3. Should a physician's duty to warn third parties at risk of HIV infection be evaluated differently if neuropsychiatric etiology is evident?

Clinical/institutional issues
1. How should patient's HIV serostatus determine the types of care rendered and the setting for care?
2. What are the advantages and disadvantages of specialized care in AIDS-dedicated units?
3. What kinds of policies are necessary for dealing with HIV-infected health care workers?
4. Should physicians, surgeons, or other health care workers be tested for HIV infection, or, if infected, for sign of neuropsychiatric illness?
5. Should HIV positive health care workers tell their patients their serologic status?
6. What types of institutional care should be available for demented persons with AIDS? How should it be funded?

Legal issues
1. As improved tests are developed for predicting the eventual development of AIDS or neuropsychiatric illness in HIV-positive individuals, should they be used to screen for employment-related purposes or to monitor employees, once hired?
2. What role does HIV-related neuropsychiatric illness play in assessing responsibility for criminal behavior?
3. What mechanisms are necessary to foster the decision-making capacity and authority of HIV-infected individuals regarding their health care?
4. How does neuropsychiatric illness effect the conflict between the duty to warn and the confidentiality of the doctor–patient relationship?

Ethical issues
1. How should medical treatment be allocated for terminally ill persons with AIDS?
2. Should the treatment refusals of questionably competent AIDS patients be honored?
3. Should a physician ever condone or assist in active voluntary euthanasia?

possible extent of cognitive deficits in the early phase of HIV infection awaits a better understanding of the neuropathological and neuropsychiatric processes in HIV infection.[7] Rather than attempting to settle this scientific score, this chapter seeks to highlight some of the public policy and ethical questions that will inevitably arise as our understanding of the impact of HIV on the CNS increases. Since most HIV-infected individuals will exhibit substantial neuropsychological impairment at some time in the course of their disease, the impact of the virus on the central nervous system and mental functioning has wide-ranging implications for clinical care and acquired immune deficiency syndrome (AIDS) policy as developed by institutions, legislatures, professional associations, and the like.

This chapter begins with a description of the forces at work in the development and implementation of public policy as it relates to AIDS. Next, follows a discussion in greater detail of proposals to screen health care workers for HIV infection and neuropsychiatric illness. Finally, a series of policy issues specifically related to HIV disease and neuropsychiatric illness are discussed.

PUBLIC POLICY AND AIDS

Policy Goals

Public health policies to control communicable disease reflect the combination of scientific knowledge with the political, economic, legal, and social factors that shape decisions regarding governmental and institutional actions. The formulation of public health policy begins with a set of goals and then asks what can be done to achieve them. The primary aim of public health intervention in a disease such as AIDS, where no cure or vaccine is available, is to modify the behaviors implicated in the spread of the causative agent, HIV. We present a set of goals we believe to be essential to achieving this aim in the health care setting (Table 2). Worksite education efforts aimed at achieving these goals are described in the chapter by Caitlin Ryan.

The high profile of AIDS in the media and among opinion leaders and the fears associated with the disease will sometimes force quick policy decisions on those entrusted with the protection of the public's health. Individuals or groups that formulate such policy need to be aware of the various forces impinging upon the process of policymaking. Of special importance are racial, ethnic, and cultural characteristics of the groups at greatest risk of HIV infection, and thus most likely to be impacted by public health policy decisions related to AIDS. Several writers[8,9] have described how effective prevention, treatment and implementation of research programs were impeded by early perceptions that AIDS was limited to specific segments of the population (i.e., gay men and intravenous drug users).

Figure 1 illustrates a proposed model for policy analysis. This model, only one of several which could be constructed, is based on the assumption that the major influences on public health policy making are public opinion and political priorities, both of which influence the perceived cost/benefit balance. If we keep in mind the general goals outlined in Table 2, we would have to consider these two major forces as they are related to each of the goals. Embedded in the information environment, in which policies are formulated and influence each corner of the policy-making "diamond," are the scientific facts and findings which inform the general public and presumably influence the attitudes and opinions of politicians and public policy makers as well. However, the model stipulates that scientific findings do not directly affect public health policy making. Scientific findings are interpreted and filtered through public opinion and the political process to influence the public policy making process.

We will now apply our model for public health policy analysis to a specific and controversial policy: the mandatory screening of HIV infection and neuropsychiatric disorders of persons in "sensitive" positions, in this case health care providers. Figure 2 elaborates the general model for policy analysis by taking into account various input sources to the screening issue.

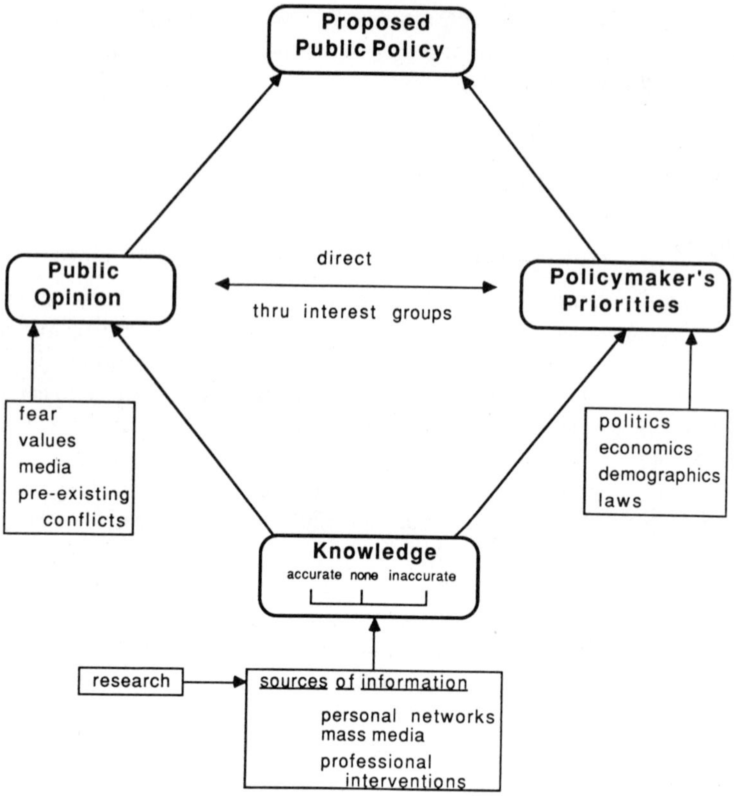

FIGURE 1. A proposed model for policy analysis.

TABLE 2. General Principles for Public Health and Regulatory Policy in Light of the Discovery of HIV-Related Organic Brain Disease

1. The overall goal in policy formulation is to produce policies which contribute to the prevention of the spread of HIV infection.
2. The secondary goal of policy is for the provision of optimal health care for individuals infected with HIV, which takes account of the special needs, requirements, and problems of patients who may have HIV-related organic brain disease.
3. Education of both health care providers and patients is essential if they are to play roles which maximize both prevention and quality of care provided.
4. The right of confidentiality and privacy of patients needs to be protected and balanced with the information needs of the public health and medical care systems in carrying out the first three principles discussed above.
5. The rights of health care workers to protection from both physical and emotional harms need to be given due consideration in any public health and institutional policies or regulations.

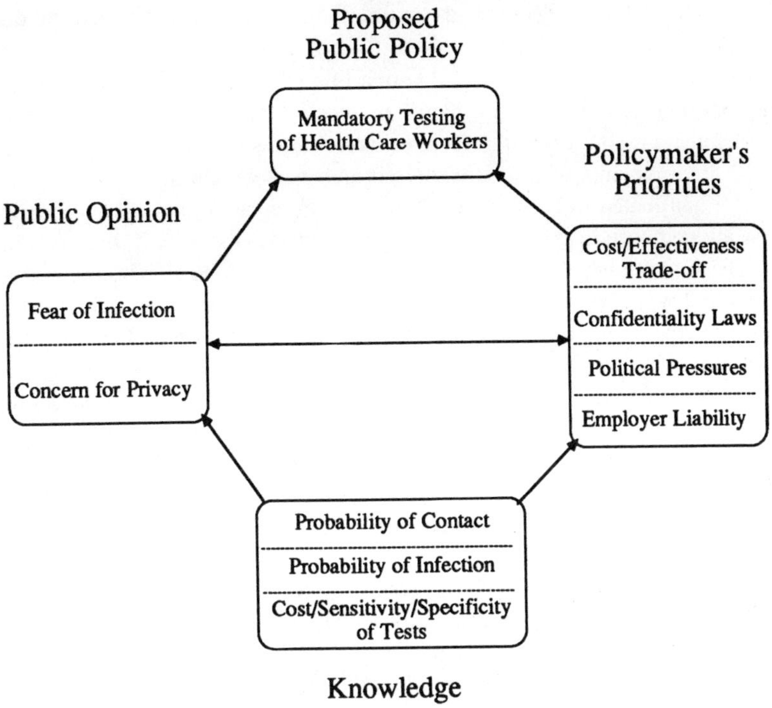

FIGURE 2. Input sources to the screening issue.

Testing and Screening

Antibody tests that determine who has been infected with HIV are widely used in both the clinical and public health arenas. Epidemiological studies have predicted that the vast majority of those infected will eventually progress to full-blown AIDS; some researchers believe that such a course is inevitable.[10,11] Yet, there is no way to predict which HIV-infected individuals will develop AIDS and at what rate. Nor are tests currently available that can predict the eventual development of cognitive deficits in HIV-infected persons. However, it is reasonable to expect that ongoing natural history and laboratory investigations will result in tests which predict with reasonable accuracy whether or not an HIV-infected individual will develop CNS illness.

Because there is no effective treatment for HIV infection of the brain, test results predicting eventual development of cognitive deficits will induce a great deal of anxiety. The ethical issues will be as serious as those surrounding the introduction of the original HIV antibody test in 1985,[12] if not more so.

The sensitivity, specificity, and actual performance levels of any of the tests that would be used in either screening for HIV infection or neuropsychiatric impairment are the threshold considerations in policy development. The parameters involved with HIV antibody testing are discussed in greater detail elsewhere.[13] The recent discovery that some persons can have HIV infection limited to macrophage cells and not produce antibodies to HIV for extended periods of time[14] has greatly complicated the determination of HIV infection based on antibody test results.

To date, there are little data available that link the types of defects seen on standardized neuropsychiatric/cognitive test batteries with actual job role performance levels. In fact, the chapters on HIV-related neuropsychiatric illness in this book reveal that many of the HIV-positive patients who demonstrate impairment in neuropsychiatric test batteries appear to be unaffected in their performance of complicated jobs.

A policy response to this issue would have to deal with at least three sets of considerations. The first is whether to screen for HIV infection among all employees, or selected groups of employees, regardless of whether or not there were any perceived or actual impairment of role performance. A second consideration in formulating a policy involves evaluation of neuropsychiatric impairments that might be more directly related to occupational role performance. A final consideration in the screening policy is how it deals with the job assignment implications of either a positive test for HIV antibodies or for any neuropsychiatric role impairments that are identified. Any screening policy which does not deal explicitly with the criteria to be used in selecting persons for testing and the consequences of positive test results will undoubtedly be seen as capricious and counterproductive.

Any screening of neuropsychiatric performance would have to consider the actual types and frequencies of CNS impairment produced by HIV, which again are quite varied and may follow different clinical courses. The frequency of testing is a concern, given the uncertain potential for shifts in clinical course, and the related issue of whether or not changes in cognitive functioning might occur at critical times in job performance. Although knowledge of the frequency of neuropsychiatric impairment in otherwise asymptomatic HIV seropositive individuals is limited, it does not appear to be a common finding when large groups of otherwise unselected seropositive persons are examined.[4,5] The World Health Organization reviewed the admittedly sparse scientific literature on neuropsychiatric aspects of HIV infection and concluded in a statement issued in March 1988[15]:

> [O]therwise healthy HIV-infected individuals are no more likely to be functionally impaired than uninfected persons. Thus, HIV screening would not be a useful strategy to identify functional impairment in otherwise healthy persons.

Treatments such as azidothymidine (AZT), in addition to having demonstrated effects on the peripheral immune system and viral replication, may in fact alter the course of HIV brain infection. New research findings include the measurements of specific viral products or products of infected lymphocytes that may themselves be neurotoxic. These measurements may, in the future, prove to be more indicative of actual or impending neuropsychiatric impairment due to HIV infection than currently available tests.[16] If there is one clear fact in the controversies surrounding the impact of HIV infection on the brain, it is that we have very incomplete yet rapidly changing scientific information on which to judge specific policy options.

Employment Policies

Such very rapid changes in scientific information complicate public policy formulation. Any policy set today may be superceded by scientific findings in the very near future. New discoveries about HIV-related organic brain disease may be used to reopen questions about employment policy and potential discrimination. Many of these questions will parallel those that have arisen in other worksite screening contexts[17–19] or the use of the recently developed test for the genetic marker for Huntington's disease.[20]

Screening programs often embrace both public health and safety goals. Drug screening, for example, recognizes that substance abuse endangers not only the user, but also third parties who might be put at risk by impaired job performance. The justifications for employee screening vary depending on the type of tests and workplace involved.[21] Medical screening commonly includes questionnaires, examinations, and laboratory tests to assess the current physical and mental health status of the individual and the ability to meet the requirements of the job. Employers may be required by law to accommodate workers with disabilities. Predictive screening is more controversial and is more likely to be subject to legal challenge. It is aimed at identifying the susceptibility of particular individuals to both occupational and nonoccupational illness that might inhibit job performance. According to ethicist Leroy Walters[22]:

> If substantial neurological compromise were conclusively demonstrated to be present in, say, 25% of asymptomatic people with HIV infection, then a strong case could be made for mandatory screening of people who are responsible for the lives of large numbers of other people, for example, airline pilots or public officials with decision-making authority over the use of nuclear weapons. However, strictly speaking, this would be a public safety rather than a public health justification.

Deciding which positions are sufficiently sensitive to warrant screening is a formidable exercise in line drawing. Professor Walters mentions nuclear weapons specialists and airline pilots. What about railroad engineers, bus drivers, or workers in the control rooms of nuclear power plants? What about anyone who drives a car or the factory workers who assemble them? Surely a mistaken judgment in any of these circumstances could result in death. Specifically, what level of role impairing deficits should trigger public concern?

Screening Health Care Workers

Employment screening issues have a special gloss when the workplace is the hospital, where health and safety issues are central. Mandatory screening for infection with HIV, already a reality for a number of population subgroups, may be proposed for health care workers, especially surgeons, nurses, and others with direct hands-on patient contact. Although there have been no reported cases of caregiver to patient transmission of HIV, the theoretical possibility exists. Proposals to screen health care workers for early cognitive deficit may be further justified by a desire to reduce the likelihood of the infliction of iatrogenic illness because of impaired performance or inappropriate clinical judgments secondary to early cognitive deficits. However, tests to screen for cognitive deficits would exacerbate already difficult problems for HIV seropositive caregivers and the institutions that employ them. What is the responsibility to inform patients of caregivers' serologic status? How should HIV-infected caregivers be monitored for possible physical or mental deterioration without unnecessarily interfering with their job performance, patient contact, or employment rights? In the absence of any accurate tests predictive of the development of CNS involvement, periodic health exams for HIV seropositive health care workers have been proposed, similar to policies for other chronic illnesses which may compromise work status. But how frequently and by whom (the employee's physician or the employer) have not been agreed on.

Any policy regarding mandatory testing of health care workers should reflect an informed analysis of costs and benefits. Costs include not only the expense of testing itself, whether for HIV infection status or neuropsychiatric performance, but also the expense of implementing any subsequent employment regulations, health status monitoring, or limiting job roles based on test results.

Another facet of the policy analysis diamond figure is public opinion. Policy-makers seek to evaluate their constituents' needs and desires. Organized interest groups lobby for policies, seeking to influence the political process. All these behaviors have characterized the debate on AIDS-testing policies and HIV. The ways in which public opinion impacts on policy formation relates to our specific example in a number of ways.

The role of fear of infection with HIV, incident to participating in the health care delivery system, will play a large part in debates about screening health care workers. This fear has a number of determinants. One issue is the difference between risk and harm, a distinction which members of the public have a great deal of difficulty in drawing.[23] This is the difference between assessing the probability of infection as opposed to the consequences of infection. Risk is itself a function of the actual or perceived probability of exposure that an individual or group may experience, modified by the degree to which they see themselves as being in intimate contact with the individual who poses that risk of transmission. There will be a continuum of levels of real or perceived fear of HIV infection in the public, determined principally by the conjoint perceptions of potential transmissibility and potential intimate contact with an HIV infected individual as illustrated in Fig. 2. This is clearly an area where perceived risk is at least as important a force in shaping public opinion as scientifically measured risk.[24]

Another fear involves potential compromise of health care. An individual may be wary of treatment by an HIV-infected caregiver. Again, one has to be concerned with both the direct and indirect impacts of policies. The consequences of delayed diagnosis and the need for counseling individuals who might be afraid to seek care are potential costs. A policy which removes HIV-infected or neuropsychiatrically impaired individuals from patient care responsibilities may impinge upon the ability of the patient to be treated by the physician of his or her choice.

Fear of transmission of HIV in the health care setting underscores the need for educating both the patient and provider. In the controversy involving the attempt of Chicago's Cook County Hospital to prevent a physician with AIDS from treating patients, misperceptions of the risk of transmission of HIV from physician to patient played a large role in the policy debate and the media coverage. The hospital's concerns included the potential financial costs if patients were to find that there was a physician with AIDS working in the hospital and seek care elsewhere. Uncertainty over what constituted potential worksite exposure led to overly restrictive limits on the physician's patient care responsibilities and, as if in reaction to those fears, excessive infection control procedures throughout the hospital.

Legal Issues

Legal protection against employment discrimination is also a critical aspect of this discussion. The recent U.S. Supreme Court decision extending the protections of Section

504 of the Federal Rehabilitation Act of 1973 to a schoolteacher with tuberculosis would seem clearly to apply to HIV-infected individuals with symptoms.[25] The Ninth Circuit Court of Appeals found that section 504 specifically applies to AIDS, finding that a schoolteacher could not be dismissed because of his illness.[26] The *Arline* court, in a footnote, explicitly reserved judgment about the how the Rehabilitation Act might apply to asymptomatic carriers of infectious diseases. The *Arline* and *Chalk* decisions could be extended readily to individuals with HIV infection and significant neuropsychiatric impairment, given the recent inclusion by the Centers for Disease Control (CDC) of neurological syndromes in category IV HIV disease.[27]

It should also be noted that the President's Commission on the AIDS Epidemic strongly recommended that federal antidiscrimination protections be extended to all persons with HIV infection. More attention needs to be given to legal protections against discrimination in private sector employment and to the special concerns that arise when the employment setting is a health care institution.

DECISION-MAKING CAPACITY ISSUES

The impact of HIV-related neuropsychiatric illness on mental functioning has many ramifications besides the issue of health-care worker screening policies. Should there be heightened scrutiny of early signs of impairment, or will increased wariness only serve to stigmatize further the HIV-infected individual and result in a self-fulfilling prophecy? In an illness as dire as HIV infection and AIDS, it is extremely difficult to determine whether depression, anxiety, or subtle personality changes are functional, situational, or organically based.[7,28] Some of the healthcare and public health policy dilemmas posed by the possibility of HIV related cognitive impairment are discussed below.

Consent to Treatment and Research

Suspicions about the mental status of the person infected with HIV call into question the individual's capacity to exercise informed, voluntary consent to treatment and research. This is of particular concern in AIDS because thc only available treatments may be invasive, irreversible, expensive, and experimental. The obligation of the physician to communicate information about treatment options and alternatives depends to a great extent on the patient's ability to understand and process such information. A physician must understand the extent to which these abilities might be impaired before attempting to secure informed consent for research or therapy.

Similar questions have arisen in the course of developing experimental treatments for Alzheimer's disease and other neurological illnesses. In addition to the neurological aspects of HIV infection that might compromise the ability to consent, AIDS is a terminal illness. In its handbook on human subjects research, the President's Commission on Medical Ethics described the ways in which a terminal illness may influence the relationship between patient and physician/investigator[29]:

> The risk of coercion and undue influence may be caused by a variety of factors. In addition to the fact that severe illness often affects a person's competence, terminally ill patients may be vulnerable to coercion or undue influence because of a real or perceived belief that participation is necessary in order to receive continuing care from health professionals as preferable to receiving no treatment. Terminally ill patients must be protected from an understandable tendency to enroll

> in research under false hopes, but IRBs [institutional review boards] should not take too protective an attitude toward competent patients simply because they are terminally ill. Some terminally ill patients may find participation in research a satisfying way of imparting some good to others out of their own misfortune—a final gift, as it were. If a terminally ill patient feels that way, he or she should not necessarily be denied that opportunity.

Foregoing Life-Sustaining Treatment

Questions of decision-making capacity are also central in determining when to honor patients' decisions to forego life-sustaining treatment. Assessments of competence are often undertaken when a patient's ability to grant informed consent is questioned, provoking both legal and psychological concerns. A patient's capacity to consent is likely to come under closer scrutiny when it is potentially compromised by underlying organic problems, as may be the case with HIV infection. Determinations of the competence of AIDS patients are confounded by the rocky course of their illness and the lucid intervals that may accompany even severe mental impairment. "Incompetency" is not a mental illness, and there is no single standard by which to judge it. In addition to a determination of the patient's "orientation times three" (to time, place, and person), an assessment of competence must also involve a searching inquiry into the person's values and attitudes prior to any mental deterioration. If the decisions of HIV-infected individuals do not concur with physicians' recommendations, those persons should not simply be presumed to be incompetent.

Legal mechanisms adopted in other contexts to foster patient autonomy should prove useful to the neurologically impaired, HIV-infected individual. "Advance directives" that allow the patient to express his or her wishes with regard to terminal care while still mentally competent are available in two types. "Living wills," or similar written documents, can be recorded to document the patient's desire to consent to a specified range of treatments in certain circumstances. These documents are expressly recognized by statutes in 38 states and the District of Columbia. In most states there are also durable power of attorney provisions for health-care decision-making that allow the patient to appoint a proxy, a spokesperson to act on the patient's behalf should he or she become incapacitated or adjudged legally incompetent.

The ability to appoint a proxy of the person's choice is especially important for gay persons with AIDS. Because current law does not generally recognize gay relationships, in the event of a conflict over treatment for an incompetent person, hospitals and courts might tend to recognize spokespersons from a patient's family of origin rather than the patient's lover or friends, especially if special arrangements had not been made in advance. Caregivers should be encouraged to discuss with patients the wishes they might have in regard to life-sustaining therapy and who they might wish to speak for them were they to become incompetent. One study of the preferences for life-sustaining therapy of gay men with AIDS found that they generally had thought about the issues and wanted to discuss them. The study also found that the physicians were not able to predict patient's preferences for care without explicit discussions.[30]

Suicide

The risk of suicide has been reported both in healthy individuals who have been identified as HIV positive and in terminally ill AIDS sufferers.[31,32] Suicide rates associated with disorders of the CNS, such as temporal lobe epilepsy, multiple sclerosis, and Huntington's disease, are at least an order of magnitude greater than for comparable illnesses not involving the CNS. Apparently, AIDS is no exception. It has been speculated that biological mechanisms may contribute to suicidal behavior in persons with AIDS. A number of drugs used to treat opportunistic infections associated with AIDS pose a risk of psychosis and delirium, perhaps further contributing to the risk of suicide. In addition, as increasing numbers of persons are tested and found to be HIV seropositive, the gloomy information about their prospects of developing AIDS may well increase the suicide rate among healthy seropositive individuals.

The issue of "rational" or "assisted suicide" has arisen within the context of AIDS. It is illegal in the United States for health care workers or others to participate in an individual's suicide. The campaign to legalize the practice of active voluntary euthanasia has been waged by the Hemlock Society in California and by counterparts in Britain and Holland. These efforts have been given further impetus by AIDS patients who have challenged the legal, ethical, and religious traditions that oppose suicide as an option for terminally ill individuals.

Finding an increased suicide risk for persons with AIDS, Marzuk and colleagues[32] concluded

> [T]he presence of concomitant psychiatric syndromes, especially depression and delirium, should lead to early psychiatric intervention. Although the illness is terminal, efforts at suicide prevention are appropriate to allow patients to rationally evaluate alternatives to treatment, to integrate their lives in terms of financial and other planning, and to allow resolution of personal friendships with family and friends.[32]

Behavioral Aspects

In the public health context, neuropsychiatric involvement may impinge on attempts to educate and alter the behavior of HIV-infected individuals. Will "recalcitrant" behavior inevitably be viewed as a manifestation of neuropsychiatric illness? Should all individuals presenting a dementia-like picture be evaluated for possible HIV infection? Public health officials and legislators may increasingly seek to use mental health facilities to "handle" persons whose sexual, drug use, or other behavior is perceived to threaten others. With the specter that such behavior may be the result of HIV encephalitis, invoking the medical or mental health model to isolate persons engaging in HIV-transmitting behavior may seem justified to some policy-makers.

HIV-related organic brain disease casts a long shadow. Consider, for example, the potential impact on the criminal proceedings where an HIV-infected individual has been charged with a crime. The requisite mental capacity (*mens rea*) to be convicted of a crime may be called into question; motivation, comprehension, and intention may each be more difficult to ascertain whenever someone is suffering from cognitive deficits. Such individuals may be found not fit to stand trial or be found to be guilty of a different or lesser offense than if otherwise impaired.

Another troubling circumstance involves the possible duty of a physician to breach patient confidentiality and warn particular third parties of possible risks of HIV exposure. This dilemma has been most frequently posed in regard to the spouse or sexual partner of the HIV-infected individual. What assurances should the doctor require that an infected patient has actually told his or her partner and plans to abstain or practice safer sex?[33]

These confidentiality and duty-to-warn questions also arise in the inpatient psychiatric unit. Patients are understandably concerned about the isolation and stigmatization that might result if their status were divulged widely to staff or to other patients. Nevertheless, for some patients who are uncooperative, irresponsible, or otherwise unable to exercise proper precautions and who put fellow patients or staff at risk of HIV infection, "the need to protect the patient community will outweigh the patient's right to confidentiality."[34] Inpatient psychiatric units and facilities for the mentally impaired present some of the most difficult settings in terms of testing and treatment issues.[35]

Clinical Trials

Another related issue in research on the neuropsychiatric aspects of AIDS is the degree to which the prospects for scientific discoveries act to deter or slow primary prevention efforts based on behavioral change. Several reports indicate that premature announcements of such technical advances as vaccines may have significant effects on educational and behavioral change efforts.[36,37]

With at least a million Americans infected with HIV,[38] there no doubt will be continued pressure for more rapid development and release of drugs with less testing. Fear of mental deterioration associated with HIV infection is likely to increase the numbers of asymptomatic individuals who seek out unproven therapies in the underground network. The research enterprise is caught between the dictates of the scientific method and the needs of a desperate and vocal population of persons at ever increasing risk of developing HIV-related disease. This will be particularly problematic in terms of developing antiretroviral therapies effective against CNS HIV infection. Clinical trials of compounds that cross the blood–brain barrier will require extensive evaluation for both efficacy and potential neurotoxicities.

PROVISION OF CARE ISSUES

Recent reports describe health care allocation issues and the ethical dilemmas posed by the care needs of AIDS patients, which will undoubtedly increase under the pressure of HIV-related cognitive impairment.[39–41] Who will pay for the long-term health care costs of brain damaged but medically stable patients, such as those whose immune systems are stabilized by drug therapy? The most useful anti-HIV treatment at this time, azidothymidine (AZT), is very costly. Many of those diagnosed with AIDS receive AZT through private or public insurance plans.[42] Reports of the beneficial effects of AZT from clinical trials of asymptomatic HIV-infected individuals will certainly increase the requests for use of this drug by patients who otherwise do not qualify for insurance coverage because they have not yet been diagnosed with AIDS.

The types and settings of care for persons with organic brain damage are quite different from those for unaffected individuals, and the ability of families and community service agencies to be involved in the care of patients is severely limited for demented individuals.

According to the Institute of Medicine in its 1988 update of *Confronting AIDS*[38]:

> Patients with dementia or other neurological disorders require a level of care that is not appropriately provided in an acute care setting. These patients frequently need custodial care more than

> treatment, and chronic care or extended care facilities are generally the setting of choice. Yet this intermediate level of care is extremely limited or even nonexistent in many cities. . . . [N]ursing homes and other long-term care facilities are reluctant to admit AIDS patients. . . . Limited reimbursement for nursing home and skilled nursing facility costs also contribute to the other problems encountered in placing patients with dementia in an appropriate care setting.

In addition to reforming skewed reimbursement systems that tend to favor acute care, other steps can be taken to provide an appropriate level of care. Unfounded fears of contagion or handling patients with infectious diseases can be dispelled for those working in institutions with little experience with HIV infection. Psychosocial interventions for the care givers, family, and close friends of such patients are important and can have a significant effect on quality of life of both patients and their families.

CONCLUSIONS

This chapter is not devoted to reaching conclusions about definitive public policy in the area of AIDS and the neuropsychiatric effects of HIV infection. Instead, this discussion has sought to illuminate the complications involved in setting and implementing policies. Finally, an attempt has been made to point out the need for constant reappraisal of scientific information and the need to update policies in the light of new findings. We have selected the issue of neuropsychiatric HIV illness because it so clearly illustrates the potential pitfalls in establishing AIDS-related public health policy. Further, the broad range of ethical issues posed by the findings described in the preceding chapters requires consideration in most, if not all, health care delivery programs. The multitude of difficult public health and ethical issues posed by the CNS complications of HIV infection will be particularly challenging to our mental health care institutions and the special therapist–patient relationships which underlie mental health care.

APPENDIX: WHO STATEMENT ON NEUROPSYCHOLOGICAL ASPECTS OF HIV INFECTION

18 March 1988

Global Programme on AIDS
Division of Mental Health
World Health Organization

In persons with the disease AIDS or in those ill with AIDS-related complex important neurological and psychiatric clinical conditions have been recognized to occur. In some cases these conditions have been linked to effects of the AIDS virus (human immunodeficiency virus—HIV) in the brain and nervous system. As a result, concern has also been expressed about whether persons infected with HIV who are otherwise healthy might experience difficulties in neuropsychological function.

A four-day Consultation (14–17 March 1988) was convened in Geneva by the WHO Global Programme on AIDS (GPA) and the Division of Mental Health (MNH) to examine currently available scientific and medical data on the neuropsychological effects of HIV infection, with particular attention to HIV infected but otherwise healthy individuals. In order to review the broad range of issues involved, 48 experts from 17 countries attended this meeting, representing the disciplines of neurology, psychiatry, psychology, neurobiology, epidemiology, social work, occupational health, ethics, clinical research, and health policy.

The consultation reported that:

> "At present, there is no evidence for an increase of clinically significant neurological or neuropsychological abnormalities in CDC Group II or Group III HIV-1 seropositive (i.e., otherwise asymptomatic) individuals as compared to HIV-1 seronegative controls. Therefore, there is no justification for HIV-1 serologic screening as a strategy for detecting such functional impairment in asymptomatic persons."

The most important outcome of these deliberations is that governments, employers and the public can be assured that based on the weight of available scientific evidence, otherwise healthy HIV-infected individuals are no more likely to be functionally impaired than uninfected persons. Thus, HIV screening would not be a useful strategy to identify functional impairment in otherwise healthy persons. Furthermore, there is no evidence that HIV screening of healthy persons would be useful in predicting the onset of functional impairment in persons who remain otherwise healthy.

The consultation recommended that as additional scientific information becomes available, this information and its policy implications should be reviewed.

The meeting also made a series of recommendations regarding the need for and types of future research and noted that the frequency of occurrence of neuropsychiatric conditions in clinically ill patients (i.e., those with AIDS related complex and AIDS) will require a review of the types of services which will be required for the care of patients.

REFERENCES

1. Wolcott DL: Neuropsychiatric syndromes in AIDS and AIDS-related illnesses, in McKusick L (ed): *What to Do About AIDS: Physicians and Mental Health Professionals Discuss the Issues*. Berkeley, University of California Press, 1987, p 32.
2. Grant I, Atkinson JH, Hesselink JR, et al: Evidence for early central nervous system involvement in the acquired immunodeficiency syndrome (AIDS) and other human immunodeficiency virus (HIV) infections: Studies with neuropsychologic testing and magnetic resonance imaging. *Ann Intern Med* 107:828–836, 1987.
3. Specter M: Early AIDS: New findings, studies suggest mind is affected first. *Washington Post,* December 18, 1987, p A-1.
4. Selnes OA, Miller EN, Becker JT, et al: Normal neuropsychological performance in healthy HIV-1 infected homosexual men: The multicenter AIDS cohort study (MACS), in *Fourth International Conference on AIDS, Stockholm, Sweden, June 12–16, 1988* abst. 8562.
5. Tross S, Abdul-Quader AS, Friedman SR, et al: Lack of neuropsychological impairment in HIV seropositive asymptomatic drug users, in *Fourth International Conference on AIDS, Stockholm, Sweden, June 12–16, 1988,* abst. 8564.
6. Janssen R, Saykin A, Kaplan J, et al: Neurologic complications of HIV infection in a cohort of homosexual men: Association with ARC but not with asymptomatic infection, in *Fourth International Conference on AIDS, Stockholm, Sweden, June 12–16, 1988,* abst. 8554.
7. Bridge TP: AIDS and HIV CNS disease: A neuropsychiatric disorder, in Bridge TP, Mirsky AF, Goodwin FK (eds): *Psychological, Neuropsychiatric, and Substance Abuse Aspects of AIDS*. New York, Raven Press, 1988, p 1.
8. Shilts R: *And the Band Played On: Politics, People and the AIDS Epidemic*. New York, St. Martin's Press, 1987.
9. Altman D: *AIDS in the Mind of America*. Garden City, Anchor Press/Doubleday, 1986.
10. Lui K-J, Darrow WW, Rutherford GW: A model-based estimate of the mean incubation period for AIDS in homosexual men. *Science* 240:1333–1335, 1988.

11. Institute of Medicine. *Confronting AIDS: Update 1988*. Washington, DC, National Academy of Sciences, 1988, pp 35–36.
12. Bayer R, Levine C, Wolf S: HIV antibody screening: An ethical framework for evaluating proposed programs. *JAMA* 256:1768–1774, 1986.
13. Saah AJ: Serologic tests for human immunodeficiency virus (HIV), in *American Medical Association: Information on AIDS for the Practicing Physician*. Chicago, AMA, 1987, pp B11–16.
14. Wolinsky S, Rinaldo C, Farzedegan H, et al: Polymerase chain reaction (PCR) detection of HIV provirus before HIV seroconversion, in *Fourth International Conference on AIDS, Stockholm, Sweden, June 12–16, 1988*, abst. 1099.
15. World Health Organization, Global Programme on AIDS. Statement on Neuropsychiatric Aspects of HIV Infection, March 18, 1988.
16. Pert CB, Ruff MR, Ruscetti F, et al: HIV receptor in brain and deduced peptides that block viral infectivity, in Bridge TP, Mirsky AF, Goodwin FK (eds): *Psychological, Neuropsychiatric and Substance Abuse Aspects of AIDS*. New York, Raven Press, 1988, pp 73–84.
17. Kolata G: Genetic screening raises questions for employers and insurers. *Science* 232:317–319, 1986.
18. Lappe M: Ethical issues in testing for differential sensitivity to occupational hazards. *J Occup Med* 25:797–808, 1983.
19. Rothstein MA: *Medical Screening of Workers*. Washington, DC, Bureau of National Affairs Books, 1984.
20. Lamport AT: Presymptomatic testing for Huntington's Chorea: Ethical and legal issues. *Am J Med Genet* 26:307–314, 1987.
21. Rothstein MA: Screening workers for AIDS, in Dalton HL, Burris S (eds): *AIDS and the Law*. New Haven, Yale University Press 1987, p 126.
22. Walters L: Ethical issues in the prevention and treatment of HIV infection and AIDS. *Science* 239:597–603, 1988.
23. Singer E, Endreny P: Reporting hazards: Their benefits and costs. *J Commun* 37:10–26, 1988.
24. Dawes RM: Measurement models for rating and comparing risks, in Sechrist L, Freeman H, Mylley A (eds): *Health Services Research Methodology: A Focus on AIDS*. Washington, DC, National Center for Health Services Research and Health Care Technology Assessment, 1989, pp. 31–44.
25. School Board of Nassau County *Florida v. Arline,* 107 U.S. 1129 (1987).
26. *Chalk v. US District Court for the Central District of California,* 840 F.2d 701 (1988).
27. Centers for Disease Control, Public Health Service: Revision of the CDC surveillance case definition for acquired immunodeficiency syndrome. *MMWR* 36:S3–57, 1987.
28. Rubinow DR, Joffe RT, Brouwers P, et al: Neuropsychiatric impairment in patients with AIDS, in Bridge TP, Mirsky AF, Goodwin FK (eds): *Psychological, Neuropsychiatric, and Substance Abuse Aspects of AIDS*. New York, Raven Press, 1988, p 111.
29. President's Commission for the Study of Ethical Problems in Medicine and Biomedical and Behavioral Research. The Official IRB Guidebook, US Government Printing Office, Washington, DC, 1983, 7G "Terminally Ill Patients."
30. Steinbrook R, Lo B, Moulton J, et al: Preferences of homosexual men with AIDS for life-sustaining treatment. *N Engl J Med* 314:457–460, 1986.
31. Glass RM: AIDS and suicide. *JAMA* 259:1369–1370, 1988.
32. Marzuk PM, Tierney H, Tardiff K, et al: Increased risk of suicide in persons with AIDS. *JAMA* 259:1333–1337, 1988.
33. Gostin L, Curran WJ: AIDS screening, confidentiality, and the duty to warn. *Am J Public Health* 77:361–365, 1987.
34. Belitsky R, Solomon RA: Doctors and patients: Responsibilities in a confidential relationship, in Dalton HL, Burris S (eds): *AIDS and the Law*. New Haven, Yale University Press, 1987 p 201.
35. Ostrow DG, Gayle TC: Psychosocial and Ethical Issues of AIDS Health Care Programs. *Qual Rev Bull* 12:284–293, 1986.
36. Ostrow DG, Eller M, Joseph J: Epidemic control measures for AIDS: A psychosocial and historical discussion of policy alternatives, in Coreless IB, Pittman-Lindeman, M (eds): *AIDS: Principles, Practices and Politics*. Washington, DC, Hemisphere Publishing Corporation, 1988, p 19.
37. Osborn JE: AIDS, social sciences, and health education: A personal perspective. *Heal Educ Q* 13:287–299, 1986.

38. Institute of Medicine. *Confronting AIDS: Update 1988*. Washington, DC, National Academy of Sciences, 1988.
39. Blank RH. AIDS as an allocation issue: Toward individual responsibility for health. Testimony presented before the Presidential Commission on the Human Immunodeficiency Virus, Nashville, March 17, 1988.
40. Lo B, Raffin TA, Cohen NH, et al. Ethical dilemmas about intensive care in patients with AIDS, in *Committee for a National Strategy for AIDS*. Washington, DC, Institute of Medicine, National Academy of Sciences, 1986.
41. President's Commission on the Human Immunodeficiency Virus Epidemic: Report of the Presidential Commission on the HIV Epidemic, Washington, DC, US Government Printing Office, June 24, 1988.
42. Buchanan RJ: State Medicaid coverage of AZT and AIDS-related policies. *Am J Public Health* 78:432–436, 1988.

19

Reactions of Medical Personnel and Intimates to Persons with AIDS

BERTRAM SCHAFFNER

INTRODUCTION

People whose lives or work bring them into close contact with victims of acquired immune deficiency syndrome (AIDS) cannot help but be deeply affected. I will try to describe some of these situations and their emotional impact, especially as they have come to view in my own practice of psychotherapy and psychoanalysis. I hope that they may, in some measure, be representative and convey the qualities of the human dilemmas and psychiatric challenges they bring with them.

PHYSICIANS' FEARS

When I first heard about AIDS, or GRID as it was then named, about 1981, it was with disbelief and the hope it was a bad dream that would soon go away. It was too frightening, and the inevitable outcome, at that time, too horrible to contemplate. The total ignorance about its cause and the nature of its transmission, naturally, aroused intense feelings of powerlessness and panic. I think I felt somewhat protected or insulated from it in my professional life, as I had no patients with AIDS or any direct contact with AIDS for at least a year. Gradually circumstances obliged me to give up the understandable hope of being spared direct experience with such danger and suffering. When an AIDS patient was referred to me for help with his depression and the planning of his remaining life-span, I could no longer live in my ivory tower with only theoretical speculations about this new illness on the world scene. Soon afterward an internist friend with a largely homosexual practice began to share with me his bewilderment over the many and strange forms that the illness took, confusions in diagnosis, inability to save the patients, difficulty in finding hospital beds for them, financial and other hardships for the young victims who were usually quite unprepared for such catastrophic events. He also described to me his own physical exhaustion and emotional depletion from having to stand by helplessly, the depression he felt over the long period of saving patients several

BERTRAM SCHAFFNER • William Alanson White Institute of Psychoanalysis and Psychology, New York, New York 10023.

times from opportunistic infections, only to see them eventually succumb to the same infection despite the use of the same medications that had worked before. He hardly mentioned the strain he was under, being in frequent close physical contact with his AIDS patients, wondering whether he himself was in danger of contagion, and having to fight off his own fears, conscious and unconscious.

Many physicians working in general hospital settings find themselves in conflict between their natural medical curiosity and their fear of contact. Some are protected by their specialties, which normally keep them from close contact with patients, for example, radiology and pathology. But the degree of dread, sometimes revulsion, felt by hospital personnel has often been demonstrated in the myriads of precautions required before entering an AIDS patient's room, or fear of touching utensils he may have used. Especially at the beginning there was widespread resistance among house staff, nurses, social workers, and ward personnel to taking care of these patients. Administrators complained about surcharges for the required private rooms, not covered by Blue Cross or Medicare; the long hospital stays, sometimes due to the nature of the illness but also often because there was no place to which they could return. Some landlords locked AIDS victims out of their apartments; some families refused to allow the patients to return home. Occasionally ambulance drivers, police, and undertakers would refuse to have anything to do with AIDS patients or their corpses.

THE PUBLIC'S FEARS

Gradually this disease has become better understood and the public more aware that AIDS is, to the best of our present knowledge, communicable mainly in a manner similar to hepatitis B: Only through blood products or through intimate, primarily sexual, contact, with direct transmission of body fluids. Fortunately, after more than 9 years of experience treating AIDS patients in hospitals, there have been no known cases of the disease appearing among health-care workers who were not exposed through either sexual or blood transmission routes. This has alleviated public panic and avoidance reactions to some degree, but the general level of fear and concern naturally continues.

MEETING PATIENTS' NEEDS

Meanwhile, the tremendous emotional and psychological damage to AIDS patients has begun to be recognized. First, because up until now the diagnosis carries with it an implicit involuntary suggestion or disclosure of a person's life-style, carrying with it a cruel social stigma, comparable to the days of *The Scarlet Letter* and in more recent times, the stigma whenever a diagnosis of sexually transmitted disease was made.

AIDS patients frequently suffer from guilt feelings for being homosexual (or drug abusers); some even view the disease as God's punishment for their sexual deviation and the sexual revolution. Sizable segments of the public at large, including members of the medical profession, have similar views and for such reasons distance themselves personally and medically from the victims as human beings, ignoring their specific personal emotional or social needs, as for example when AIDS patients were not allowed to have any visitors but their biological families, with whom they were not necessarily close, and were thus shut off from their lovers or friends, with whom they might be on closer terms. A real emergency arose over the question of how to provide adequate psychiatric care to patients with AIDS, which was first given wide attention in 1982 and responded to primarily by the Gay Men's Health Crisis, which mobilized a group of largely homosexual social workers, psychologists, and a few psychiatrists.

MY FIRST AIDS PATIENT

My first contact with a severely ill AIDS patient came about when a young man of 32 was referred to me for follow-up after his discharge from a psychiatric ward at a general hospital. His illness had been diagnosed 7 months previously. A fiercely self-reliant workaholic, he needed to deny his illness, was determined to fight it off and to survive, concealed his symptoms, and tried to repress all his feelings as well. He had to be hospitalized when he became hypomanic. This subsided after medication in the hospital. I wondered if he would now develop a depressive mood swing. When he arrived, I saw only a severely undernourished individual, defiantly independent, trying to communicate an air of strength and well-being, impatient to return to his work as an artist, mentioning only in passing that he was having difficulty with his vision. I was so involved in determining his psychiatric state and how to meet his needs that I did not notice at all what I might be feeling. After all, I had only shortly before read that although nurses, doctors, and laboratory workers who care for AIDS patients are the most obviously exposed persons, and would be expected to be the first casualties if the disease were spread easily by touch, coughing, or sneezing—so far there had been no cases among health workers, unless there were direct sexual contact, sharing of needles by drug abusers, or transfusions of blood or blood products. So far as I was aware, I did not feel any fear at the time of the first two interviews. However, after a few weeks, when the patient's condition rapidly deteriorated, his visual difficulty turned into virtual blindness, his body shrank further in volume, and he was noticeably weak, I began to feel overwhelmed by the tragedy unfolding before me, its unstoppability, and the futility of help through conventional psychiatry at this juncture. I began to concentrate all my energy to persuade him to accept rehospitalization, and I was grateful when he agreed. He used the bathroom and left my office.

FEARS OF CONTAGION AND PUBLIC EXPOSURE

The patient after him, who had observed him as he was leaving, said to me, "I'm no doctor, but if anyone asked me, I'd say that your last patient has AIDS. He has just used your bathroom. I don't want to lose you, and of course I don't want anything to happen to myself. I hope you are taking due precautions." The patient's words penetrated through to the feelings I had not yet dared to recognize in myself because he was so open and direct in dealing with his own fears. His simple expression of the fear of death, which we doctors have been traditionally trained to ignore, opened a floodgate of emotions in me. Fear of my own possibly becoming infected, of dying, reminded me that being a doctor does not confer immunity. I also permitted myself for the first time to recall that there could be a possible threat to my own practice and livelihood. What if patients were to become afraid to come to my office because I had permitted an AIDS patient to sit on my office chair? Or even be on the premises? I recalled that the tenants of one New York City apartment building had actually sued, though unsuccessfully, to evict an immunologist from his office because his practice included patients with AIDS. It began to haunt me that the patient had told me, just before he returned to the hospital, that he could no longer read the elevator buttons and had managed to reach my floor by asking other passengers to push the correct button for him. Whom had he spoken to? What did they make of his condition? What was their reaction? Might there actually be an attempt to restrict my practice, or worse? I began to see in my own quickly rising fears, the irrational degree to which fright can lead one.

RESPONSIBILITY TO THE AIDS PATIENT

A psychotherapist colleague without a medical background described his dilemma upon learning, after 3 months of treatment of a male patient, that the man had just been diagnosed as having AIDS. Recognizing his unfamiliarity with the area, the therapist made it his business to learn as many medical facts as possible. He consulted his peers and older colleagues, familiarized himself with the help available through Gay Men's Health Crisis and other agencies. Naturally, he also discussed with his wife his concern for her health and that of their young children. His first reaction was to put the health needs of his own family first, but he was also convinced that AIDS was not easily transmittable, because of the small numbers of cases as compared to the huge numbers of people in the "at risk" categories, who were much more intimately exposed than he would be. He decided to take all reasonable precautions and to continue to treat the patient, because "I could not respect myself as a person if I were to abandon this human being. When you take someone on, you do it for the long haul." He went on to tell me, "The first big test came when the patient asked if he could use my bathroom. I asked myself whether I could tell him that he could not. Remembering my convictions, I gave him permission. But despite all my rationalizing, when he left I gave the bathroom a scrubbing such as it had never had before. For weeks I could not even put his checks among my other papers." Subsequently he was relieved to learn from a research worker in the field of the retrovirus, that the life of the virus is extremely fragile, it dies as soon as it dries, and is easily destroyed by the use of soap, water, and a 1 : 10 solution of chloride bleach.

PATIENT ABANDONS THERAPY

However, my colleague had also discovered what is frequently encountered with AIDS patients—the difficulty in trying to apply usual psychiatric method with them. Now this patient became so preoccupied with his new reality situation, that he was less interested in dealing with his subjective feelings. For a few weeks they tried to work on his attitudes toward the future, but when the patient had to cope with the loss of his roommate, moving to a more expensive apartment that he could not afford, fears of his co-workers finding out, and so forth, he felt he could no longer continue therapy. The therapist reduced his fee drastically and offered more frequent sessions to tide him over the crisis, but at this point the patient abruptly stopped treatment. My colleague commented, "I think I was almost more upset about his state than he was. The thought of his own death seemed almost to relieve him, while I had to deal with my own feelings of frustration and that somehow I had failed. I felt that the patient whom I could not think of abandoning, had abandoned me."

EMOTIONAL PRESSURES UPON DOCTORS

Treating these patients is bound to put the doctors involved under powerful stress. AIDS patients' emotional equilibrium needs careful attention. It is well known that the results of all treatment are considerably affected by the patient's ability to keep a sense of purpose and to see some positive role in his remaining lifespan. Therefore the real emotional responses of the therapist toward the AIDS patient are an integral part of the management of the case. But physicians' feelings vary widely, from compassion and dedication to private condemnation or rejection, depending on the physician's own attitudes and background, especially when he or she is particularly moralistic and judgmental. The self-disparaging AIDS patients cannot survive additional disapproval from their physicians. The essential compassionate awareness and involvement with the AIDS patient's life situation may be a difficult departure from the strict objectivity once considered to be the *sine qua non* of "scientific psychotherapy." It calls for the physicians and psychotherapists involved to adopt an approach usually associated with the "family physician." But they also have to be on guard against overinvolvement, overidentification, and other intense emotions that may be released.

How does the physician cope with his or her own feelings? One told me, "We've been trained for so long to ignore and suppress our own feelings, certainly not to show them, that we may unintentionally try to suppress patients' feelings as well, and resent it if they call upon us to feel along with them. Especially since learning from Kübler–Ross of the importance of helping the dying to share their feelings, we must take time to listen to the patient, and to ourselves as well. But I find that becoming more personally involved with the patient's life and mortality, though very rewarding, takes it emotional toll on me." Another very empathic physician stated, "How can I help having strong feelings? When you treat a young person so frequently over a 2-year period, you do get involved in a sense of kinship and friendship. Sometimes I have wept together with a patient, I'm not sure that did him any harm. Still, as I was trained as a physician not to show my feelings, I wonder afterward if it was appropriate. I also wonder, as the number of AIDS patients in my practice increases, what it is doing to me. It is almost impossible to keep my therapeutic optimism. You simply can't deny the hopelessness of the disease so far, it has not yet established boundaries, one day it may include myself." How did he deal with his own fears? He said, "I think my overcoming my fear was coincidental with reaching out more to my patients, in trying to help *them* keep up their spirits and to help them die in dignity. When they do die, I know I feel grief, but sometimes I don't even have the time to grieve, or the right person to share my grief with."

Physicians who themselves are members of the groups at risk, are likely to become very anxious about their own health, because of frequent physical proximity to AIDS patients and daily reminders of its symptoms. In 1987, homosexual physicians formed a large percentage of those rendering primary care to these patients, especially in large urban areas like New York and San Francisco. One hospital-based neurologist working with these patients observed to me, "Homosexual physicians and personnel have been notably courageous in taking active roles in the care of AIDS patients. Maybe they are responding to their identification with the patients, or feel a strong sense of community and the need to protect their own from a hostile environment." He also commented, "Homosexual physicians who have not yet 'come out of the closet' or who are afraid for their status or position in case of exposure of their life-style in the hospital, may go through intense conflicts and guilt, for example, for failing to be assertive in case of inappropriate remarks or actions by a co-worker toward an AIDS patient." One resident who did show his concerns in such an instance, was chided by a colleague who asked him, "Why do you care so much about this guy with AIDS? He's going to croak anyway," followed by insinuations about the resident's own sexual orientation.

Physicians naturally suffer from physical strain as well. A female internist with strong maternal feelings, whose practice includes a large number of gay male patients, wept in talking to me, "I can't believe the degree of stress I am under. Seeing so many young people die, as well as the hours of care they need, you can't imagine the number of days and nights that I am called upon. It's not just the hours, although I hardly have time to be with my own family. It's the feelings that mount up. The worst is wondering if you are a failure as a doctor. I know with my head that I am not, still when you see so many of your patients die, you stop being rational."

A young male physician stated, "We all seem to be able to accept death more easily in older people. It's an entirely different matter when you deal with people in their 30s whom you've first seen as creative, brilliant, vital. It is such a sense of waste and loss. This young group is usually not prepared to die. Often they get very angry about it, even refuse to cooperate with treatment. They also raise uncomfortable issues that I don't like dealing with, such as their right to commit suicide or to have euthanasia. It's very rough, because sometimes emotionally I agree with them."

Another physician told me, "Seeing so many patients with AIDS is affecting me with a more global fear. I find myself worrying about a possible major change in society's attitude toward sexual mores. Lately society has been more tolerant of sexual freedom but now there may be more intolerance, or outright prohibition. This could alter my entire personal future and civil rights. Worrying about this, it is hard to remain detached and unaffected. I've almost become afraid to make another diagnosis of AIDS. I feel devastated by each new case."

The same internist said, "I used to think I had more energy than anybody, but now I'm finding that I have to take off at least one day a week, and do you know, I am feeling guilty about it!" Some doctors also feel overwhelmed by their inability to do anything about the severe economic plight of many AIDS patients. If self-employed they may not be eligible for unemployment insurance, may not have adequate medical insurance or savings to take care of themselves during a protracted illness. Fortunately, in 1985 AIDS patients became automatically eligible for Social Security disability payments, once the diagnosis had been established.

The list of pressures upon doctors would not be complete without mentioning the large group of patients known as "the worried well" whose needs are quite insistent and draining. These patients are not demonstrably ill, but keep requiring proof that they are not ill, while also seeming to insist that they must be. They need many hours of study and reassurance, which can be not only fatiguing but irritating to physicians more at home with purely physical disease. Fortunately they can refer such patients to interested psychiatrists and psychotherapists who may be better prepared to deal with obsessive worriers.

RELIEVING THE TENSIONS

Also fortunately, physicians dealing with AIDS patients have recently found ways to cope better with the heavy feelings aroused in them, by sharing and expressing their reactions to colleagues going through similar experiences, in small physicians support groups. (It has also become increasingly common in recent months for physicians in frequent contact with AIDS patients to enter psychotherapy themselves.)

SUPPORT GROUPS

These doctors in small groups usually begin by admitting their profound sense of unsureness professionally in dealing with AIDS patients. The courses of the various forms of the illness are so uncharted; medications work differently in different patients, depending on factors not yet discovered or defined. The outcomes of the treatments are so unpredictable, and this can be profoundly disturbing to a professional person, especially a younger one, who feels the need to be adequate to the responsibility for the welfare of a patient, when there may actually be no effective or even clear course of treatment to follow. Support-group members often derive considerable relief from realizing that these feelings of professional frustration, uneasiness, or even confusion, are normal under the circumstances and shared by others.

Support group members may also assist each other in practical coping with difficult medical situations they have just been through by sharing new information or discussing methods they have just learned about. This can go a long way to counteract the sense of isolation, inadequacy, or personal failure, especially for doctors who work in separate individual practices or in different hospitals. There is emotional relief through sharing medical knowledge with colleagues as well as sharing the sense of bewilderment at the complications of the disease, but also often a sense of relief at being able to express such feelings out loud to persons willing and able to understand what they have been going through. They feel close again, in a sympathetic group, accepted once more in a world that they may have begun to sense as unfriendly to them. They sometimes derive a sense of success from seeing the relief they are giving to each other.

In a support group members can air their own sense of devastation over seeing their patients deteriorate. Different physicians have differing styles of adjusting to the stress of coexisting with a dying patient and trying to endure the person's chronic decline and the final moment of the actual death of the patient. Some doctors try to protect themselves against overwhelming emotions, possibly by anticipating the death far ahead of time, as if to be prepared against any surprises and to remain detached and controlled as possible.

Others allow themselves to identify more personally with the patient, and to participate more actively in the patient's feelings. Perhaps they trust themselves to cope with the inevitable shock and sense of loss when the patient enters the final phase of his illness.

AMBIVALENCE TOWARD AND FROM PATIENTS

Physicians' distress over AIDS patients are not always connected with warm feelings of identification. Sometimes support-group members are called upon to help each other with patients they do not like or, with patients who do not like the doctors. AIDS patients are often angry—angry at their illness, angry at the world, their fate, the social and economic difficulties they must contend with—and frequently these resentments are expressed toward their doctors. The conscientious caring doctor may be especially vulnerable to attacks by a patient. Some angry patients become highly critical, belittling the doctor's abilities or the services provided, demanding unreasonable or excessive attention and commitments of time; or they try to involve the doctor in tricky or unanswerable questions. Doctors may have difficulty tolerating the criticism, especially when unjustified, or in dealing with or challenging the often clearly irrational accusations and complaints. It can be especially hard to deal with patients by whom they feel intimidated. Here small support groups play an especially useful role in helping physicians to ventilate their consternation and indignation to other physicians rather than possibly doing so injudiciously to the irritating patient, thus helping to discharge and resolve their feelings, and assisting them to feel comfortable in setting limits with the unreasonable patient.

Small support groups have also played useful roles in dealing with guilt feelings that the individual physician often experiences, not only when a patient has died despite all the physician's efforts, but guilt feelings toward a patient when the doctor was not present at the time of the patient's death. Some physicians put themselves under undue pressure by promising greater availability to the patient than they are able to deliver. For example, one doctor, in a gesture of sympathetic understanding and generosity, promised to allow a patient to die at home rather than in a hospital; and he later regretted the impossible task he had undertaken of trying to provide adequate medical care in the home setting that was not equipped to deal with medical emergencies. Support groups may also be used to guard members from overinvolvement professionally in a patient's welfare, by helping physicians recognize what the overinvolvement could do to the emotional well-being of their own families and loved ones, and to help them maintain a workable balance between them, as well as looking out for their personal needs and sustenance as well.

ADVICE REGARDING SUPPORT GROUPS

A few words about the form of such support groups: Groups may vary from quite structured to totally unstructured, with or without a leader, with or without a psychiatrist as therapist or participant observer. Generally, support groups meet at regular intervals. The only truly essential requirement is the strictest observance of confidentiality. It has also been found quite helpful to make sure that doctors feeling special needs for help indicate their needs clearly at the beginning of the session, to make sure that they are not left stranded and their problems undealt with at the end of the session. Of course it goes without saying that the ideal size of such support groups is small. Four has been found to be a very useful number.

DENTISTS' EXPERIENCES

To turn briefly to other medical personnel with whom the AIDS patients come in contact, one must have great sympathy for the position of the dentist, who often sees himself as at very great risk of accidental infection, since his work brings him in direct contact with several body fluids: blood and saliva and possibly nasopharyngeal secretions and tears. From the first announcements that the HIV virus was occasionally present in saliva and tears, both dentists and dental patients have had a noticeably higher degree of anxiety about contamination and worries about breakdowns in antiseptic techniques. Dentists now routinely wear protective goggles and gloves and many frankly refuse any patient known to have HIV blood antibodies. Dentists fear having patients with visible signs of AIDS in their waiting rooms. The consequent difficulties that AIDS patients have had in obtaining dental care, have given rise to special dental clinics catering only to AIDS patients, such as the Lambda Center for Dental Health in New York City, opened in 1987.

REACTIONS OF NURSES AND OTHER HOSPITAL PERSONNEL

Nurses have very similar fears, since they are frequently in contact with body fluids from AIDS patients. Some AIDS patients may require such frequent and repeated nursing care, as for example when they need their beds changed as often as 20 times in one day, that the nurses' anxiety about AIDS may express itself in protests against the physical strain, excessive work, and health risks. This may be exacerbated when the nurse is pregnant or planning to have a child, in today's atmosphere of fear of giving birth to an infant with AIDS. Male nurses may be variously affected, depending on their own sexual orientation or ambivalence toward homosexuals and drug users. Many hospitals now routinely include anxiety-reducing sessions for nurses, to educate them in personal safety precautions to reduce their particular fears about contact with AIDS patients. These have by and large been successful, and there has been a remarkably low incidence of hospital personnel acquiring any AIDS-related illness through contact with patients. Nevertheless, some nurses may be so phobic that they refuse to care for AIDS patients, posing a problem for hospital administrators. Each case is usually decided individually. The tendency now is to determine whether there is any scientific basis for regarding the nurse's exposure as potentially dangerous to her, and to learn whether her previous life experience had given her any special basis for her particular fear. In general, younger women have been more likely to dread close nursing contact, while older or more maternally oriented women have often shown greater ease in caring for them.

Ward personnel's fears closely parallel those of nurses, since they too handle equipment and eating utensils, and so forth, that have been in contact with the AIDS patients. Fortunately group discussions with ward personnel have often proved successful in coping with their worries. I have participated in such ward discussion groups and found the personnel refreshingly open, direct, perceptive and responsive. Frequently they are easily accepting of AIDS patients.

Hospital administrators have been hard hit, especially in recent years, caught between the Federal government's efforts to reduce costs by cutting hospital appropriations, and the rapidly increasing numbers of AIDS patients in hospitals, by the number of hours of daily medical attention they require, the high cost of the newer drugs becoming available to deal with the complications of AIDS, and the increasing lengths of hospital stays. Naturally they may develop resentment toward AIDS patients, which are occasionally felt by the already oversensitive AIDS patients as rejection. Methods are being constantly sought to reduce hospital stays or nursing care, e.g., in Cooperative Care units in which patients' families or companions substitute for nurses, by teaching family and friends to give medical care at home. Hospital social workers are also caught up in rapidly increasing pressures to cope with bureaucracy to obtain funds and placement for AIDS patients when they become able to leave the hospital.

REACTIONS OF FAMILY AND OTHER INTIMATES

Now to turn to reactions I have encountered among intimates of persons with AIDS. This group embraces close friends, co-workers, and especially families, including those of biological origin, marriage, and lover relationships. The reaction of intimates is often crucial to the physical and psychological stability of the AIDS patient. If they desert him, it can only increase the patient's sense of being a social pariah and his tendency to withdraw from society, even to barricade himself against family, friends, and medical help. If a patient tends in this direction, much may depend upon the intimates' personal courage, knowledge of self-management during the disease, and his previous attitudes toward contact with illness in general.

One patient of mine illustrated her inability to surmount the fear of illness: She has customarily avoided any visits to medical facilities or friends in hospitals. When a very close friend of hers was diagnosed as having AIDS, she said, "I keep putting it off. It may be better to go 3 weeks from now. Maybe I should go to the funeral and not have to see him suffer. I know others who have it too, but I don't even want to think about it. It's all too much to bear."

REACTIONS OF EMPLOYERS AND CO-WORKERS

Employers and co-workers often struggle with mixed feelings when a fellow employee comes down with AIDS. There are moving reports of executives of large corporations who have been retained in their positions and protected financially, with a minimum of disturbance suffered by the patient or his co-workers. This situation may be more difficult when the patient works in a smaller enterprise, depending upon how closely he works with other employees, the quality of their previous interpersonal relationship, and the degree of openness or secrecy with which he has lived his personal life-style.

One employer consulted me because of conflict between his personal friendship and loyalty to an employee with AIDS who was essential to his business, and his uncertainty as to how to deal with clients who ordinarily come into close contact with the patient, who happened to be in charge of marketing and sales. The patient was a fastidious, hypersensitive, perfectionistic individual, already in a severe depressive reaction to having AIDS. He was particularly fearful of losing his one source of personal security, his very good appearance, due to impending chemotherapy and possible baldness. He was also under stress that week, planning to reveal to his family for the first time both his homosexuality and the fact that he had AIDS. At that very moment the employer, a compassionate individual but highly tense over his own personal marital and financial problems, attempted to remove pressure upon the patient by telling him that he would now be relieved of his salesman duties and could work unseen in another part of the office. The employer's offer was the last straw for the employee, who abruptly left the office for home and took his life.

TWO COUPLES WITH AIDS

When a patient is first diagnosed with AIDS, his lover naturally goes through shock as well. For many established lovers, awareness of the eventual loss of the loved one is uppermost, next to awareness of the potential physical suffering and emotional agonies that they will be sharing. The lover may know that he is headed for a prolonged period of extraordinary self-sacrifice in emotions, energy, time, stress, and usually money, for which he may not be at all prepared, sometimes even at the expense of his own livelihood. Only too often neither member of a homosexual couple is in a secure financial position; they may have managed only by combining their incomes, and the loss of one or both may be devastating.

One patient of mine, whose lover has had AIDS with recurring infections for the past 2 years, was referred to me because of a paralyzing depression. The first reality factor to be dealt with was that he had been nursing his ailing lover himself almost 16 hours daily, sleeping poorly on improvised bedding, awakened frequently by the lover's coughing. When temporary voluntary and paid medical assistants were brought in five nights per week, my patient recovered from his physical exhaustion sufficiently for us to begin to deal with psychological issues. He was naturally living with the dread of contracting AIDS himself, but trying to assuage his fears by reminding himself that he and his lover had been living together for 5 years before the lover came down with AIDS and that so far he himself had no hematologic or other suggestive symptoms. Still, it was a constant effort for him to control his worry. In addition, he uncovered deep feelings of resentment toward his lover for acquiring the dread disease and spoiling what he had regarded as a perfect relationship. Previously they had lived the so-called "open relationship" life-style until the advent of AIDS, at which time they promised each other to be completely faithful. As the lover got sicker, he felt the need to confess to my patient that he had not been able to live up to the promise of fidelity and asked for forgiveness. Until the time of treatment, my patient had not been able to forgive him, precipitating deep depression. As a sickly child, he himself had learned to live by a personal code of protecting others from the burdens of his illness, and had expected the same from his lover. He felt deeply betrayed, and I tried to help him make the major adjustment of accepting his lover's human frailties, and even to become a parental figure to the person who had formerly been a parental figure for him. He recovered from his depression, regained his energy and warm feelings toward his lover, and even found ways to salvage the business that he had jeopardized by devoting all of his waking hours to the lover with whom he had been angry.

In a different situation, a homosexual couple came to me for joint therapy, when AIDS complicated an already difficult relationship of 3 years. Their neurotic conflicts had resulted in a virtual cessation of sexual intimacy and a real danger of separation. The one with the illness had long been pushing to solidify a kind of intensely romantic marital type of bonding, and was unaware how much he had been pressuring his partner to a degree of closeness that the partner could not bear. They had never been able to discuss psychological problems together, although they had tried, so the roots of their difficulties were unclear to them. When AIDS entered the picture, the situation called for emergency clarification. The uninfected partner, who felt less adequate and competent than the one with AIDS, was deeply concerned about the amount of responsibility he would be assuming, and also about the resentment he felt. He was beginning to feel trapped, and withdrew further from the patient who in turn clung even more.

Joint therapeutic sessions made it possible for the AIDS patient to become aware of his interpersonal operations to hold his lover, and for the lover to come to terms with the reasons underlying his withdrawal, to recognize that his sense of inadequacy actually antedated their relationship, helping to reduce the blaming and friction between them. The sick one is now accepting his partner's need for growth and individuation, and is relieved that they can now communicate and that therefore he will not be abandoned at this critical time of his life.

REACTIONS OF FAMILIES TO AIDS PATIENTS

The reactions of the patient's biological family also play a tremendous role, the importance of which cannot be overestimated. When the biological family has already known of their relative's life-style, they may be better able to accept the new shock of the discovery that he has AIDS. Discovering both at once can sometimes be too much for a family to assimilate and to remain positive toward the person. The lover of one AIDS patient told me, "I don't know how I would have survived without my family. They have been wonderful. They call often, ask about my lover, they offer all kinds of support, to fly up and be with us, or to send money if needed. It is all very frightening to them, but they do not plague me with their fears."

Some families, even when they have already made peace with a son's homosexuality, may still be beset with fears of public disclosure that their son has this disease. In a recent example, one family tried to conceal it by forbidding the son with AIDS to tell his friends, and will not agree to his request that his obituary include a request for donations to the Gay Men's Health Crisis, from whom he had received much physical and moral support.

Public health education and reduction of panic and prejudice does not extend far enough from the larger urban centers into smaller towns or agricultural areas of this country. When one of my patients wrote to his parents in the southern part of the United States that he was planning to visit them, they replied, "You may come to visit but you will have to stay in a hotel; we have read that gays carry AIDS germs and your mother and I do not wish to run the risk of contracting it."

Another patient of mine suffered tremendously when he asked to visit his home in the midwest. His mother replied, "On second thought, I don't guess it would be a good idea for you to come, especially if you told everybody what you have. I'm sure they would feel uncomfortable." My patient reacted, feeling crushed and bitter, "I believe she is ashamed of me. You know, she really believes that I am being punished by God for being gay."

FEARS OF AIDS IN A HETEROSEXUAL FAMILY

The last example from my practice is that of a husband and wife who are struggling with the unanswerable questions, fears, and imponderables of this formidable disease-complex: They report that theirs has been a reciprocally happy marriage, and only in the last few years during which the husband was undergoing enormous stress at work, has he resorted to occasional relief of tension through casual homosexual experiences in movie houses. He has had no known contact with any one with AIDS, but he has been overcome with feelings of guilt and remorse, is convinced that he must already have the disease, and worst of all, is convinced he must have already transmitted it to his wife and especially to his youngest daughter. Fortunately all tests for signs of AIDS have proven negative, but he is still compulsively examining himself for early symptoms and becomes agitated whenever his wife or child becomes ill. He has a detectivelike mind, reads everything available about AIDS, but cannot find peace because he literally "knows too much" and inevitably draws the most self-punitive conclusions. A deeply religious person since childhood, he has been filled with guilt and condemnation of his homosexual experiences, and says his worst fear is of the disgrace he will bring upon the family when AIDS finally makes its appearance. In treatment, his depression has lifted somewhat, especially after he took his wife into his confidence. Her warmth, understanding, and nonjudgmental reaction have served to relieve the panic to some degree. In joint sessions with her, he is able to explore the origins of his childhood fearfulness and his turning to males for emotional support. In the joint therapy he is discovering that it is safe to reveal one's needs to a female and that she can genuinely give him her full love and support without losing respect for him.

CONCLUSION

I have tried to give you an overview of some of the reactions to AIDS that I have been privileged to observe among my colleagues and among my patients and their families. I have had to learn new aspects and dimensions of the practice of medicine and psychiatry, and to change some of the methods I had been taught. Above all I have learned that one has to have courage, and that one must find a new way in therapy, a judicious mixture of both psychotherapy and friendship. Still, it is necessary to be on guard not to incorporate the fears and emotional reactions of the patient to the point that one's own requisite stability is endangered.

Lastly, one needs to ask in what way is the treatment of AIDS patients different from the treatment of any other of the fatal illnesses to which mankind is prone? I think the primary differences are its newness, severity, the unsolved mysteries of transmission and cure. But, in addition, there is the special situation of powerful social bias against sexually transmitted diseases in general, and against the two groups thus far most afflicted, homosexuals and drug abusers. These biases have made it far harder for patients, their families, lovers and physicians to handle, and also made it easier for the untouched segments of the population to distance themselves from AIDS patients as people, even to view them with indifference or neglect, to treat them as less than human.

However, the gradual widening of the incidence of AIDS in the general population, the unforeseeable dimensions or end of the disease, are slowly penetrating into our awareness. One reason that the treatment of AIDS differs from the management of other fatal or plague-like illnesses in the past, is that we as a people have been able to live in denial of the seriousness and danger of AIDS. We have not really allowed ourselves to comprehend that we are living in a pandemic, worldwide, affecting 165 countries in the world. We have not allowed ourselves to experience fully the peril in which we are living. We have not realized that we ought to be fully engaged in a major national, or international, endeavor to conquer AIDS, before it destroys us all. We have not had candor and courageous leadership in either the political or the medical field, with the exception of the lone voice of our Surgeon General Koop. We have delayed taking brave actions because of traditional mores, values, and prudishness. We have quibbled over what words we may or may not say out loud on television, or at what age to be sexually explicit with schoolchildren. We have not faced the fact that this is a time of dire emergency, such as a war, and that our fight against AIDS is really the equivalent of war for human survival. We have been clamoring to preserve many cherished individual values, forgetting that if we do not temporarily give them up, as in war, we may not be here to reclaim them when the war against this disease is over.

We are living through a very dark moment in medical and social history, in which it is of the utmost importance to cultivate one's faith in the positive forces in human nature, and to demonstrate one's faith by living it.

20

The Training and Support of Health Care Professionals Dealing with the Psychiatric Aspects of AIDS

CAITLIN C. RYAN

INTRODUCTION

Over the past 8 years of the acquired immune deficiency syndrome (AIDS) epidemic, health care providers have been affected as definitively as patients. Many have reported feeling overwhelmed by their caseloads of young terminal patients or perhaps inspired by the courage and resourcefulness demonstrated by their patients in responding to the illness. Some have been appalled at the level of discrimination and social sanction endured by patients and their family members. Still others have personally experienced a level of ostracism or social isolation from colleagues, as a result of "AIDS phobia" and prevailing fear about the disease.

Medical schools have reported concern and anxiety among some students about working with AIDS patients, along with a reluctance to select such specialities as internal medicine where practitioners work more intensively with AIDS.[1] Media reports of providers who quit or were fired rather than treat AIDS patients have mirrored the public fear that has prevailed since AIDS was first identified.

In high incidence areas, providers who initially treated AIDS patients when appropriate services were limited or unavailable, graphically describe that experience[2]:

> The sudden onslaught of AIDS has forced all of us on the frontline to become "experts" in a very short period of time. We have developed new skills and stretched ourselves beyond what we ever thought possible—compelled by the new faces, names and problems that come before us each day. From the onset until now, working with AIDS has been like fighting a war. The enemy is a disease that has so far thwarted our most sophisticated technology. Beyond its physical toll, AIDS exacts an emotional price as well. Service providers and survivors alike suffer a form of post-traumatic stress syndrome—from the loss, the fear, the incredible suffering and indignities that the disease and discrimination call forth. I can certainly say that AIDS has changed me. In the near future, it will have touched us all.

Clearly, AIDS has challenged providers on a personal level at the same time as it is initiating long term changes in the American health care system. Rather than decreasing

CAITLIN C. RYAN • AIDS Policy Center, Intergovernmental Health Policy Project, George Washington University, Washington, D.C. 20007.

the need for professional education and support, however, the AIDS epidemic is only illuminating tremendous gaps in these areas. From the emergence of AIDS until now, the need for training, the need for acknowledging and managing providers' fears and emotional responses to this highly fatal modern "plague" remains substantial.

This chapter identifies basic factors that can inhibit a practitioner's work with AIDS affected patients; identifies key elements that promote and prevent burnout among staff; and provides recommendations for designing and implementing employee AIDS education programs.

HISTORICAL FACTORS THAT INFLUENCE THE NEED FOR TRAINING AND SUPPORT

As a newly identified infectious disease that was apparently transmitted through "body fluids" or sexual contact, AIDS quickly became sensationalized. The complex nature of the disease was difficult to convey in short media reports or news articles. Early on, both health care workers and the general public were, in fact, uncertain how AIDS was spread and factual knowledge was not readily available. Professional training at that time, was limited to direct patient experience. Anecdotal reports along with a few initial studies indicate that comfort level and feelings of competency have increased in proportion to the numbers of patients that providers have cared for.[3,4] Because so much of the early professional expertise was gained from treating patients directly and few published articles were available until more recently to guide clinical practice and training, significant numbers of health care providers have not received specific AIDS education or training, nor have they had an opportunity to work with an AIDS-affected patient. The lack of consistent, standardized AIDS training materials and curricula for professional schools as well as continuing education programs has made it difficult for providers to receive comprehensive AIDS education.

Furthermore, a federally funded interdisciplinary provider education program was not initiated until 1987, and each discipline has responded to the training needs expressed by their individual members with varying degrees of urgency and allocation of resources. (See Appendix I for a list of HRSA and NIMH AIDS training programs for health care providers.)

Public policy statements, issued by a number of professional associations and specialty groups, have offered some guidance in defining a provider's ethical responsibility to their patients and clients. Nevertheless, actual training, both in terms of curricula and the development of educational materials has been slow to emerge from most professional groups, with perhaps the exception of the American Psychiatric Association and the American Psychological Association initiatives.[5] On a state level and more frequently in collaboration with the state health department and state professional associations, training is being made available to some health care providers (usually public employees) in approximately two thirds of the states.[6] Training is also increasingly available through local health departments in higher incidence cities.

BARRIERS TO AN APPROPRIATE CAREGIVER RESPONSE

Several factors that characterize the transmission and prognosis of AIDS as well as the populations initially observed to be at risk for HIV infection have made it difficult for many health care professionals to respond appropriately in providing quality patient care:

1. Demographics of initially identified risk groups which include gay and bisexual men, IV drug users and minorities and the lack of familiarity with the characteristics, special needs and concerns of these groups
2. Attitudes and values about identified risk groups that affect patient care, in particular, homophobia (an irrational fear and prejudice towards homosexuals) and racism
3. Sexual transmission of HIV and attitudes toward human sexuality
4. Rapid progression of disease and grim prognosis once AIDS has been diagnosed
5. Practitioner's discomfort in working with terminally ill patients
6. Young age of patients
7. Fear of infection
8. Need to alter procedures substantially to provide for appropriate infection control practices, testing, and counseling guidelines

Discrimination as a Barrier to Patient Care

The initial identification of AIDS with socially stigmatized groups affected the public's response and, not surprisingly, the response of many health care providers. Discrimination in service delivery has been reported by many patients and family members as well as by colleagues of reluctant and fearful providers, often to state agencies and advocacy groups.[7] Because individuals in these groups have historically been underserved, many were suspicious and fearful themselves in presenting for treatment and care. Moreover, since many of these patients were in a relatively young age group, their family members and significant others frequently had no previous experience with chronic or life threatening illness, and were thus uninformed of patients' rights or unaware of how to advocate on the patients' behalf. Longstanding difficulties in serving gay men, IV drug users, and minorities compounded their difficulties in receiving appropriate care.

Racism and Cultural Biases Affect Care

Racism and cultural biases that affect appropriate health care delivery have been documented in the literature.[8] These include such attitudes as "blaming the victim" for their stigmatized or low socioeconomic status or for their behaviors such as IV drug use. They may also include assigning negative characteristics to minority patients or clients. Racism can be associated with providing poor quality care or with reluctance or refusal to work with minority patients and clients. Recent AIDS specific literature has identified cultural barriers in treating black Americans who are reported to be at higher risk for HIV infection than whites.[9,10] Although few articles have been published on working with other minorities at risk for AIDS, an understanding of cultural differences, help-seeking behaviors and how different cultures affect an individual's capacity to use professional services are essential to providers working with minorities at risk of HIV infection.[11]

The literature documenting provider reluctance to treat IV drug users is less prevalent, although anecdotal reports from social workers, nurses, and physicians confirm the extent of the problem. The issue of IV drug use is further complicated by such factors as race, ethnicity, low socioeconomic status, and prevalence for relapse among patients.

Homophobia Affects Care

Since the mid-1970s, researchers have documented homophobic attitudes among service providers that have interfered with the provision of quality care to gay men and lesbians.[12–14] Increasingly, researchers have focused on the responses of providers to AIDS patients, in particular those who are gay men. Because caring for AIDS patients may be a provider's first experience in dealing with openly gay patients, emotional responses can be critical in determining their reaction to AIDS in general.

In studies measuring the attitudes of nurses, physicians, and medical students toward patients, all evidenced a significant level of homophobia and many felt that the patients were to blame for their illness. Douglas and Kalman's early study revealed that more than half their sample of hospital-based physicians and nurses "feel more negatively about homosexuality since the emergence of the AIDS crisis." A similar percentage agreed with the statement, "In the hospital, patients with AIDS receive inferior care compared with patients with other illnesses." Even more disturbing was their finding that 15% of the doctors and nurses sampled agreed with the statement, "Homosexuals who contract AIDS are getting what they deserve."[15]

Kelly's studies of both medical students and physicians presented four identical vignettes to participants. In each, the patient was identified as either having leukemia or AIDS and as being either homosexual or heterosexual. In both studies, AIDS patients were regarded as being much more deserving of what happened to them, dangerous to others, deserving to lose their jobs or to be quarantined. Moreover, regardless of which disease was involved, the homosexual patients were viewed as being more responsible for their illness, more dangerous to others and suffering less pain than heterosexual patients. In all areas, both medical students and physicians were less willing to interact, even in the most casual manner, with an individual identified as homosexual, than with one identified as heterosexual. They were also much less willing to engage in conversation with an AIDS patient, socialize with, continue a friendship or renew a lease with someone who had AIDS.[16,17]

Issues of Sexuality

Coupled with homophobic attitudes among some practitioners is their generalized discomfort in dealing with sexuality and with a disease that is sexually transmitted. Limited attention is given to human sexuality in many professional schools so that providers are often reluctant or embarrassed to discuss sexuality, even as it pertains to diagnosis or treatment.[18] Inadequate sexual history taking is an issue for all mental health providers though generally only physicians or physician assistants have been sampled for this information. In a follow-up of their 1984 study of California physicians on AIDS related competence, Lewis, Freeman, and Corey reported inadequate sexual history taking in 65% of their respondents, even though 66% had patients at risk for HIV infection.[19]

A particularly alarming result of inadequate sexual history taking was suggested by researchers in a study of hospital-based HIV testing at the St. Paul-Ramsey Medical Center in St. Paul, Minnesota where almost one half of physician-ordered HIV-antibody tests were administered without a sound medical reason or without the patients' consent. According to the study, of all antibody tests administered in the hospital over a 15-month period, only 10% fulfilled all the criteria for an appropriate test. In a *New York Times* interview, Dr. Keith Henry, a co-investigator, suggested that most physicians probably found it easier and less time consuming to administer the test, rather than to take an accurate sexual history.[20]

This generalized discomfort with human sexuality has implications for treating HIV-affected patients. Currently, 69% of diagnosed AIDS patients are gay and bisexual men (including those who also use IV drugs). In addition to working with patients, special sensitivity to the needs of their biological family members—many of whom may not be aware that their son is gay—is required, to assist families with their coping and grieving process. Many who learn simultaneously that their son is gay and has AIDS face two life crises. Some will meet their son's significant other or lover for the first time in the hospital setting. If providers are unable to accept their patients' sexuality, they will also have difficulty responding to the needs and potential caregiving roles of their patients' support system.[21–25]

Because much of the home care for AIDS patients is provided by their biological family as well as by their support system, providers will need to work with other gay individuals in planning necessary extended or outpatient care.[26] Joanne Lynn, a noted medical ethicist and gerontologist, has observed that more than two thirds of the care for the elderly is provided by their families.[27] Although estimates are not available for AIDS- and HIV-affected patients, one can assume that at least two thirds and perhaps more of the care required by these patients is offered by their families, lovers, significant others, and community volunteers, a sizable percentage of whom are gay and lesbian. This percentage is no doubt even higher with AIDS, since so few nursing homes and long-term care facilities have been willing to accept AIDS-related patients.[28] Practitioners who are not familiar with gay patients and their family systems are advised to contact gay-related professional associations for consultation, information on training conferences, and the availability of appropriate educational materials to assist them in working with this population. (See Appendix III for a listing of reference organizations.)

Issues Related to Terminal Illness

Practitioners have often reported their difficulty in treating patients who will not recover. Even though mental health providers, in particular, work extensively with patients grieving many losses including relationships, behaviors, and so forth, many professional schools do not provide adequate training in grief and bereavement and death-and-dying issues. Health care professionals, in general, unless they receive specialty training, do not routinely receive sufficient education in working with terminally ill patients. In working with AIDS patients, many of whom deteriorate rapidly, providers have expressed negative emotions including anger, depression, frustration, and hopelessness about "not being able to do what we were trained to do." The stress of working with large numbers of terminally ill patients and with those who are often in the same peer group as their health care providers (due to the relatively young age of most AIDS patients) is frequently described as being overwhelming.[29]

BURNOUT PREVENTION AND MANAGEMENT

Burnout has become a concern in higher incidence areas and increasingly, professional associations and community based AIDS organizations are offering seminars on avoiding overload and caring for the caregivers of AIDS patients. Characterized as a severe physical and emotional response to chronic stress by specialist Martha Bramhall, burnout is often the inevitable result of overworked staff and overburdened agencies.* Given the multiple challenges of serving AIDS-affected patients and clients who are often debilitated, without the necessary resources or placements, socially stigmatized and emotionally demanding as a result of extensive psychosocial needs, burnout is an increasingly prevalent response of providers and community volunteers in settings that serve a large number of AIDS related patients. In a multihospital study measuring social workers attitudes toward working with AIDS patients, burnout was identified as the workers' chief concern in serving this population.[30]

Prevention

Burnout prevention is as much an administrator's responsibility as it is an individual employee's responsibility, particularly since situational stress factors—those inherent in the job—are perhaps the basic causes of burnout.[31] For the employee, mastering the skills of time management, stress management and self-care (including the ability to set limits appropriately) are key factors in avoiding potential burnout.

Ironically, employees at highest risk of burnout are often those who are most idealistic and dedicated as well as those with very high standards and a commitment to providing quality patient care. In stressful work settings, which can include inadequate staffing and resources, potential funding problems, high turnover, high caseloads, and insufficient time to meet the need for personal support—burnout prevention becomes the shared responsibility of management and staff.

Administrators will need to incorporate burnout prevention into the work setting[32] which includes the following:

- Providing training for both new employees and veterans on burnout prevention and identification
- Reducing situational stress within the agency that can promote burnout
- Providing ongoing support groups for staff
- Developing a system to treat acute burnout among staff

*The author gratefully acknowledges the assistance of Martha Bramhall, LCSW, psychotherapist and stress management specialist, in researching this section.

Administrators and clinical directors can actively help to prevent burnout by implementing a series of practical tasks:

1. Becoming familiar with the signs and symptoms of burnout so they can identify affected workers early and assist them in mitigating its effects
2. Helping newly hired staff to set realistic expectations, to identify their own motivations, personality needs and coping styles, while assisting staff in setting priorities
3. Assisting staff in varying their caseload so that it is not overloaded with end stage AIDS patients, HIV-infected families, or other patients who may require extensive services and care
4. Implementing "time-out" work-related activities, apart from direct clinical service and care, such as committee work, teaching opportunities, lunch time discussion groups, continuing education programs, and special projects to give staff a break from high-intensity, stressful, and emotionally draining work
5. Involving family members and significant others in orientation and training programs that include AIDS education and prevention information to reduce their fear of their partner's risk of infection, and to assist them in understanding job related pressures and demands
6. Sponsoring and encouraging fitness and wellness programs for staff
7. Encouraging staff to participate in outside activities that diverge from work-related demands
8. Developing morale building activities such as staff retreats, awards dinners, opportunities for public recognition for the staffs' contributions and family events

Support Groups

A consistent recommendation for health care settings that provide services to HIV-affected patients has been to establish support groups that can give workers an opportunity to ventilate feelings, to share resources, and to deal with the untimely death of their patients. Certainly providers will express fears and misconceptions *before* working with AIDS patients. Nevertheless, it is normal for practitioners, even those, who have worked with AIDS-affected clients for a considerable period of time, to experience fantasies about contagion or to dream about developing AIDS or of becoming infected with HIV. These are coping mechanisms for working with clients who face life threatening situations and for managing the generalized fear that exists with regard to AIDS. This prevalence of a subconscious response to working with AIDS was reported in a study of young physicians conducted at San Francisco General Hospital where one in three male physicians reported having nightmares about AIDS.[33] In many studies of health care workers' concerns about AIDS, fear of contagion has been repeatedly expressed, even among well-informed and knowledgeable practitioners. This consistent finding suggests that ongoing support is a critical factor in assisting providers during the epidemic, both to avoid burnout and to maintain mental health.

The support of co-workers, in particular, but also the availability of support from supervisors, significant others, and spouses, is associated with low levels of burnout and other mental health problems related to job stress.[34] The availability of staff support in a busy clinical setting is generally erratic and often requires individual staff to seek out peer support either briefly during their workday or after hours and on weekends. An increasing sense of isolation, lack of contact with others experiencing similar problems and concerns, and limited opportunities to express negative or emotionally charged feelings all contribute to burnout. Agency and clinical directors in settings that serve HIV-affected patients must implement support groups to enable staff to manage countertransference issues, fears, ethical concerns, and a variety of related issues that will arise when working with this population. Unfortunately, in some areas support groups have not been given priority by administrators so they are not viewed as being essential to workers and may only be offered after work hours or on a volunteer basis. In higher incidence areas where caseloads and time pressures are especially demanding, workers may feel torn between taking care of their own needs by attending these groups or attending to the multiple needs of their patients and clients.

To alleviate these additional pressures, administrators should:

1. Incorporate staff support groups into the routine work week during regular hours
2. Set aside a consistent time for the session (support groups may be longer but generally 1 hr/week will help staff focus and express critical feelings and concerns
3. Encourage *all* employees to attend and assist staff in managing their responsibilities so they are able to do so

Various models have been suggested, and administrators may choose to experiment with different types of groups until they find what works best in their setting. Examples include a leaderless support group, similar to a rap group; a group led by an outside and neutral professional; or a group led by the staff supervisor. The regularity of the sessions is perhaps the most important factor, in addition to their inclusion within a time frame accessible to everyone.

In providing worker support, special sensitivity is needed in managing the fears and concerns of spouses and other family members who may lack sufficient information about HIV transmission and prevention and who are frightened that providers may become infected and transmit HIV to other family members, particularly children. For example, 8 of 10 social workers surveyed in one large urban study reported that their family and friends would be concerned that they were working with AIDS patients, and 44% felt that their families would be frightened.[35] In another study, more than one third of rural southern physicians reported that their families were concerned that they could contract AIDS as a result of providing patient care.[36] Some facilities have responded to these concerns either by inviting family members to attend staff AIDS training and orientation sessions or by conducting special family AIDS education programs.

Identifying Burnout and Recovery

Identifying the signs and symptoms of burnout can help supervisors and staff intervene early with themselves or with co-workers suffering from it. It is possible to recover from burnout and to continue working in the same profession, even with similar patients and clients. However, recovery requires a commitment to changing some of the behaviors that contributed to burning out, such as overwork, insufficient attention to personal needs including recreation, outside interests, companionship, diet and exercise, unmanageable caseloads, and taking on too much responsibility, often through difficulties in setting limits or prioritizing.

Acknowledging that one is burned out is the first step to recovery. The following list includes some signs and symptoms associated with burnout:

- Lethargy
- Sense of meaninglessness
- Chronic fatigue
- Somatic complaints, i.e., headache, backache, stomach problems
- Difficulty feeling motivated or finishing tasks
- Feeling overwhelmed
- Frequent feelings of anger, impatience or irritation
- Agitated depression
- Difficulty sleeping
- More frequent use of alcohol, drugs, tobacco, or food
- Sense of emotional numbness
- Finding it more difficult to empathize or care for clients' problems
- Spiritual depletion
- Reluctance to socialize
- Feeling emotionally depleted or drained
- Reluctance to get out of bed or go to work
- Realization that most time is spent working

Recovering from burnout involves assessing how burnout occurred, i.e., how behaviors, attitudes, values, and the work setting contributed to burning out, and then changing those factors. Many of the recommendations for preventing burnout can help an individual recover, but the individual must also acknowledge his or her condition to their supervisor, co-workers, and friends and enlist their help in recovery. Cutting back the normal workload significantly, setting priorities that include personal time, time for recreation and exercise, meditating or meeting spiritual needs, getting sufficient rest, and eating well are key components in recovering from burnout.[37]

AIDS TRAINING ISSUES

Multiple barriers exist to providing appropriate services to patients affected by AIDS that present significant challenges to health care workers. As caseloads increase, meeting the need will challenge the entire health care delivery system. The implications for training in professional schools, in continuing education programs and in clinical settings are clear. In order to respond to the growing number of patients requiring services, which include identified patients and their families and support systems as well as individuals at risk, all health care settings must offer or make available comprehensive provider education.

Goals for implementing on-site AIDS training are similar for all settings: (1) to train providers and staff at *all* levels to decrease fear and increase worker competence, (2) to decrease discrimination in various levels of service delivery and to increase quality patient care, (3) to increase appropriate utilization of infection control guidelines, and (4) to keep staff up to date on recent scientific developments as they pertain to treatment and patient management. For mental health providers, AIDS training must also focus on integrating psychosocial and medical aspects of AIDS, preventing burnout among staff and assisting providers in understanding life-style and cultural aspects of groups at risk of HIV infection.

Although the length of time available to train staff may vary, three components are essential in providing appropriate AIDS education. These include (1) factual scientific information on transmission, patient management, and infection control; (2) an emotional component to identify providers' fears, feelings, and biases, with time to process them; and (3) an ethical and legal component, articulating the providers' responsibility in responding to general dilemmas that AIDS will introduce.

Few evaluative models for training health care providers have been published, although education and training are described as helpful and as increasing worker competence by many attending such sessions. On the basis of training experiences with more than 40,000 individuals since 1983, almost two thirds of whom were health care providers, the author has consistently experienced this response.

Of the studies published on training health care providers to deal with AIDS, all show clear improvement in workers' attitudes toward patients and their comfort level in providing services to AIDS patients after training was administered. These include a study of 237 staff members at Boston's New England Deaconness Hospital,[38] an attitudinal study of 22 registered nurses at Pennsylvania State University,[39] a Massachusetts state-funded study of 1247 health care providers (including nurses, support staff, physicians, and laboratory technicians) in hospital-based training sessions,[40] and a second consecutively administered Massachusetts study of more than 200 health care providers.[41]

Improvements in accuracy of medical and technical knowledge were evidenced, as demonstrated by significant increases in correct responses in the Massachusetts state study. These include improved awareness of infection control procedures as well as routes of transmission. What this study and others suggest, however, is that repeated exposure to factual AIDS training (e.g., medical, infection control guidelines) coupled with opportunities to express feelings, and to explore biases and prejudice in nonjudgmental environments, are essential to increase providers' comfort level in working with AIDS affected patients, and conversely, to decrease discrimination and inappropriate care. In the experience of the author, one-time training is not sufficient for most individuals to learn the facts, expose myths and misconceptions, identify personal biases, and ventilate feelings. For optimal learning and integration, AIDS-related information, including an opportunity for discussion, must be repeated over a period of time. Nevertheless, both hospital administrators and agency and clinic directors must begin somewhere (1) to introduce AIDS education, and (2) to provide a baseline of knowledge for all staff members. Some may avoid initiating training by claiming that one session is inadequate to train all staff or perhaps contend that it would be too difficult to schedule training for everyone. Even in settings with a high incidence of AIDS where providers tend to be more knowledgeable about AIDS issues, staff can benefit from attending an AIDS training session. Content can be varied to update staff on new scientific developments, community resources, stress management and burnout prevention. On any given day, crises will prevent attendance by all staff who were invited to participate, so that videotaping or repeating a session for workers on different shifts can make this important information available to those who need it.

In the author's experience, hospital and agency administrators or department chairs generally order AIDS training for "professional" staff only. Others, who have frequent direct patient contact, such as LPNs, janitorial and dietetics staff, and attendants, rarely get the opportunity they need to learn about AIDS and to process their own fears and concerns. Because professionals often have supervisory or perhaps direct authority over these staff members, and thus will have to respond to patients' complaints of excessive garbing or verbal and physical abuse which can arise as a result of fear and uncertainty, it is important that *all* staff receive training.

Training Content

In-Service Training

In training health care providers to work with the psychiatric aspects of AIDS, a one day session, with ongoing support as a follow-up, is ideal. In addition to incorporating a medical and psychosocial overview, the session should include emotional responses of staff, working with IV drug users and chemically dependent patients, legal and ethical issues, community resources, and at least one speaker or a panel of speakers representing the patient's perspective. This would include HIV-affected individuals, their family members and significant others.

Brief Training on Specific Topics

Although no particular change has been noted in providers' attitudes through involvement of patients in brief training sessions (of 1½ hr each), it is the author's observation after conducting hundreds of training sessions, that having patients as speakers serves to enhance the training experience by (1) humanizing AIDS and helping providers personalize the epidemic; (2) reducing fears of what patients may look or act like; and (3) normalizing the providers' experience with stigmatized groups initially identified with AIDS by allowing them to converse directly, ask questions and have an opportunity to re-examine personal biases. It is also the author's observation that no apparent studies have measured providers' attitudes and knowledge after full-day training sessions, in particular, where patients, family members and significant others have participated as speakers.

One-Day Training

The author has trained in 1-hr, 2-hr, 5-hr, and 8-hr to 2-day and entire course contexts. A 1-day format allows providers to develop some degree of comfort in a group setting where they may feel more willing to express fears and examine biases. It also allows repeated exposure to AIDS information and an opportunity to ask questions in a variety of ways.

A particularly effective full-day training was developed by the author for chemical dependency treatment programs where patients and staff generally work in a milieu setting. This involves medical and psychosocial content, content on staff feelings and community resources, in addition to a 2-hr modified psychodrama session in which two HIV-affected patients interact with staff in a circle, acting out everyday experiences with their parents, employer, lover, or spouse.* Providers and patients are asked to exchange roles and to speak from the perspectives of the other individual. An additional group exercise in which providers are organized into four to five subgroups representing staff from various community agencies that serve AIDS patients, gives providers a hands-on experience of the complexity of multiple needs AIDS-related patients have as well as how those needs are often overlooked, how patients are discriminated against or underserved. These groups include community-based AIDS organizations; religious organizations, clinics, or hospitals; mental health providers or agencies; and social service workers. In this exercise, providers are assigned to a particular group, while receiving a list of attitudes and responses with which they will address the patient when he or she presents for services. Attitudes range from frustration over not being able to help the patient due to overwhelming caseloads, to fear and anxiety, to hostility, to acceptance. These exercises are especially effective in combination and should only be used during full-day sessions due to their length and the provocativeness of the material. Immediately following these two sessions, providers and patients join one another in the circle and share their individual responses to the exercises.

An inclusive 1-day training program for mental health practitioners should include the following content:

- Medical overview
  - Discussion of HIV infection
    - Transmission
    - Infection control
    - Prevention and risk reduction
  - Use of HIV-antibody test
    - Counseling seronegative and seropositive patients
  - Discussion—concept of risk behaviors versus risk groups
  - Special populations
    - Women, children, minorities, gay and bisexual men, IV drug users, hemophiliacs
- Psychosocial overview
  - Patient responses to stages of HIV infection
    - At risk, seropositive, ARC, AIDS
  - Ethnic, racial, and cultural issues
    - Practical concerns (housing, benefits, etc.)
  - Counseling issues
    - Differences and similarities with traditional practice
    - Psychopharmacology
    - Individual, couple, and family issues
  - AIDS dementia
  - Loss and bereavement
  - Death and dying
  - Confidentiality and discrimination
  - Safer sex

*The author gratefully acknowledges the contribution of James Enneis, former Chief of Psychodrama, St. Elizabeth's Hospital, Washington, DC, in developing this training format.

Issues in working with chemically dependent patients
- Psychodynamics of chemically dependent patients
- Treatment issues
- Staff issues and concerns
  - Myths and misconceptions
  - Fears and feelings
  - Life-style issues of patients—personal belief systems and values
  - Support

Legal and ethical issues
- Federal and state antidiscrimination laws
- Patients and employees' rights
- Advocacy
- Ethical dilemmas and responsibilities

Community resources
- Support services and home care
- Mental health services
- Legal services
- Spiritual counseling
- Community organizations

Panel of PWAs and HIV-affected individuals, including family members and significant others

Group discussion

Special Training Considerations

In planning and implementing AIDS training for mental health practitioners, several features deserve special attention. Although training on the medical and psychosocial aspects can be provided in a brief didactic session, it is the observation of the author and of many colleagues that training must be long enough to allow participants to process their fears and feelings, absorb new information, and understand the rationale for practicing specific interventions and procedures.

Infection Control Procedures

A clear problem area for practitioners has been a lack of consistency in maintaining appropriate infection control practices with patients. Generally speaking, infection control guidelines are required to protect both health care workers and patients from infections that either could carry and spread, e.g., hepatitis B. Infection-control practitioners have often noted that it is difficult for some health care workers to regularly follow these procedures. Failure to comply with routine infection-control guidelines predates AIDS, yet fear of AIDS has increased anxiety among providers that they could potentially become infected through routine patient contact. Even though specific infection-control guidelines to prevent HIV infection have been in effect since 1982, many workers are still uncertain about some of these practices[42] or fail to practice them routinely.[43] A study of infection-control knowledge and practice among Wisconsin dentists, for example, indicated that approximately three fourths of the more than 1500 dentists responding used gloves during patient contact either occasionally or never.[44] Frequency of needlestick injuries and mucosal exposures appear high among some groups of providers, as reported by 94 of 175 health care workers at San Francisco General Hospital and 36% of medical residents at two New York hospitals. Fear of contagion is a consistent concern among providers. More than one half of the health care workers in the New England Deaconness study, for example, agreed with the statement, "AIDS makes my job a high risk occupation."[45] In a study of AIDS-related knowledge and attitudes among rural Georgia physicians, fear of contagion was significantly correlated with negative attitudes toward AIDS patients.[46] Concern about transmission was an issue for 35% of the more than 400 social workers surveyed in 12 major teaching hospitals who were worried about the possibility of developing AIDS through direct patient contact.[47] In a Minnesota-based hospital study of more than 600 nurses, half worried about getting AIDS at least once a week, while 25% thought about it daily.[48]

Awareness of the prevalence of providers' fear and the need to include content on the use of infection-control guidelines are important factors in planning AIDS training. Many providers will assert that using gloves, in particular, is too time consuming or perhaps interferes with their ability to properly examine patients. Nevertheless, available data and anecdotal information suggest that subconscious fear is a prevailing concern for a significant number of practitioners. Appropriate use of infection-control procedures can help to bind this fear and ultimately, to provide better patient care.

Increasingly, states are mandating procedures to require health care workers to utilize infection-control procedures and to require employers to provide appropriate training and infection-control materials. Between 1983 and 1988, at least 15 states adopted legislation requiring specific education on infection-control precautions. Some states, such as Florida and Washington, are linking AIDS education to licensure.[49]

Behavioral Change Issues

For many practitioners, the direct behavioral interventions required with patients as a result of AIDS are new or perhaps significantly different than traditional, nondirective psychotherapeutic practices. Because AIDS is transmitted by high-risk sexual behaviors, mental health providers must assist patients in identifying these behaviors, grieving their loss, and replacing them with low-risk activities. These interventions and sexual behavioral strategies may be uncomfortable for some practitioners who are unused to dealing with sexual material directly or openly during therapy, or who may not themselves generally introduce this content into the sessions. Some guidelines for helping patients explore these issues have been suggested for work with both individuals and groups.[50–52] Practitioners must also learn to work with chemically dependent patients and those whose addictive behaviors can increase their risk of infection through impairing their judgment or by further challenging their immune systems. Practitioners will often need training on specific strategies and interventions to use with patients both in terms of their specific behaviors and their alcohol and drug usage.

Community Resources

Special training on the use and inclusion of community-based services can help practitioners, especially in lower incidence areas where these resources may be more difficult to find. Often, patients and their family systems can best be helped with support groups, patient empowerment groups, pastoral care, home care, respite, or legal services. In order to make this information available, providers must be aware of what programs exist and how patients can access them. Resources available through the national educational organizations listed in Appendix III can help providers locate and use these services.

Ethical Dilemmas and Legal Considerations

Perhaps some of the most immediate questions providers face in working with AIDS-affected patients are the ethical and legal challenges raised by the epidemic. These include issues of prolonging life in treating a technology-dependent condition, confidentiality, ethical responsibility to patients and to one's profession, conflict with personal biases, duty to warn a spouse or sexual partner, as well as some of the dilemmas raised in research with experimental drugs. On a very general level, many of these issues are already addressed in a health care provider's professional code of ethics. Specificity to some of the dilemmas introduced by AIDS have been broadly responded to by public policy statements issued by the American Medical Association, the American Psychological Association, the American Psychiatric Association, the American Nurses Association and the National Association of Social Workers (See Appendix II). Nevertheless, while these statements often remind providers of their ethical and professional obligations, they do not deal directly with providers' fears, emotions, and personal feelings about working with socially stigmatized groups. As a result, many providers may feel caught in a double bind, and without the necessary outlets to discuss their concerns—in outlets that would provide training, peer support and supervision.

CONCLUSION

The training and support of health care professionals dealing with the psychiatric aspects of AIDS—an area frequently overlooked by administrators and agency directors—has taken on increased urgency as the epidemic spreads. Health care professionals are in a unique position to quell panic and reduce fear among the general public. Mental health providers, in particular, can assist at-risk individuals in making the necessary behavioral changes to reduce their risk of infection. They can help HIV-infected individuals develop appropriate coping skills, as well as avoid transmission and reinfection. They can help colleagues and staff confront their feelings, fears, and negative emotions. Given the disturbing case projections made by the Public Health Service by 1991, when significantly increased numbers of sick and dying patients are anticipated, it is critical that specialized training be developed and implemented to assist health care professionals respond appropriately and compassionately to AIDS.

APPENDIXES

Appendix I: NIMH AIDS Training Programs*

First Generation of Contractors

American Psychiatric Association

Carolyn B. Robinowitz, M.D.
Principal Investigator
AIDS Education Project
1400 K. St. NW
Washington, DC 20005
(202) 682-6331

Mr. John A. Bonnage
Project Director
AIDS Education Project
1400 K St. NW
Washington, DC 20005
(202) 682-6104

Ms. Carol Svoboda
Education & Training Specialist
AIDS Education Project
1400 K St. NW
Washington, DC 20005
(202) 682-6147

Ms. Lorna Charles
Project Coordinator
AIDS Education Project
1400 K St. NW
Washington, DC 20005
(202) 682-6143

University of California, Los Angeles

Charles Lewis, M.D., Sc.D.
Principal Investigator
UCLA AIDS Educational Training for Health Care Providers
School of Medicine
Los Angeles, CA 90024
(213) 825-6709

Arlene Fink, Ph.D.
Evaluator
UCLA AIDS Educational Training for Health Care Providers
School of Medicine
Los Angeles, CA 90024
(213) 394-9791

University of California, San Francisco

Leonard S. Zegans, M.D.
Principal Investigator
AIDS Professional Education Project
Langley Porter Psychiatric Institute
Box F-0984
401 Parnassus Avenue
San Francisco, CA 94143
(415) 476-7520

Margaret Grade, Ph.D.
Project Director
AIDS Professional Education Project
36 Farnsworth Lane
San Francisco, CA 94117

Jeffrey S. Mandel, Ph.D., M.P.H.
Education Development
AIDS Professional Education Project
36 Farnsworth Lane
San Francisco, CA 94117
(415) 476-7880
(415) 775-1666

*Reprinted from *Contractors for the Training of Health Care Providers to Address Acquired Immune Deficiency Syndrome (AIDS)* (Bethesda, MD, NIMH).

George Washington University

Jeffrey S. Akman, M.D.
Project Director
AIDS Education Project
Department of Psychiatry and Behavioral Sciences
2150 Pennsylvania Avenue, N.W.
Washington, DC 20037
(202) 994-1567

Ms. Victoria L. Herzberg
Coordinator
AIDS Education Project
Department of Psychiatry and Behavioral Sciences
2150 Pennsylvania Avenue, N.W.
Washington, DC 20037
(202) 994-1567

Ellen Gerrity, Ph.D.
Project Evaluator
AIDS Education Project
c/o Center for Family Research
2300 I Street, N.W. Room 613
Washington, DC 20037
(202) 994-2624

University of Miami

Carl Eisdorfer, Ph.D., M.D.
Principal Investigator
Comprehensive AIDS Program
P.O. Box 01696 (D-90)
Miami, FL 33101
(305) 549-6327

Rick Zimmerman, Ph.D.
Training Contract Evaluator
Comprehensive AIDS Program
P.O. Box 248162
Coral Gables, FL 33124
(305) 284-6762

Mr. Richard Iacino
Training Contract Coordinator
Administrative Director
Comprehensive AIDS Program
School of Medicine
P.O. Box 016960 (D-90)
Miami, FL 33101
(305) 547-6535

Mr. Mario Rodriguez
Training Associate
Comprehensive AIDS Program
P.O. Box 016960 (D-29)
Miami, FL 33101
(305) 547-6535

New York University

Patricia M. Hurley, Ph.D., R.N.
Principal Investigator–NIMH Contract
NYU Regional AIDS Education and Training Center
50 West 4th Street
532 Leon Schimken Hall
New York, NY 10003
(212) 998-5334

Erline P. McGriff, Ed.D., R.N.
Principal Investigator–HRSA Grant
NYU Regional AIDS Education and Training Center
50 West 4th Street
532 Leon Schimken Hall
New York, NY 10003
(212) 990-5335

Arnold Grossman, Ph.D.
Assistant Director
NYU Regional AIDS Education and Training Center
429 Shimkin Hall, Washington Square
New York, NY 10003
(212) 998-5332

Barbara Hummel-Rossi, Ph.D.
Director of Evaluation
NYU Regional AIDS Education Center
429 Shimkin Hall, Washington Square
New York, NY 10003
(212) 998-5332

State University of New York at Stony Brook

Rose A. Walton, Ed.D.
Project Director
AIDS Education and Resource Center
School of Allied Health Professions
HSC L-2, Room 052
Stony Brook, NY 11794-8204
(516) 444-3241

Joseph A. Rukeyser, Ph.D.
Associate Project Director
AIDS Education and Resource Center
School of Allied Health Professions
HSC L-2, Room 075
Stony Brook, NY 11794-8204
(516) 444-2403

Ms. Kerry L. Knauf
Administrative Assistant
AIDS Education and Resource Center
School of Allied Health Professions
HSC L-2, Room 075
Stony Brook, NY 11794-8204
(516) 444-3209

Barbara Mautner, RN, CSW
AIDS Educator (part time)
AIDS Education and Resource Center
School of Allied Health Professions
HSC L-2, Room 075
Stony Brook, NY 11794-8204
(516) 444-3208

Northwestern University

Kathleen Sherdan, J.D., Ph.D.
Co-Director
AIDS Mental Health Education and Evaluation Project
Deputy Director, Comprehensive AIDS Center
Northwestern University Medical School
303 E. Superior, Passavant 528B
Chicago, IL 60611
(312) 908-7190

John P. Phair, M.D.
Director
Comprehensive AIDS Center
303 E. Chicago, Searle 3-447
Chicago, IL 60611
(312) 908-8196

Harold M. Visotsky, M.D.
Co-Director
AIDS Mental Health Education and Evaluation Project
303 E. Superior, 5 East
Chicago, IL 60611
(312) 908-8049

University of Washington

Lewayne D. Gilchrist, Ph.D.
Principal Investigator
AIDS Training Project
School of Social Work
4101 15th N.E. JH-30
Seattle, WA 98195
(206) 543-5640

Heather Andersen, RN, MN
Project Director
AIDS Training Project
820 N.E. 45th XD-20
Seattle, WA 98105
(206) 543-9750

Maura A. Kirkham, Ph.D.
Evaluator
AIDS Training Project
820 N.E. 45th XD-20
Seattle, WA 98105
(206) 543-9750

Second Generation of Contractors

Abt Associates Inc.

Mr. Vincent Scardino
Project Director
55 Wheeler Street
Cambridge, MA 02138
(617) 492-7100

Mr. Raymond Glazier, Jr.
Logistical/Training Support
55 Wheeler Street
Cambridge, MA 02138
(617) 492-7100

Ms. Anne Marie Silvia
Education Department
Director
AIDS Action Committee of Massachusetts
661 Boylston Street
Boston, MA 02116
(617) 437-6200

D. Earl Brown, Jr., M.D.
Technical Advisor
55 Wheeler Street
Cambridge, MA 02138
(617) 492-7100

Mr. Ronald Autry
Program Manager and Trainer
AIDS Action Committee of Massachusetts
661 Boylston Street
Boston, MA 02116
(617) 437-6200

Mr. Denis James
Professional Health Educator
AIDS Action Committee of Massachusetts
661 Boylston Street
Boston, MA 02116
(617) 437-6200

David Connell, Ph.D.
Director of Research and Evaluation
55 Wheeler Street
Cambridge, MA 02138
(617) 492-7100

American Psychological Association

Ms. Jean C. Kelleher
Administrative Coordinator
AIDS Community Training Project
1200 17th Street, N.W.
Washington, D.C. 20036
(202) 955-7744

James Jones, Ph.D.
Interim Executive Director
Public Interest
AIDS Community Training Project
1200 17th Street, N.W.
Washington, D.C. 20036
(202) 955-7699

Mr. Walter Batchelor
Acting Director
AIDS Community Training Project
1200 17th Street, N.W.
Washington, D.C. 20036
(202) 955-7744

John R. Anderson, Ph.D.
Assistant Director
AIDS Community Training Project
1200 17th Street, N.W.
Washington, D.C. 20036
(202) 955-7744

University of Arizona

James A. Allender, Ph.D.
Psychologist and Co-Director
AIDS Education Projects
3113 E. First Street
Tucson, AZ 85716
(602) 323-2437

Kay A. Bauman, M.D., MPH
Principal Investigator and Director
AIDS Education Projects
3113 E. First Street
Tucson, AZ 85716
(602) 323-2437

Pam Reid Duffy, Ph.D., RN
Clinical Specialist
AIDS Education Projects
3113 E. First Street
Tucson, AZ 85716
(602) 323-2437

Susan E. Moher, M.Ed.
Health Educator and Curriculum Coordinator
3113 E. First Street
Tucson, AZ 85716
(602) 323-2437

Irene K. Sassoon
Health Educator and Administrator
AIDS Education Projects
3113 E. First Street
Tucson, AZ 85716
(602) 323-2437

California State University, Long Beach

Nancy H. Corby, Ph.D.
Director
AIDS Prevention Project
City of Long Beach
Department of Public Health
635 Cedar Avenue
Long Beach, CA 90802
(213) 495-2330

Fen Rhodes, Ph.D.
Director
AIDS Education Project
1250 Bellflower Blvd.
Long Beach, CA 90840
(213) 985-7508

Ms. Katrina Billingsley
Director
Professional Education Program
AIDS Education Project
Psychology Department
1250 Bellflower Blvd.
Long Beach, CA 90840
(213) 985-7508

David Martin, Ph.D.
UCLA School of Medicine
Research and Education Institute, Inc.
AIDS Education Project
Harbor/UCLA Medicine Center
1124 W. Carson Street
Torrance, CA 90502-2064
(213) 533-3196

Cornell University

Milton Viederman, M.D.
Program Director
Payne Whitney Clinic
The New York Hospital–Cornell Medical Center
525 East 68th Street
New York, N.Y. 10021
(212) 472-6271
(212) 472-6270

Jimmie Holland, M.D.
Co-Program Director
Memorial Sloan-Kettering Cancer Center
1275 York Avenue
New York, N.Y. 10021
(212) 794-7051

Nathan Kravis, M.D.
Assistant Program Director
Payne Whitney Clinic
The New York Hospital–Cornell Medical Center
525 East 68th Street
New York, N.Y. 10021
(212) 472-8323
(212) 472-6467

Jonathan Polan, M.D.
Assistant Program Director
Payne Whitney Clinic
The New York Hospital–Cornell Medical Center
525 East 68th Street
New York, N.Y. 10021
(212) 472-6549
(212) 472-6467

Samuel Perry, M.D.
Co-Program Director
Payne Whitney Clinic
The New York Hospital–Cornell Medical Center
525 East 68th Street
New York, N.Y. 10021
(212) 472-6899

Mary Jane Massie, M.D.
MSKCC Psychiatrist Coordinator
Memorial Sloan-Kettering Cancer Center
1275 York Avenue
New York, N.Y. 10021
(212) 794-8010

University of Hawaii at Manoa

John McDermott, M.D.
Project Director
AIDS Education Project
John A. Burns School of Medicine
Department of Psychiatry
1356 Lusitana Street
Honolulu, HI 96813
(808) 548-3420

Peter Guay, Ph.D.
Assistant Professor of Psychiatry
AIDS Education Project
John A. Burns School of Medicine
Department of Psychiatry
1356 Lusitana Street
Honolulu, HI 96813
(808) 548-3420

Paul Landers, M.A.
Instructor of Psychiatry
AIDS Education Project
John A. Burns School of Medicine
Department of Psychiatry
1356 Lusitana Street
Honolulu, HI 96813
(808) 548-3420

Charles Mueller, Ph.D.
Assistant Professor of Psychiatry
AIDS Education Project
Kapiolani Medical Center for Women and Children
Department of Psychiatry
1319 Punahou Street
Honolulu, HI 96826
(808) 947-8375

Frank Gowaty, M.D.
Assistant Professor of Psychiatry
AIDS Education Project
John A. Burns School of Medicine
Department of Psychiatry
1356 Lusitana Street
Honolulu, HI 96813
(808) 548-3420

Myra Johnson, M.S.S.W.
Instructor in Psychiatry
AIDS Education Project
John A. Burns School of Medicine
Department of Psychiatry
1356 Lusitana Street
Honolulu, HI 96813
(808) 548-3420

Jane Waldron, Ph.D.
Co-Project Director
AIDS Education Project
Kapiolani Medical Center for Women and Children
Department of Psychiatry
1319 Punahou Street
Honolulu, HI 96826
(808) 947-8375

Health Education Resource Organization

Ms. Andrea Wilson
Project Director
AIDS Training for Health Professionals
101 West Read Street
Suite 812
Baltimore, MD 21201
(301) 685-1180

Ms. Jackie Yancey
Administrative Assistant
AIDS Training for Health Professionals
101 West Read Street
Suite 812
Baltimore, MD 21201
(301) 685-1180

Mr. Andrew Lentz
Training Coordinator
AIDS Training for Health Professionals
101 West Read Street
Suite 812
Baltimore, MD 21201
(301) 685-1180

JSI Research & Training Institute, Inc.

Patricia Fairchild, MA
Project Director and Vice President
210 Lincoln Street
Boston, MA 02111
(617) 482-9485

Ms. Linette Liebling, M.S.P.H.
Training Specialist
210 Lincoln Street
Boston, MA 02111
(617) 482-9485

Rima Rudd, MSPH, Sc.D.
Evaluation Specialist
Massachusetts College of Pharmacy
179 Longwood Avenue
Boston, MA 02115
(617) 732-2901
(617) 482-9485

Stephen Wroblewski, M.Div. LSW
Project Coordinator
210 Lincoln Street
Boston, MA 02111
(617) 482-9485

Lori Kiel, A.B.
Administrative Assistant
210 Lincoln Street
Boston, MA 02111
(617) 482-9485

University of Louisville

Roger A. Bell, Ed.D.
Project Director
AIDS Health Education Program
Medical-Dental Research
Room 512
Department of Psychiatry
School of Medicine
Louisville, KY 40292
(502) 588-5393

Robert L. Frierson, M.D.
Assistant Director
AIDS Health Education Program
Ambulatory Care Building
Department of Psychiatry
Louisville, KY 40292
(502) 588-5867

Ms. Jean Kuntz
Program Assistant
AIDS Health Education Program
Medical-Dental Research Building
Room 513
Department of Psychiatry
School of Medicine
Louisville, KY 40292
(502) 588-5393

Theodore B. Feldmann, M.D.
Co-Director
AIDS Health Education Program
Medical-Dental Research
Room 516
Department of Psychiatry
School of Medicine
Louisville, KY 40292
(502) 588-5393

Judi Phillips, M.Ed.
Project Coordinator
AIDS Health Education Program

Medicine-Dental Research Building
Room 529
Department of Psychiatry
School of Medicine
University of Louisville
Louisville, KY 40222
(502) 429-6517

Michigan State University

Terry S. Stein, M.D.
Principal Investigator
AIDS Education Project
A-233 East Fee Hall
East Lansing, MI 48824
(517) 353-9245

Mary McCormack, Ph.D. (Cand.)
Education and Resource Program Director
AIDS Education Project
B-321 West Fee Hall
East Lansing, MI 48824
(517) 355-9324

Lynda J. Farquhar, Ph.D.
Student Education Coordinator
College of Human Medicine
A-101 East Fee Hall
East Lansing, MI 48824
(517) 353 8856

Rebecca Henry, Ph.D.
Evaluation Coordinator
OMERAD
A-202 East Fee Hall
East Lansing, MI 48824
(517) 353-2037

Wanda Lipscomb, Ph.D.
Project Manager
AIDS Education Project
A-236 East Fee Hall
East Lansing, MI 48824
Research Associate
B-320 West Fee Hall
(517) 483-2750

Mr. Eric Zook
Research Associate
AIDS Education Project
B-320 West Fee Hall
East Lansing, MI 48824
(517) 337-2307
(517) 355-9324

Reynard Bouknight, M.D., Ph.D.
Co-Principal Investigator
AIDS Education Project
College of Human Medicine
B-338 Clinical Center
East Lansing, MI 48824
(517) 355-9633

Robert Richard, Ph.D.
Continuing Education Coordinator
GRAMEC
220 Cherry, S.E.
Grand Rapids, MI 49503
(616) 459-2872

David Solomon, Ph.D.
Evaluation Coordinator
OMERAD
A-206 East Fee Hall
East Lansing, MI 48824
(517) 353-8856

Mr. John Curtis
Research Associate
AIDS Education Project
B-320 West Fee Hall
East Lansing, MI 48824
(517) 351-7503
(517) 355-9324

Ms. Ruth Greenbaum
Research Associate
AIDS Education Project
B-320 West Fee Hall
East Lansing, MI 48824
(517) 483-2750
(517) 332-2263

University of Rochester

Judith Landau-Stanton, MB, ChB, DPM
Principal Investigator–Project Director
AIDS Training Project
Department of Psychiatry
300 Crittenden Boulevard
Rochester, NY 14642
(716) 275-5693
(716) 275-2718

Colleen Clements, Ph.D.
Co-Investigator–Ethicist
AIDS Training Project
Department of Psychiatry
300 Crittenden Boulevard
Rochester, NY 14642
(716) 275-5693
(716) 275-2718

Gloria Horsley, RN, MS, CS
Co-Investigator–Project Coordinator
AIDS Training Project
Department of Psychiatry
300 Crittenden Boulevard
Rochester, NY 14642
(716) 275-5693
(716) 275-2718

William Valenti, M.D.
Co-Investigator–Medical/Infectious Disease Advisor
AIDS Training Project
Department of Psychiatry
300 Crittenden Boulevard
Rochester, NY 14642
(716) 275-5693
(716) 275-2718

Ann Zettelmaier, M.D.
Co-Investigator–Psychiatric/Neuropsychiatric Advisor
AIDS Training Project
Department of Psychiatry
300 Crittenden Boulevard
Rochester, NY 14642
(716) 275-5693
(716) 275-2718

Robert Cole, Ph.D.
Co-Investigator–Coordinator of Research and Evaluation
AIDS Training Project
Department of Psychiatry
300 Crittenden Boulevard
Rochester, NY 14642
(716) 275-5693
(716) 275-2718

M. Duncan Stanton, Ph.D.
Co-Investigator–Research and Internal Systems Advisor
AIDS Training Project
Department of Psychiatry
300 Crittenden Boulevard
Rochester, NY 14642
(716) 275-5693
(716) 275-2718

Wayne State University

Fredericka P. Shea, Ph.D., RN
Principal Investigator
AIDS Training Program for Health Care Providers
College of Nursing
Wayne State University
5557 Cass Avenue
Detroit, MI 48202
(313) 577-4134

Joel W. Ager, Ph.D.
Program Evaluator
AIDS Training Program for Health Care Providers
Department of Psychology
71 W. Warren
Detroit, MI 48202
(313) 577-2826
(313) 577-4134

Ali M. Naqvi, Ph.D.
Project Director
AIDS, Research, Training and Education Program

AIDS Training Program for Health Care
Providers
Department of Psychology
71 W. Warren
Detroit, MI 48202
(313) 577-5549
(313) 577-4134

Appendix II: AIDS Activities and Policy Statements of National Professional Associations

American Psychiatric Association

AIDS Education Project

The AIDS Education Project began in the fall of 1986 after the APA was awarded a contract from the National Institute of Mental Health (NIMH) to provide training and education to health care professionals on the spectrum of neuropsychiatric and biopsychosocial conditions and psychological consequences of AIDS and HIV infection. The work of the Project is guided by a 12 member Steering Committee on AIDS, chaired by Dr. Stuart Nichols. The Education Project has trained nearly three thousand health care professionals to date, including psychiatrists, psychologists, social workers, nonpsychiatric physicians, medical residents, nurses, occupational therapists, and community volunteers. It currently offers programs on immunology, virology, epidemiology, prevention, coping, antibody testing, public policy, ethics, the neuropsychiatric aspects of AIDS, psychopharmacology and management, psychoimmunology, psychotherapy, and counseling. To best address the needs and interests of various health care professionals, the Project staff conducts a training survey to assess individual learning needs. The results of the survey guide the content and structure of its educational activities and programs. Each program is also evaluated on its usefulness and quality; the results of these evaluations are then used in planning future educational programs.

In addition to these efforts, APA has identified a large cadre of nationally recognized experts on AIDS, and developed a myriad of educational materials including, but not limited to, an *AIDS Primer*, containing information on the medical and neuropsychiatric aspects of AIDS and HIV infection; Case Management Units, offering a series of clinical vignettes focusing on the needs of patients; Training Modules, addressing 10 different topics related to HIV infection, including transmission, virology, medical diagnosis, and treatment; a Fact Sheet on AIDS providing a general overview on AIDS and answers to some of the more frequently asked questions (English and Spanish translations are available); an instructional videotape containing brief vignettes each of which highlights a specific affective as well as cognitive AIDS-related issue and serves to stimulate interactive group discussion; and a computerized self-help test on the psychiatric aspects of AIDS which includes questions on epidemiology, neuropsychiatry, psychopharmacology, clinical assessment, antibody testing, drug therapies, and psychosocial issues.

Many of the people involved in the Project serve as consultants for planning other AIDS training projects. The staff also keeps information on file of psychiatrists who have expertise in a specific AIDS-related field and are available to serve as speakers on various topics. Having this information allows our staff to make appropriate referrals and/or answer requests for information. The Project also serves as a contact point for APA District Branch AIDS activities.

Commission on AIDS

In addition to its educational activities, the APA is also actively involved in the development of AIDS policies and guidelines. Through the work of the Ad Hoc Committee on AIDS Policy (serving a one year term), the APA has released its guidelines on confidentiality and disclosure, inpatient and outpatient services, psychiatrists who are HIV infected, and two policy statements on AIDS and HIV infection (see attached). These documents were issued to provide some guidance to members of the profession as they struggle to honor their duty to preserve the confidences of their patients while taking adequate precautions to protect others who may be at risk of contracting the disease.

In December 1988, a 15-member Commission on AIDS was established replacing the Ad Hoc Committee on AIDS as well as the Committee on the Psychiatric Aspects of AIDS. This Commission includes representation from individuals with expertise in AIDS research, education, drug abuse, clinical care, and the policy aspects of HIV infection. The Commission's charge includes advising the Assembly and the Board of Trustees about AIDS priorities; planning and implementing a comprehensive program on AIDS; promoting collaboration with other medical specialists to ensure adequate attention to the neuropsychiatric and psychosocial aspects of HIV infection; expanding current APA AIDS professional and public education activities at all levels; and ensuring appropriate psychiatric consultation in the development of policies related to economics, law, and governmental action.

The Commission is currently developing (1) a 'white paper' concerning the role of psychiatrists in HIV issues for publication in APA journals; (2) a model document for general physicians on counseling HIV-infected persons and those at risk; and (3) an assessment instrument for determining the degree of cognitive impairment of HIV infected persons.

For more information about the APA AIDS Education Project or the Commission on AIDS, contact Carol Svoboda, Project Director, at (202) 682-6104.

*American Psychiatric Association Position Statement on Human Immunodeficiency Virus (HIV) Related Discrimination**

The American Psychiatric Association (APA) recognizes that individuals may develop and maintain anxiety and/or unjustified fears such as have occurred in reaction to HIV-related issues.

These fears should not be the basis of discriminatory actions nor prevent access to medical care, housing, public transportation, employment, education, and life, medical or disability insurance.

Specifically, the APA considers it a priority to educate its members, other health care professionals, and the general public to reduce these reactions to HIV conditions.

The APA shall respond to instances in which such reactions to HIV conditions lead to discriminatory practices or become the basis of unjustified public policy.

American Psychiatric Association Position Statement on AIDS†

Introduction

The Human Immunodeficiency Virus (HIV) is thought to cause the Acquired Immune Deficiency Syndrome (AIDS), AIDS Related Complex (ARC) and probably other disease states. In the following statement the term HIV disease is used to refer to the entire range of clinical conditions in adults and children which may be produced by this virus.

Position Statement

1. Psychiatrists should work actively and effectively to counteract inappropriate reactions to HIV disease in their communications and professional activities.
2. Psychiatrists have a responsibility to educate themselves, their patients and their communities with regard to the neuropsychiatric and psychosocial aspects of HIV disease including its biological and psychiatric clinical manifestations, the psychosocial reactions to the illness and the appropriate treatment modalities available to patients. To this end, psychia-

*Adopted December 1986.
†Adopted December 1986.

trists should integrate their efforts with those of other medical disciplines and work conjointly with them.

3. Psychiatrists and other physicians have an obligation to become educated about the legal and ethical aspects of HIV disease and to help patients make informed and rational decisions, for example, in the areas of confidentiality, privacy, informed consent, living wills, and durable powers of attorney.
4. Educational activities should be undertaken to prevent the spread of HIV disease.
5. Activities which attempt to reduce risk-associated practices should be based upon knowledge and understanding of the complex and sensitive nature of this effort.
6. It actively supports efforts to eliminate medical, psychiatric, social, economic, occupational, legal, educational, and other forms of discrimination which is based on the fear of HIV disease.
7. The confidentiality of persons undergoing HIV serologic testing for clinical or research purposes should be protected, and all information obtained including identifying data and test results should be used only for the purposes explicitly stated in the informed consents and releases of information. When testing is performed for clinical or research purposes, attention to the psychiatric implications must be considered pre- and post-testing and the possible adverse consequences of serologic testing be explicitly stated in the informed consent.
8. Knowledge of serologic test results may have beneficial or adverse psychiatric effects. Currently, there is insufficient information to support the assumption that knowledge of one's serologic status necessarily leads to risk-reduction behavior change. Research is needed to clearly identify the psychiatric ramifications of serologic HIV testing and to define appropriate criteria for its use.
9. There is urgent need for research on the psychiatric presentations and complications of HIV infection.

*American Psychiatric Association AIDS Policy: Interim Guidelines for Outpatient Psychiatric Services**

I. Patient Care

In the medical setting, all available evidence indicates that AIDS is a disease of low transmissibility. Education and counseling regarding HIV transmission continue to be needed and should be available to physicians and other medical personnel. Historically, medical personnel have been exemplary in the treatment of patients, even in situations of personal risk. It is expected that this tradition will continue.

1. All psychiatric patients shall be treated based on their clinical condition; neither HIV infection, serologic status, nor suspicion that the patient is at risk of HIV infection shall, in and of itself, impede the delivery of appropriate medical-psychiatric treatment.
2. In therapeutic relationships the psychiatrist should work with patients to reduce risk behavior regardless of serologic status.
3. HIV serological testing should be performed on a case-by-case basis with informed consent when medically indicated. HIV serological testing should not be performed solely for the purpose of routine screening or staff awareness.
4. If a patient known to be HIV infected engages, or threatens to engage, in behavior which is known to transmit HIV disease, the psychiatrist shall assure that, in addition to education, appropriate clinical steps are taken to attempt to modify the behavior.
5. Regardless of HIV serologic status, all outpatients should be considered potentially at risk

*September 10, 1988.

for transmitting or receiving HIV infection. A minimal standard of care for outpatient clinics should include:

a. implementation and monitoring of infection control procedures as outlined by current CDC standards; and
b. appropriate management of affective, cognitive and behavioral disturbances to ensure risk reduction for both patients and personnel.

6. AIDS education should play an important role in the treatment of all psychiatric patients. Appropriate education and supportive services for patients, family and staff should be available. Appropriate services might include:
   a. printed educational materials readily available for patients and staff;
   b. education regarding behaviors which place an individual at risk for HIV infection; and alternative behaviors;
   c. evaluation of a patient's behavior for assessment of risk to self or others; and
   d. discussions of, indications for and consequences of testing for HIV where appropriate.
7. Individuals who undergo HIV testing shall receive:
   a. appropriate support services before and after testing to interpret test findings and deal with consequences of test findings, including the possibility of test errors; and
   b. appropriate support services to deal with concerns about or consequences of HIV infection.
8. All mental health facilities need to provide appropriate support and education services to enable staff to carry out CDC infection control guidelines.

II. Disclosure

In a situation where a particular patient is known to be HIV infected, deciding whether to disclose a patient's HIV infection to other staff is a delicate clinical question. The responsible physician should disclose the information to appropriate staff only after discussions with the patient, when the physician determines that appropriate treatment of the patient requires such disclosure.

*American Psychiatric Association AIDS Policy: Confidentiality and Disclosure**

Introduction

The AIDS epidemic presents difficult and perplexing issues, many of which involve conflicts between the rights of infected individuals and the society's interest in containing the epidemic. Because these questions are highly controversial, and because so many important scientific questions about the disease remain unanswered, a definitive public health strategy has not yet emerged.

Physicians have an important role to play in controlling HIV infection. However, for physicians, the care and treatment of individual patients is of the utmost importance. Patients must be confident that issues discussed with their physicians are private and will not be unnecessarily divulged. Certainly any breach of confidentiality should be a last resort, only after scrupulous attention has been given to all other alternatives.

At the present time, the operational public health strategy promotes voluntary testing while eschewing programs of contact tracing, surveillance, segregation, and other measures that could discourage people from seeking testing. Many troublesome ethical and clinical questions arise in the context of dealing with individual patients, and the purpose of this document is to provide some guidance to members of the profession as they struggle to honor their duty to preserve the confidences of their patients while taking adequate precautions to protect other persons who may be at risk of contracting the disease.

Physicians should be aware that state laws may restrict some of the actions recommended in these guidelines. Where conflict exists, attempts should be made to modify laws in accordance with the principles expressed herein.

*December 1987.

Confidentiality

Physicians have an ethical obligation to recognize the rights to privacy, to confidentiality, and to informed consent of all patients. During the initial clinical evaluation, the physician should usually make clear the general limits of confidentiality. If the physician has reason to suspect the patient is infected with HIV (e.g., seropositive) or is engaging in behavior that is known to transmit HIV disease, the physician should notify the patient of the specific limits of confidentiality. Further, if the physician intends to inquire specifically about a patient's HIV status, the physician should, in such instances, notify the patient about the limits of confidentiality in advance of asking such questions.

II. Notification of Third Parties

In situations where a physician has received convincing clinical information (based on the patient's own disclosure of test results or on documented test records) that the patient is infected with HIV, the physician should advise and work with the patient either to obtain agreement to terminate behavior that places other persons at risk of infection or to notify identifiable individuals who may be at continuing risk of exposure. If a patient refuses to agree to change behavior or to notify the person(s) at risk, or the physician has good reason to believe that the patient has failed to or is unable to comply with this agreement, it is ethically permissible for the physician to notify an identifiable person whom the physician believes to be in danger of contracting the virus.

III. Disclosure to Third Parties

Most states now require physicians to report cases in which they diagnose AIDS to a public health agency, while only a few require the reporting of cases in which individuals test positive for HIV. It is ethically permissible for a physician to report to the appropriate public health agency the names of patients who are determined by convincing clinical information (based on the patient's disclosures of test results or documented test records) to be HIV infected and whom the physician has good reason to believe are engaging in behavior which places other persons at risk of HIV infection. Although we recognize that public health agencies have varying responses to the problem at the present time, provision of this information will allow them to take whatever measures they regard as appropriate.

*American Psychiatric Association AIDS Policy: Guidelines for Inpatient Psychiatric Units**

I. Patient Care

In the medical setting, all available evidence indicates that AIDS is a disease of low transmissibility. Education and counseling regarding HIV transmission continue to be needed and should be available to physicians and other medical personnel. Historically, physicians and other medical personnel have been exemplary in the treatment of patients, even in situations of personal risk, and it is expected that this tradition will continue.

1. All psychiatric patients shall be treated based on their clinical condition; neither HIV infection nor serologic status shall, in and of itself, impede the delivery of appropriate medical-psychiatric treatment.
2. HIV serological testing should be performed on a case-by-case basis with informed consent when medically indicated. HIV serological testing should not be performed solely for the purpose of routine screening or staff awareness.
3. Regardless of HIV serologic status, all inpatients should be considered potentially at risk for transmitting or receiving HIV infection. A minimal standard of care should include:
   a. Implementation and monitoring of infection control procedures as outlined by current CDC standards;

*September 10, 1988.

b. Appropriate management of affective, cognitive and behavioral disturbances to ensure risk reduction for both patients and personnel;
c. Appropriate education and supportive services for patients, families and staff.

4. If a patient known to be HIV infected engages, or threatens to engage, in behavior that places other individuals at risk, the responsible physician shall assure that appropriate clinical steps are taken to control the behavior, and, if necessary, isolate and/or restrain the patient.

II. Disclosure

Once a patient has been hospitalized on a psychiatric unit and responsibility for the patient's care has been assumed, a need to protect other patients and staff from foreseeable dangerous behavior arises. In the situation where a particular patient is known to be HIV positive, the following additional guidelines are recommended:

1. Deciding whether to disclose a patient's HIV infection to other staff is a delicate clinical question. The responsible physician should disclose the information to appropriate staff only after discussions with the patient, when the physician determines that appropriate treatment of the patient requires such disclosure.
2. If the patient engages in behavior likely to transmit the virus and there is a significant risk that such behavior cannot be controlled by other measures, then disclosure of a patient's infectious condition to other patients at risk is permissible. Disclosure is not a substitute for adequate clinical care, and it is usually inappropriate for the physician or staff to disclose a patient's HIV infection to other patients.

III. Discharge

At the time when discharge is otherwise clinically appropriate, and the patient represents a substantial risk of danger to others by virtue of behavior known to transmit the virus, and this danger is not related to a specific mental condition, it is inappropriate to retain the person in the hospital solely for the purposes of quarantine or preventive detention.

American Psychiatric Association AIDS Policy: Interim Guidelines for Psychiatrists Who Are HIV Infected

I. Introduction

HIV infected individuals must be treated with compassion and with due respect to rights, privacy and confidentiality. However, because of the physician's professional obligation to do no harm, guidelines are needed in the event that psychiatrists are unable to perform professional duties due to HIV disease. Psychiatrists, like all physicians, should be aware of and comply with the U.S. Centers for Disease Control (CDC) Guidelines for Preventing Transmission of Infection with HIV when dealing with body fluids. Clinical evidence indicates that HIV infection is not a disease spread by casual contact. The clearly defined modes of transmission are: direct exposure to HIV infected blood or direct exposure to HIV infected semen.

Physicians should be aware of state laws restricting some of the actions recommended in these guidelines. Where conflict exists, attempts should be made to modify laws in accordance with the principles expressed herein.

II. Clinical Competency

Recognition of impairment of clinical competency from any illness should be the responsibility of the individual treating the physician, as well as supervisors, peers and family. Restriction of clinical privileges on the basis of HIV infection alone is clearly unwarranted. When observation of the psychiatrist's behavior indicates that impaired clinical competence, the APA Guidelines for Intervention with Impaired Physicians should be followed and appropriate authorities notified.

III. Confidentiality

Public health reporting of HIV infection should be no different for psychiatrists than for other infected individuals. All reporting requirement should maintain an individual's rights to privacy and confidentiality insofar as possible. APA's Guidelines relating to confidentiality and disclosure of individuals who are HIV infected should also apply to psychiatrists.

IV. Discrimination

There is no indication for mandatory HIV testing for physicians. Discrimination solely on the basis of HIV status in licensing, hospital privileges, or admission to medical training programs is inappropriate.

National Association of Social Workers

Acquired Immune Deficiency Syndrome: A Social Work Response*

Background

Acquired immune deficiency syndrome (AIDS) is a complicated disorder that impairs the human body's immune system and renders it vulnerable to rare and most often fatal diseases such as Kaposi's sarcoma, pneumocystis carinii, and other opportunistic infections. Since the National Centers for Disease Control began its enumeration of diagnosed cases in 1981, there have been more than 44,000 persons in the United States diagnosed as having AIDS.

It is predicted that by 1991, 270,000 Americans will have been diagnosed as having AIDS, and more than 179,000 Americans will have died from AIDS. By 1991, AIDS is expected to become the 10th leading cause of death in the United States.

To date, the only known modes of transmission for human immunodeficiency virus (HIV) infection, which can develop into AIDS, are the exchange of blood, semen, and vaginal secretions through anal, vaginal, and possibly oral sex; the use of contaminated needles and syringes; contact with contaminated blood or blood products; intrauterine exposure before, during, or shortly after childbirth; and possibly an infected mother's milk.

The psychological and social repercussions of AIDS, AIDS-related complex (ARC), and HIV infection are similar to those of other life-threatening, catastrophic illnesses. Social isolation, discrimination, anxiety, depression, concern about body image, finances, loss of control, and a confrontation with one's own mortality are among the critical issues challenging people with AIDS and HIV infection. In addition, many of these individuals, persons assumed to be infected, and those closely associated with them have met extreme rejection and have experienced isolation resulting from the public's panic over the contagion of AIDS. People with AIDS, ARC, and HIV infection, and those who only have sought diagnostic screening for the disease have been terminated from employment, discharged from military service, evicted from their homes, denied health and social services, and have been targets of harassment and violence. When an irrational fear of AIDS is compounded by homophobia, people with AIDS, ARC, and HIV infection, or persons assumed to be infected, may find themselves rejected by families, friends, and co-workers. Both children and adults infected with HIV or diagnosed as having AIDS have been denied access to foster care placement, residential placement, long-term care facilities, and hospices. Thus, they are bereft of essential social and emotional supports.

*Policy statement approved by the NASW Delegate Assembly, November, 1987. For further information contact the National Association of Social Workers, Inc., 7981 Eastern Avenue, Silver Spring, Maryland 10910; telephone: (301) 565-0333.

Statement of Issues

AIDS, ARC, and HIV infection represent an international public health crisis that affects all people and must be addressed by social workers at all organizational levels. AIDS has been found in all segments of the population, including heterosexual men and women and children. HIV-infected persons are disproportionately members of minority communities. HIV testing should be voluntary and not mandatory; testing should be anonymous and with strict confidentiality when required for medical reasons. Informed consent should be required. Social workers should protect the civil and human rights of people taking antibody tests. Because of the emotional stress associated with the testing process, pre- and postcounseling is a necessary component of all testing programs. Whenever possible, skilled professional social workers should conduct pre- and posttest counseling.

The social work profession must take an active political role in seeking solutions to the complex problems that AIDS, ARC, and HIV infection present to individuals and to our society. Social workers are mandated by the National Association of Social Workers *Code of Ethics* to respond to the social impact of AIDS and have demonstrated strong leadership since the beginning of the epidemic.

Because of the complex biopsychosocial issues presented by AIDS, ARC, and HIV infection, social workers, with their special knowledge, skills, and sensitivity, can make a unique contribution to the management of this crisis by pursuing action in eight areas:

1. *Research.* Basic research, including epidemiological, clinical, and psychosocial studies, is imperative. Social workers, particularly in the area of psychosocial research, have a special contribution to make. They have been at the forefront of issues relating to AIDS and have demonstrated significant leadership in identifying critical issues and needs and have a responsibility to continue in these research efforts.

2. *Public Education and Dissemination of Information.* Accurate information about AIDS; HIV infection control measures; prevention; treatment; and medical, financial, and psychosocial resources available should be widely distributed. The fears of caregivers and the general public must be addressed with appropriate education and interventions. Adequate public funds must be authorized for educational efforts among the general public to reduce the fear of AIDS, ARC, and HIV infection and the stigmatization of persons assumed to be at risk for infection. Adequately funded public education programs should encourage prevention, early treatment, and formulation of new behaviors to reduce the risks of HIV infection. Professional health care organizations, training programs, and continuing education programs should incorporate the latest information and address especially the needs of minority groups, adolescents, women, infants and children, the developmentally and physically disabled, and the chronically mentally ill. Education and training programs must accommodate differences in culture and ethnicity among people. Program materials must be clear and explicit and targeted to individuals of all sexual orientations. Social workers should work cooperatively with existing AIDS-related educational, treatment, and research organizations. Especially important, social workers should be educated and updated on all AIDS-related issues, including prevention strategies, and should play major roles in reducing public hysteria and prejudice.

3. *Psychological and Social Support.* Comprehensive psychological and social support is necessary to help persons with AIDS, ARC, and HIV infection and all individuals close to them. Extended families, including domestic partners and significant others, represent rich resources of emotional and social support, just as they represent a network of persons likely to be affected by the disease-related changes, including death, of persons with AIDS and HIV infections. All care providers should respect the individuality of people with AIDS, ARC, and HIV infection and the importance of the individual's relationships with family, domestic partners, and close friends.

The diversity of interpersonal relationships and support systems should be recognized, nurtured, and strengthened. Supplemental services, including support groups, counseling, and therapy, should be made available to people with AIDS and AIDS-related conditions and their loved ones as well as to others who feel vulnerable. In addition, all providers of care should have access to support groups and related services to alleviate the stress inherent in assisting persons with AIDS-related conditions. All AIDS-related service organizations should provide for support, supervision, respite, and recognition of social workers engaged in the emotionally demanding work of serving people with AIDS.

4. *Service Delivery and Resource Development.* A comprehensive service delivery system to respond to AIDS based on a case management model must include suitable housing, adult-child foster care, home health and hospice care, appropriate, affordable health care, access to legal services, and transportation services. Children needing foster care should be provided care at the least restrictive level in nonsegregated settings. Traditional health and social welfare agencies including income maintenance programs must become responsive; eligibility requirements and coverage by health insurance and income maintenance should be adapted to meet the rapid onset and catastrophic effects of AIDS. The health status of people with AIDS-related disorders may vary daily. Currently, service delivery systems do not take health care needs and work requirements into consideration. Systems should be more flexible in providing services for individuals with AIDS-related disorders.

Adequate funding both from public and private sources should be provided to assist alternative health and social services that deal with AIDS and AIDS-related conditions in various communities. Such services, many of which are complementary to and cooperative with mainstream services, help broaden and strengthen the range of traditional supports available to persons with AIDS and AIDS-related conditions. Social workers should be encouraged to be involved in the initiation of—and serve as membership on—local, statewide, regional, and national AIDS task forces.

5. *Civil Rights.* No person should be deprived of civil rights or rights to confidentiality because he or she has been diagnosed as having contracted AIDS, is infected with HIV, or is assumed to be at risk for infection. Nondiscrimination laws should be extended and existing legal protection should be vigorously enforced to protect individuals with AIDS, ARC, and HIV infections from being presumptively deprived of health care, employment, housing, and immigration rights.

6. *HIV Testing.* Social workers should be concerned particularly with the violation of human rights and the psychosocial consequences to people taking HIV antibody tests. Given the potential for serious discrimination, all testing should be voluntary, anonymous, and conducted with informed consent. Social workers should make certain that the limits of the predictive value of such testing are known in advance by clients. Appropriate pre- and post-test counseling must be offered by social workers or other skilled professionals. Social workers are mandated to protect client confidentiality.

7. *Professional Accountability.* The helping professions and appropriate licensing authorities should use their full range of persuasive and regulatory powers to ensure that people with AIDS, ARC, and HIV infection and their significant others are not discriminated against in their eligibility for or receipt of services because of their illness or lack of financial or social resources.

8. *Political Action.* Social workers, individually and organizationally, should participate with other groups to lobby actively at local, state, and federal levels on behalf of people with AIDS in order to improve their quality of life; protect their civil liberties; and to advocate for increased funding for appropriate education, prevention, interventions, treatment, services, and research.

The National Association of Social Workers (NASW), as the organizational arm of the profession, must help coordinate a response to AIDS, ARC, and HIV infection by pursuing the multifaceted strategy outlined in this policy statement.

*AIDS and the Schools: A Position Statement from the NASW Commission on Education**

Acquired immune deficiency syndrome (AIDS) is a growing threat to the public health in America. As of August 10, 1987, the Centers for Disease Control reported 40,051 cases of AIDS of whom 715 (1.8%) were under age 20. The total number of reported deaths is 23,165. AIDS is currently the third leading cause of death among women ages 15 to 19 in New York City. It is estimated that 1 to 1.5 million Americans are currently infected with the virus that causes AIDS - the Human Immunodeficiency Virus (HIV). By 1991, the Public Health Service has projected that the cumulative number of cases in the U.S. will total over 270,000 while the total number of deaths from AIDS will have reached over 179,000. Three thousand of the projected cases of AIDS are estimated to be among children.

AIDS is an infectious disease that is ultimately fatal in its end stage when individuals become susceptible to a broad range of unusual malignancies and rare infections. The virus that causes AIDS (HIV) is transmitted in three ways: through sexual intercourse (anal or vaginal); by the exchange of blood through sharing needles or drug paraphenalia; or by the exchange of contaminated blood or blood products, including transmission from mother to developing fetus. AIDS is *not* transmitted by casual contact. Adolescents are at particular risk of becoming infected with HIV and potentially developing AIDS through sexual activity and experimentation with alcohol and drugs which can affect judgement and behavior.

Statistics indicate that over 70% of teenagers have had sexual intercourse by the age of twenty, many with more than one partner. Nearly one half—5 to 10 million—of all sexually transmitted disease patients are under 25 years. The National Institute of Drug Abuse found in a 1986 study that 1.1% of U.S. high school seniors reported that they had used heroin. Runaways and teenage prostitutes are at particular risk, as are minorities of color. Nationally, 40% of all cases and 80% of pediatric cases are black and Hispanic. Since developing a cure or an effective vaccine is still years away, education about risk reduction is our primary prevention strategy currently available.

AIDS Education in the Schools

The National Association of Social Workers' Commission on Education expresses its strong support for Surgeon General Dr. C. Everett Koop's policy recommendation that schools must play a major role in educating children and adolescents about the disease, its transmission and its prevention.

In the Surgeon General's report on AIDS published late in 1986, the Public Health Service called for information and education to change behavior as these are "the primary ways to stop the epidemic of AIDS" (p. 4). Citing adolescents and preadolescents as those whose behavior we wish especially to influence because of their vulnerability when they explore their own sexuality (heterosexual and homosexual) and perhaps experiment with drugs, the Surgeon General asserts that education about AIDS should start in early elementary school and at home. This affords parents the opportunity to discuss with their children their own moral and ethical standards, according to Dr. Koop.

NASW's Commission on Education offers the following guidelines for AIDS curriculum, instruction and counseling in schools:

1. In developing curricula and teaching materials, schools should provide for collaboration with parents, students and community groups.
2. AIDS curricula must be taught in the context of broader courses on sex education and family life education which stress that sex is one component of human relationships and that it has both positive aspects and risks.

*August 1987.

3. AIDS education should begin in the 3rd grade and must be appropriate to the child's age and developmental stage.
4. From the 6th grade onwards, information must be explicit, including the transmission of the virus through homosexual and heterosexual sex and intravenous drug abuse, and practicing safe preventive sex through the use of condoms. Girls and boys must understand that intercourse can cause pregnancy or infection with a sexually transmitted disease, including AIDS. Sex with intravenous drug users and prostitutes can also cause infection with HIV and other sexually transmitted diseases.
5. The acquisition of sexual knowledge and understanding is a gradual and cumulative process. Many young adolescents do not know what their adult sexual preference will be or do not think that they could become addicted to drugs, particularly intravenous drugs. AIDS curricula should therefore continue throughout the secondary school years as the stage of behavioral exploration heightens and young people are confronted daily with decision-making options.
6. Special provision must be made to inform non-English-speaking students, students with low levels of literacy and students with handicapping conditions.
7. Dropout prevention and reentry programs should provide AIDS education and information.
8. Parent education and training should be provided to enable parents to discuss with their children accurate factual information within the context of their own family values.
9. Because the goal is to affect or change behavior, instruction alone is not sufficient. Counseling students and parents about feelings, behavior and making decisions should be available to supplement factual information.
10. School social workers should be available to provide counseling and referral for more intensive mental health and social services to students and their families. AIDS has serious mental health implications. Young people faced with the knowledge that they have tested positive for HIV or have developed AIDS-related conditions face anxiety and depression from lack of accurate information, fear of social isolation, sickness, suffering and death. The peers and classmates of students with AIDS, their parents and school staff will feel anxiety and grief as the disease progresses. As the number of diagnosed adults increases, more children in school will be affected by AIDS in their families.
11. Staff training and case consultation when appropriate must be provided to teachers, administrators and pupil services personnel.
12. Schools should provide information on local and national resources such as AIDS information centers, hotlines, clinics, and other services.
13. Curricula should be modified over time as new information becomes available.

AIDS Policies in the Schools

NASW's Commission on Education supports the Surgeon General's recommendations regarding cases of children with AIDS in the schools. "No blanket rules can be made for all school boards to cover all possible cases of children with AIDS" he states.

None of the identified cases of AIDS in the United States are known, or are suspected to have been, transmitted from one child to another in school, day care or foster care settings. The Centers for Disease Control guidelines for workplace and school settings state that AIDS is not transmitted by casual contact. Routine safety procedures for handling blood or other body fluids, which should be standard for all children in schools, would be effective in preventing transmission of the virus from children with AIDS to other children in school. Moreover, a study of HIV-infected children with hemophilia attending school with non-HIV-infected children who participated in the same activities and interacted daily, determined that *none* of the non-infected children became infected with HIV.

NASW's Commission on Education therefore reinforces the guidelines developed both by the Surgeon General and the National Education Association which emphasize that each case should be considered separately and individualized to the child and the setting, as would be the procedure for any child with a handicapping condition. The Commission asserts that the child's emotional, social and family situation should also be considered in the decision-making process, after a home visit and assessment by the school social worker and involvement of the parents (NASW's policy guidelines are available to provide further details).

In planning to implement the Early Intervention Program for handicapped infants legislated by the Education of the Handicapped Act Amendment of 1986, State Education Agencies and collaborating agencies should provide for the needs of infants and toddlers with the AIDS virus. As of August 10, 1987 children under 5 formed 68% of all reported cases under twenty years of age. It is estimated that approximately 60% of the babies born to HIV-infected mothers will in time develop the disease and die. Pregnant women most at risk are intravenous drug users or the sexual partners of HIV-infected drug users, or the sexual partners of other men who are infected with the virus. The number of HIV-infected babies is also expected to increase.

In Summary

The NASW Commission on Education

1. Supports the Surgeon General's recommendations on full, accurate factual AIDS education within the schools.
2. Urges school social workers to seek continuing education on all aspects of AIDS including community resources and referral.
3. Recommends that school social workers
   - support and contribute to the development of AIDS curricula for students, parents and teachers in regular and special education
   - provide information and counseling for students on AIDS issues and referral to appropriate community resources
   - collaborate with school administrators and special education directors in planning services to students infected with the AIDS virus and to the schools these students attend
   - provide case management as needed to facilitate and ensure comprehensive services for students and their families
   - offer guidance, consultation and accurate information to local school boards and parent groups
   - develop in-service training programs and discussion groups for school staff

Appendix III: National Lesbian and Gay Health Professional Associations

American Association of Physicians for Human Rights
2940 16th Street #309, San Francisco, CA 94103; (415) 558-9353

Annual national conference, referral information and position statements on health and AIDS related issues.

National Lesbian and Gay Health Foundation
P.O. Box 65472, Washington, D.C. 20035; (202) 797-3708

Annual national conference and national AIDS forum, referral information, research and publication of resource material including a national directory of health care providers for lesbian and gay patients and clients.

REFERENCES

1. Specter M: Medical profession confronts new generations' AIDS fear. *Washington Post* January 20, 1988, p 1.
2. Ryan CC: A day in the life of an AIDS health worker. National Association of Social Workers AIDS Public Information Campaign, 1988, pp. 10–13.
3. Wiener L: An attitudinal study of social work responses to the AIDS patient population. Dissertation, New York University School of Social Work, 1988.
4. Wertz DC, Sorenson JR, Liebling L: Knowledge and attitudes of AIDS health care providers before and after education programs. *Public Health Rep* 102:248–254, 1987.
5. Hendee WR, Rapoza NP, Rinaldi RC: The American Medical Association's program on HIV infection and AIDS. *JAMA* 258:1519–1520, 1987.
6. Intergovernmental Health Policy Project, Washington, DC, 1988.
7. Rowe MJ, Ryan CC: Medical care and potential discrimination, in *AIDS: A Public Health Challenge—State Issues, Policies and Programs.* Washington, DC, Intergovernmental Health Policy Project, 1987.
8. Thomas A, Sillen S: *Racism and Psychiatry.* Secaucus, New Jersey, Citadel Press, 1972.
9. Mays VM, Cochran SD: Acquired immune deficiency syndrome and black Americans: Special psychological issues. *Public Health Rep* 102:224–231, 1987.
10. Rogers MF, Williams WW: AIDS in blacks and hispanics; implications for prevention. *Issues Sci Technol* 3(3):89–94, 1987.
11. Jue S: Identifying and meeting the needs of minority clients with AIDS, in Leukefeld C, Fimbres M (eds): *Responding to AIDS—Psychosocial Initiatives.* Silver Spring, Maryland, National Association of Social Workers, 1987, pp 65–79.
12. Garfinckle EM, Morin SE: Psychologists' attitudes toward homosexual psychotherapy clients. *J Social Issues* 34:101–111, 1978.
13. DeCrecenzo TA: Homophobia: A study of attitudes of mental health professionals toward homosexuality. *J Social Work Hum Sex* 2:115–136, 1984.
14. Matthews WC, Booth MW, Turner JD, et al: Physicians' attitudes toward homosexuality: Survey of california county medical society. *West J Med* 144:106–110, 1986.
15. Douglas CJ, Kalman CM, Kalman TP: Homophobia among physicians and nurses: An empirical study. *Hosp Community Psychiatry* 36:1309–1311, 1985
16. Kelly JA, St. Lawrence JS, Smith S, et al: Medical students' attitudes towards AIDS and homosexual patients. *J Med Ed* 62:549–556, 1987.
17. Kelly JA, St. Lawrence JS, Smith S, et al: Stigmatization of AIDS patients by physicians. *Am J Public Health* 77:789–791, 1987.
18. Wiebe C: Professional demands, human frailties—Doctors respond to AIDS. *New Physician* 35(1):14–17, 1986.
19. Lewis C, Freeman H, Corey C: AIDS related competence of california's primary care physicians. *Am J Public Health* 77:795–799, 1987.
20. AIDS testing without consent. *New York Times,* January 9, 1988, p 7.
21. Morin S, Batchelor W: Responding to the psychological crises of AIDS. *Public Health Rep* 99:4–9, 1984.
22. Furstenberg AL, Olson NM: Social work and AIDS. *Social Work Health Care* 9(4):45–62, 1984.
23. Christ G, Wiener L: Psychosocial issues of AIDS, in Devita V, Hellman S, Rosenberg SA, (eds): AIDS: *Etiology, Diagnosis, Treatment and Prevention.* Philadelphia, JB Lippincott, 1985, pp 275–297.
24. Ferrara AJ: My personal experience with AIDS. *Am Psychol* 39:1285–1287, 1987.

25. Carl D: AIDS: A preliminary examination of the effects on gay couples and coupling. *J Marital Family Ther* 12:241–247, 1986.
26. Mailick M: The impact of severe illness on the individual and family: An overview. *Social Work Health Care* 5:117–128, 1979.
27. Swick T: Joanne Lynn—Views on the care of the elderly and dying. *ACP Observer* pp 16–17, 1987.
28. Rowe MJ, Ryan CC: Medical care, in *AIDS: A Public Health Challenge—State Issues, Policies and Programs*. Washington, DC, Intergovernmental Health Policy Project, 1987.
29. Okie S, Carton B: The stresses of treating AIDS: with limited options, health professionals seek small victories. *Washington Post,* January 19, 1988, p 1.
30. Wiener L: An attitudinal study of social work responses to the AIDS patient population. Dissertation, New York University School of Social Work, 1988.
31. Bramhall M, Ezell S: How burned out are you? *Public Welfare* 39(1):23–27, 1981.
32. Bramhall M, Ezell S: How agencies can prevent burnout. *Public Welfare* 39(3):33–37, 1981.
33. Colburn D, Thompson L: Treatment risks, difficulties foster young doctors doubts. *Washington Post,* June 5, 1987.
34. Davis-Sacks ML, Jayaratne S, Chess W: A comparison of the effects of social support on the incidence of burnout. *Social Work* pp 240–244, 1985.
35. Wiener L: An attitudinal study of social work responses to the AIDS patient population. Dissertation, New York University School of Social Work, 1988.
36. Smith MU, Godean RE, Katner HP: Knowledge and attitudes of rural Georgia physicians concerning AIDS, in *The Fifth International Conference on AIDS, Montreal Canada, June 1989.*
37. Bramhall M, Ezell S: Working your way out of burnout. *Public Welfare* 39(2):32–39, Spring 1981.
38. DeNoon D: AIDS takes it psychological toll on the health care community, *In These Times* October 14–20, 1987, pp. 6–7.
39. Young EW: Nurses' attitudes toward homosexuality: Analysis of change in AIDS workshops. Unpublished manuscript, Pennsylvania State University.
40. Wetrz DC, Sorenson JR, Liebling L, et al: Knowledge and attitudes of AIDS health care providers before and after education programs. *Public Health Rep* 102:248–254, 1987.
41. O'Donnell L, O'Donnell CR: Hospital workers and AIDS: Effects of in-service education on knowledge and perceived risks and stresses. *NY State J Med* 87(5):278–280, 1987.
42. Wertz DC, Sorenson JR, Liebling L, et al: Knowledge and attitudes of AIDS health care providers before and after education programs. *Public Health Rep* 102:248–254, 1987.
43. DeNoon D: AIDS takes it psychological toll on the health care community. *In These Times* October 14–20, 1987, p 7.
44. Jones RB: Wisconsin dentistry survey—Infection control practices, knowledge and beliefs, in *The American Association of Public Health Dentistry Annual Meeting, October, 1987.*
45. DeNoon D: AIDS takes it psychological toll on the health care community. *In These Times* October 14–20, 1987, pp 6–7.
46. Smith MU, Godean RE, Katner HP: Knowledge and attitudes of rural Georgia physicians concerning AIDS, in *The Fifth International Conference on AIDS, Montreal Canada, June 1989.*
47. Wiener L: An attitudinal study of social work responses to the AIDS patient population. Dissertation, New York University School of Social Work, 1988.
48. Campbell S, Maki M, Willenburg K, et al: Knowledge of HIV transmission and attitudes about AIDS among 629 registered nurses at a Minnesota hospital, in *The Fifth International Conference on AIDS, Montreal, June 1989.*
49. Rowe M, Keintz R: State AIDS Legislation Related to Worker Notification and Exposure: 1983–88. AIDS Policy Center, Intergovernmental Health Policy Project, The George Washington University, Washington, DC, 1989.
50. Shernoff M, Palacios-Jiminez L: AIDS: Prevention is our only vaccine available. *J Social Work Hum Sex* 6:135–150, 1988.
51. Shernoff M: How to integrate AIDS prevention into clinical practice. Unpublished manuscript, 1986.
52. Palacios-Jiminez L, Shernoff M: Facilitators' Guide to Eroticizing Safer Sex: A Psychoeducational Workshop Approach to Safer Sex Education. New York, Gay Men's Health Crisis, 1986.

V

Conclusion

21

Future Studies in Psychoneuroimmunology

T. PETER BRIDGE and LORING J. INGRAHAM

INTRODUCTION

While the presence of a chapter on the future of psychoneuroimmunology in a book concerning the acquired immune deficiency syndrome (AIDS) suggests that the two areas are coextensive, they are not. Nonetheless, there is a great deal of overlap between the two areas. The progress that must be made in combatting AIDS needs to include the expertise of neuroscientists and immunologists knowledgeable in the interface of the immune system and central nervous system (CNS). Presented here then are a review of psychoneuroimmunology and suggestions for the future.

PAST AND FUTURE STUDIES

Arguably, the progress made to date in the fight against AIDS results from the rapid utilization of data from the field of retrovirology. Thus, we now know the etiologic agent for the disease, human immunodeficiency virus (HIV), and have a rapid screening test to detect antibodies to HIV in blood.[1,2] More specific, but time consuming, culture procedures are also available to confirm the results of the antibody test.[3] As we have become aware of the presence of HIV dementia, become sensitized to the possibility of cofactors for HIV infection, and focused on the psychological concomitants of AIDS, the field that suggests that it next needs to be applied in the fight against AIDS is psychoneuroimmunology.

Certain aspects of the immunologic effects of HIV infection as well as the virology of HIV must be reviewed as background to considering the relevant aspects psychoneuroimmunology to AIDS. Opportunistic infections in AIDS patients clearly indicate the underlying collapse of their immune system and subsequent inability to defend against illnesses such as *Pneumocystis carinii* pneumonia or Kaposi's sarcoma.[4,5] By infecting the T4 or helper lymphocyte, and ultimately destroying them, HIV infection exacts a profound immune disregulation setting the stage for the opportunistic infections and conditions that

T. PETER BRIDGE and LORING J. INGRAHAM • Intramural Research Program, National Institute of Mental Health, Bethesda, Maryland 20892.

are ultimately fatal for the AIDS patient. As a result of this lymphotropism and cell destruction, there are overall decreases in the total number of lymphocytes, with specific losses of the T4 cells.[6] In contrast, the number of T8 suppressor cells remains relatively constant, leading to a reversal of the usual T4/T8 ratio from nearly two to less than 0.5. As well, there is a loss of cutaneous hypersensitivity to a variety of antigens such as tetanus toxoid, PPD, or candida.[4] Because HIV selectively infects and destroys the T4 lymphocyte and the monocyte/macrophage, perturbations in the production, release, or endorgan sensitivity/depletion of immunotransmitter compounds are likely correlates in HIV illness.

HIV is an RNA containing virus that is specifically trophic for certain cells, including T4 lymphocytes, monocytes, glial and neural cells, as well as cells in the kidneys, lungs, and gut.[4] The virus has been identified in multiple body fluids including blood, semen, CSF, urine, tears, saliva, and could theoretically be found in any body fluid or organ of an AIDS patient. HIV uses an enzyme unique to the strain of retroviruses, reverse transcriptase, that allows the virion to encode its genetic material into the genome of the infected cell.[8] The virus is also characterized by the capacity to mutate spontaneously, usually in its envelop protein. To date, more than 200 separate isolates of the virus have been made.[9] The most immunogenic portion of the envelop protein, an glycoprotein labeled gp120, is being studied extensively for its ability to have vaccines raised against it.[10] The isolation of HIV from brain tissue of AIDS patients and the capacity of that brain tissue to transmit the virus to susceptible cell lines during cocultivation make the point that the brain can serve as a reservoir for the infection.[11] The relative paucity of CNS histopathology detected to date associated with HIV infection of the brain make the effect of HIV on neurons uncertain. Further, there are few data available to predict the effects of the encoding of HIV genomic material on neurons.

The neurotropic nature of retroviruses predicts the association of CNS symptoms with HIV infection. As well, neurotropic characteristics of HIV infection are also predicted by the entry receptor protein shared by the CNS and the immune system.[11,12] Of broader interest than the molecular basis of HIV neurotropism are the considerable interdigitations of the central nervous and immune systems. Our rapidly expanding understanding of the interface between these two physiologic systems makes the application of this expertise in the fight against AIDS a compelling opportunity. Little is known about the precise psychoneuroimmunologic disregulation that is exacted by the natural course of HIV infection in man. In contrast, a considerable knowledge base has developed concerning the impact of HIV infection on the immune system. As a result of the intensive study of the immunodisregulating effects of HIV, there are sufficient data to generate scientific controversy; e.g., the primacy of the infection of the T4 lymphocyte or the monocyte/macrophage by HIV.[13] As established as the clinical data are regarding the cognitive, motor, and affective impact of HIV on the CNS, the neurophysiologic basis of HIV in the brain is currently a developing area of investigation.[14,15] Analogous to the application of retrovirology in the fight against AIDS, the time is at hand to apply the knowledge base in the field of psychoneuroimmunology in that effort.

Observations that behavior and behavioral choices have an impact on health status date back at least to the work of Engel.[16] Contemporaneous to this approach, the work of Holmes operationalized measures of life event impact on health status, thus estimating that impact by empirical methods.[17] While methodological debate ensued regarding the conceptualization of "stress" as either a dependent or an independent variable in models estimating the effects of life events on health status, other scientists were identifying the molecular relationships between the immune and central nervous systems underpinning these observations.

With any homeostatic system, such as is conceptually represented by the summated functions of the immune, central nervous and endocrine systems, the entry point of analysis is somewhat arbitrary. Beginning, therefore, with those elements of shared or reciprocal structure between the immune and nervous systems, it can be reasoned that it is through these shared elements that communication between the two systems exists. Further, it will be actions mediated through these common elements that would lead one to the expectation that perturbations in the shared function of one system will have similar effects alternate system. It will be a corollary expectation that those events initiating a response (e.g., cognitive vs. immunologic stimuli) in that system will be to some degree unique to that system, influencing a reciprocal response from the other system by the communicating elements (e.g., neurotransmitters, immunotransmitters) that they share. Finally, given this dynamic conceptualization of the interrelationships of these two systems, it can be expected that responses to the system specific stimuli will be system specific as well (e.g., behavior, affective state, vs. blastogenic response, chemotaxis).

Although the historical perspective may be obscure as to which observations initiated a persuasive set of data that behavior and immunomodulation are interconnected, the behavioral concomitants of adrenocortical hormones are pivotal in this history. Appreciation of the anti-inflammatory effects of adrenocortical hormones led to the production of synthetic corticoid preparations. As these preparations were used, and overused, exogenous Cushing's syndromes appeared. Symptomatically similar to endogenous Cushing's, but different in some significant behavioral ways, the affective correlates of corticoid administration drew considerable research interest. Reversing the logic of these antiinflammatory neurohumoral effects, researchers began to observe that affective disorders were often, but not invariably, associated with aberrant adrenal function.[18] Like endogenous Cushing's syndrome, the exogenous forms demonstrated affective symptomatic lysis when hormonal function was normalized. Not surprisingly, the alterations in adrenal function in affective disorder also returned to normal in the face of efficacious treatment for the mood disorder.[19] Further work in this area led to a voluminous body of research documenting frequent, but not invariable, abnormalities in the hypothalamic–pituitary–adrenal (HPA) axis in mood disorder.[20]

While clinical and epidemiologic research were establishing links between behavior and immunity, research was also moving forward to establish the molecular connections between these phenomenon. Results of this work have established that both the immune and central nervous systems produce peptide compounds capable of influencing the alternate system and that both systems share receptors in common for these transmitter compounds. It has been shown, for example, that a variety of immunostimulant events (viral infections, tumor cells, and bacteria) result in the production of the neurohumoral compounds ACTH and endorphins by peripheral blood lymphocytes (PBL).[21] PBL ACTH and endorphins were shown to be identical across a variety of biochemical parameters to their neurohumoral counterparts.[22] Subsequent work demonstrated that PBLs were capable of producing other peptide hormones, including TSH,[23] VIP,[24,25] and somatostatin.[26] Extrapolating, Blalock and colleagues exposed PBLs to CRF and found that the central hormone was capable of eliciting ACTH secretion in PBLs.[27] Corticosterone production by PBL then inhibited further CRF and ACTH secretion. Thus it is demonstrated that PBLs are responsive both to peripheral and central peptides in their production of corticosteroid compounds, analogous to the mechanisms that control centrally mediated production of corticosteroids.

Humorally based transmitter compounds are also secreted by cells of the immune system. Known as lymphokines (e.g., interleukin-2, γ-interferon); cytokines (e.g., ACTH, TSH, B-endorphin, alpha interferon) produced by activated T cells; and cytokines (e.g., interleukin-1, B-interferon) produced by B cells and monocytes, these compounds have immunoregulatory roles as well as having central effects in the brain. When examined by shared function, considerable overlap exists in neurohumoral and lymphokine function.[28]

Interferons (α, β, γ) are produced by PBL, fibroblasts, and activated T cells with both immunologic and neuropsychiatric activity.[21,22,28,29] Animal research has provided evidence that interferon has multiple neurohumoral-like actions. These include (1) stimulation of corticosteroid production[30,31]; (2) increased melanin synthesis[30]; (3) opiate receptor binding[32]; and (4) increased iodine uptake in thyroid cells.[33] In addition, norepinephrinelike activity by interferon has been observed in myocardial cells.[34] Research has also shown that familiar neuropeptide antagonists interfered with the activity of interferon in the brain. For example, naloxine reduced the opiate receptor binding by interferon, without affecting its antiviral activity.[35] Dexamethasone administration also counteracted interferon's ACTH-like activity without altering its immunologic actions.[36] The separability of the immune and neuropsychiatric actions of these lymphokines suggests strongly that some common mechanism exists to turn on these systems, while potentially distinct receptors permit differential blockage of the immune and neuropsychiatric effects.[28]

Clinical data relevant to the neuropsychiatric effects of interferon are beginning to accumulate as various clinical trials with the compound are under way. As well, interest in viral etiologies of neuropsychiatric disorders propel studies from that perspective. Early trials of alpha interferon indicate that a fatigue–asthenia syndrome is a common side effect of that therapy in cancer patients.[37] A pre-/posttherapy study of alpha interferon's effects on behavior, cognition, and affect in cancer patients indicated widespread neuropsychiatric effects of the therapy. Following therapy there was increased fatigue, psychomotor slowing, and cognitive impairment paradoxically associated with substantial improvement in mood. Interestingly, the administration of dopaminergic agonist and antagonist drugs were reported to attenuate/alleviate this fatigue–asthenia syndrome.[37] Recent data also indicate that evening administration may attenuate many of the fatigue–asthenia symptoms.[38] This is noteworthy in light of animal work indicating the α-melanocyte stimulating hormone (MSH) activity of interferon.[30] Looking at serum interferon levels in psychiatric patients, high titers of α-interferon were seen in 25% of psychotic patients examined.[39] This contrasts to elevated serum interferon levels in less than 2% of the control subjects. While intriguing, other studies of CSF interferon found no such elevations in psychiatric patients.[40,41]

Interleukin-1, produced by macrophages and the B lymphocytes, and interleukin-2 produced by the activated T lymphocyte, are now having neuropsychiatric effects documented. Common to both is the glucocorticoid inhibition of their secretion.[34,42] Variously hydrocortisone,[34] dexamethasone,[34] and ACTH[42] have inhibitory actions for both interleukins, as well as for interferon. Recent data relying on hypophysectomy and/or adrenalectomy indicate that the pituitary–adrenal axis is integrally involved in this system. As with interferon, the interleukins also show reciprocal relationships with glucocorticoid compounds. Thus, exogenous administration of interferon or either interleukin results in glucocorticoid release in a homeostatic effort.

Clinical data indicate a role of interleukin 1 in promoting slow-wave sleep and stimulating hypothalamic thermoregulatory centers.[43] Initial results of clinical trials with interleukin-2 are reporting fatigue-asthenia side effects similar to interferon.[44] In healthy normal subjects, an increase in plasma interleukin-1 is associated with the onset of slow wave sleep, while an increase in plasma interleukin-2 follows and is greatest during non-REM sleep and nighttime wakefulness.[45] The association between substances involved in immune responses and sleep has led Krueger and Karnovsky to suggest that "sleep may indeed by intimately involved in processes that counter infections" (p. 510).[46]

Other evidence for the interconnections of the immune and central nervous systems are the immunosuppressive effects that have been observed with various psychoactive medications. It has long been observed that intravenous drug users are prone to a greater incidence of infectious illness, although such observations cannot fix causality with the drug of abuse, the life-style of the drug user, or other factors. Consequently, animal and in vitro research has been used to examine the issue that the "abused" drug may by immunosuppressive in its own right. Such examinations have been extended to licit psychoactive agents as well. In a series of experiments with THC, Friedman and colleagues observed that THC reduced monocyte chemotaxis in culture, inhibited blastogenesis following mitogen stimulation, inhibited natural killer cell activity, and suppressed interferon and interleukin one and two production.[47] Phencyclidine (PCP) has also demonstrated reduction in interleukin 1 production, suppressing radiolabelled thymidine incorporation in T4, T8, and B lymphocytes.[48] Alcohol in vitro shows reductions in lymphocyte mitogen response as well, while alcoholics frequently show reduced total lymphocyte numbers.[49] Observations that interferon administration is often associated with neutropenia, and that lithium carbonate has been observed to be effective in reversing neutropenia, led investigators to examine the effects of lithium administration upon the ability of interferon to block granulopoietic differentiation. While interferon normally blocks granulopoiesis, lithium administration prevents this effect.[50] In contrast, lithium has been observed to increase lymphocyte blastogenesis to mitogen stimulation in manic-depressive patients treated with lithium.[51] In another study, chlorpromazine administration was associated with increasing brain interferon levels in mice.[52] Other studies have suggested that haloperidol magnifies delayed hypersensitivity in mice, leading to the speculation that this effect may be mediated through dopamine receptors located on lymphocytes.[53]

In addition to neurotransmitter modulating drugs being associated with immunologic effects, other investigators have studied the effects of neurotransmitters on the immune system directly. The observations that hypothalamic lesions in rats were associated with a variety of transient immunomodulatory effects in lymphocyte number, natural killer cell activity, or lymphocyte mitogen response led to the speculation that these transient effects might be neurotransmitter mediated.[54] Further studies indicated that serotonin, perhaps mediated through a glucocorticoid route, decreases both IgM and IgG response to sheep red blood cell (SRBC) antibody response.[54] Using intracisternal 6-hydroxydopamine injections in mice, resultant central noradrenergic depletion resulted in decreased IgG and IgM SRBC antibody response. Other studies detail immunomodulatory roles for other neurotransmitters, such as substance P, somatostatin, and vasoactive intestinal peptide (VIP).[24–26] Presumably, the ability of these neurotransmitters to affect immune function rests on the presence of receptors for these peptides on lymphocytes.[26] Substance P modulates phagocytosis and stimulates lymphocyte proliferation, while somatostatin and VIP inhibit lymphocyte proliferation.[26,55] VIP inhibits both lymphoblastic transformation and lymphocyte chemotaxis.[24] The inhibitory neurotransmitter, γ-amino butyric acid (GABA) is elevated in response to lymphokine release in the SRBC test.[56]

In considering the fullest range of the reciprocal influences of the immune and central nervous systems, attention must be paid as well to the potential influence of behavior and affective state on immune function. Behavior and affective state have clearly both efferent and afferent relationship to brain function, and given all that has been discussed, would at least be expected to have some indirect relationship to immune function. In a most elegant study, Ader and Cohen used classic conditioning to modify immune function in mice.[57] The Glasers and their colleagues have observed that psychosocial variables, such as loneliness and life events, were associated with reductions in natural killer cell activity and reductions in IgA in the context of naturally occurring stressors.[58] Affective syndromes, with their attendant behavioral expression, are associated with immunosuppression and potentially with the progression of HIV disease.[44,59]

SUMMARY AND FUTURE DIRECTIONS

As this review makes apparent, there are numerous data focused on the immunologic defects associated with HIV disease. In contrast, we have fewer data on the CNS aspects of HIV disease, and those that we do have are confusing. Potentially the most destructive aspect of this illness is the neurotropic nature of the virus with its early and potentially slow onset of neuropsychiatric impairment and the potential for the CNS to serve as a reservoir for the virus by protecting it behind the blood-brain barrier. Were this an illness similar to Alzheimer's with obviously identifiable tissue destruction associated with the illness, the degree of symptomatology would seem comprehensible. Furthermore, if analogous tissue destruction were present in CNS HIV disease, it would have been observed by now. It has not, and the degree of brain pathology found at *post mortem* examination has presented etiologic enigmas. While the hoped-for end point of any AIDS research agenda must be the prevention and/or cure for AIDS, we are not close to those points at present.

As a first step, considerable progress in understanding the neurophysiologic processes that underlie the CNS HIV symptomatology is needed. That understanding must be based on examination early in the course of the illness, in individuals being treated with antiviral and immunorestorative therapies,[60] and on the longitudinal comparison of physiologic parameters across patients and within individuals. The recent review by Price et al.[61] provides a current overview of this area.

Important relationships that need further investigation over the course of HIV infection include the effect of psychological variables such as social support or depressive symptomatology on immune function, the relationship between immune function and neuropathology, and the effect of current pharmacotherapy on neuropsychological function. As our understanding of these phenomena grows, we will then be able to build and begin empirical investigation of models that more accurately reflect the complex interactions among psychological, immunological, and neurological variables in HIV infection. An example of careful model building and the presentation of testable hypotheses is Solomon's[62] postulates proposed for CNS–immune interaction. Although it may be tempting to speculate at this point that social support can alleviate depression, less depression can then protect immune function, protected immune function can then militate against the neurotoxic effects of HIV, such speculation is premature. As Darko[7] points out, facing death is a wrenching enough experience without worsening the burden with guilt from not having tried hard enough to accept or give emotional support.

In summary, empirical approaches to the tremendously complex potential interactions of neurological, psychological, and immunological aspects of HIV infection may best begin by focusing on individual strands in the psychoneuroimmunological net. As our knowledge of simple unidirectional bivariate relationships builds, models that incorporate multivariate predictors and reciprocal effects can be built on an empirical, rather than speculative, base. We must focus on psychoneuroimmunological contributions to health and improved function in as well as to pathological processes and disease. Finally, we should not be so fascinated by relationships among psychological, neurological, and immunological events as to neglect searching for the mechanisms underlying these phenomena.

REFERENCES

1. Gallo RC, Salahuddin SZ, Popovic M, et al: Frequent detection and isolation of cytopathic retroviruses (HTLV-III) from patients with AIDS. *Science* 224:500–502, 1984.
2. Weiss SH, Goedert JJ, Sarngadharan MG, et al: Screening test for HTLV-III antibodies. *JAMA* 253:221–225, 1985.
3. Levy JA, Hoffman AD, Kramer SM, et al: Isolation of lympocytotrophic retroviruses from San Francisco patients with AIDS. *Science* 225:840–842, 1984.
4. Fauci AS, Masur H, Gelmann EP, et al: The acquired immunodeficiency syndrome: An update. *Ann Intern Med* 102:800–813, 1985.
5. Centers for Disease Control: Revision of the case definition of acquired immunodeficiency syndrome for national reporting—United States. *MMWR* 34:373–375, 1985.
6. Fauci AS, Macher AM, Longo, DL, et al: Acquired immunodeficiency syndrome. *Ann Intern Med* 100:92–106, 1984.
7. Darko DF: A brief tour of psychoneuroimmunology. *Ann Allergy* 57:233–238, 1986.
8. Hoffman AD, Banapour B, Levy JA: Characterization of AIDS associated retrovirus reverse transcriptase and optimal conditions for its detection in virions. *Virology* 147:326–335, 1985.
9. Coffin JM: Genetic variation in AIDS viruses. Background paper. Washington, DC: Committee on National Strategy for AIDS, 1986.
10. Gartner S, Markovits P, Markovitz DM, et al: Virus isolation from and identification of HTLV-III/LAV-producing cells in brain tissue from a patient with AIDS. *JAMA* 256:2365–2371, 1986.
11. Dalgleish AG, Beverley PCL, Clapham PR, et al: The CD4 (T4) antigen is an essential component of the receptor for the AIDS retrovirus. *Nature (Lond)* 312:763–767, 1984.
12. Pert CB, Hill JM, Ruff MR, et al: Octapeptide deduced from the neuropeptide receptor-like pattern of antigen T4 in brain potently inhibit human immunodeficiency virus receptor binding and T cell infectivity. *Proc Natl Acad Sci USA* 23:9254–9258, 1986.

13. Gartner S, Markovits P, Markovitz DM, et al: The role of mononuclear phagocytes in HTLV-III/LAV infection. *Science* 233:215–219, 1986.
14. Stoler MH, Eskin TA, Benn S, et al: HTLV-III Infection of the central nervous system. *JAMA* 256:2360–2364, 1986.
15. Chiodi F, Asjo B, Fenyo EM, et al: Isolation of HIV from CSF of antibody positive virus carrier without neurological symptoms. *Lancet* 1:1276–1277, 1986.
16. Engel G: A unified concept of health and disease. *Perspect Med Biol* 3:459–485, 1960.
17. Holmes TH, Treuting T, Wolff HG: Life situations emotions, and nasal disease. *Psychosom Med* 13:71–82, 1951.
18. Carroll BJ: The hypothalamic pituitary adrenal axis: Functions, control mechanisms and methods of study, in Davies B, Carroll BJ, Mowbray RM (eds): *Depressive Illness, Some Research Studies*. Springfield, Illinois, Charles C Thomas, 1972, pp. 23–68.
19. Sachar AJ, Asnis G, Halbreich U, et al: Recent studies in the neuroendocrinology of major depressive disorders. *Psychiatr Clin North Am* 3:313–326, 1980.
20. Targum SD, Sullivan AC, Byrnes SM: Neuroendocrine interrelationships in major depressive disorders. *Am J Psychiatry* 139:282–286, 1982.
21. Blalock JE, McMenamin DH, Smith EM: Peptide hormones shared by the neuroendocrine and immunologic systems. *J Immunol* 135:858s–861s, 1985.
22. Blalock JE, Smith EM: Human leukocyte interferon. *Proc Natl Acad Sci USA* 77:5972–5974, 1980.
23. Smith EM, Phan M, Coppenhaver D, et al: Human leukocyte production of immunoreactive thyrotropin. *Proc Nat Acad Sci USA* 80:6010–6011, 1983.
24. Giachetti A, Goth A, Said SA: VIP in rabbit platelets and mast cells. *Fed Proc* 37:357–361, 1978.
25. O'Dorisio MS, O'Dorisio TM, Cataland S, et al: VIP as a biochemical marker for polymorphonuclear leukocytes. *J Lab Clin Med* 96:966–971, 1980.
26. Lygren I, Revhaug A, Burhol PG, et al: VIP and somatostatin in leukocytes. *Scand J Clin Lab Invest* 44:347–349, 1984.
27. Smith EM, Morrill AC, Meyer WJ, et al: CRF induction of leukocyte derived immunoreactive ACTH and endorphins. *Nature (Lond)* 321:881, 1986.
28. Blalock JE: Relationships between neuroendocrine hormones and lymphokines. *Lymphokines* 9:1–13, 1984.
29. Hall NR, McGillis JP, Spangelo BL, et al: Evidence that thymosins can function as neuroactive immunotransmitters. *J Immunol* 135:806s–811s, 1985.
30. Blalock JE, Harp C: Interferon and ACTH induction of steroidogenesis. *Arch Virol* 67:45–49, 1981.
31. Chany C, Rousset S, Bourgeade MF: Regulatory effects of interferons in various cells. *Ann NY Acad Sci* 350:254–265, 1980.
32. Smith EM, Blalock JE: Human lymphocyte production of CRF and endorphin. *Proc Natl Acad Sci USA* 78:7530–7534, 1981.
33. Friedman R: Interferon interaction with thyroid cells. *J Interferon Res* 2:387, 1982.
34. Blalock JE, Stanton J: Common pathways of interferon and hormonal action. *Nature (Lond)* 283:406–408, 1980.
35. Blalock JE, Smith EM: Human leukocyte interferon. *Biochem Biophy Res Commun* 101:472–478, 1981.
36. Kelso A, Munck A: Glucocorticoid inhibition of lymphokine secretion. *J Immunol* 133:784–791, 1984.
37. Adams F, Quesada JR, Gutterman JU: Neuropsychiatric manifestations of human leukocyte interferon therapy in patients with cancer. *JAMA*, 252:938–941, 1984.
38. Abrams PG, McClamrock E, Foon KA: Evening administration of alpha interferon. *N Engl J Med* 312:443–444, 1985.
39. Preble O, Torrey EF: Serum interferon in patients with psychosis. *Am J Psychiatry* 142:1184–1186, 1985.
40. Roy A, Pickar D, Ninan P, et al: A search for interferon in CSF of schizophrenics. *Am J Psychiatry* 142:269, 1985.
41. Rimon RH, Halonen P, Lebow P, et al: Antibrain antibodies and interferon in the serum and the cerebrospinal fluid of patients with schizophrenia, in Mozorov P (ed): *Research on the Viral Hypothesis of Mental Disorders*. Basel Karger, 1983, pp 161–167.
42. Besedovsky H, Del Rey A, Sorkin E, et al: Immunoregulatory feedback between interleukin 1 and glucocorticoid hormones. *Science* 233:652–654, 1986.
43. Krueger J, Walter J, Dinarello CA, et al: Sleep promoting effect of interleukin 1. *Am J Physiol* 246:994–999, 1984.

44. Rubinow DR, Joffe RT, Brouwers P, et al: Neuropsychiatric impairment in patients with AIDS. *Adv Biochem Psychopharm* 44:111–115, (1988).
45. Moldofsky H, Lue FA, Eisen J, et al: The relationship of interleukin-1 and immune functions to sleep in humans. *Psychosom Med* 48:309–318, 1986.
46. Krueger JM, Karnovsky ML: Sleep and the immune response. *Ann NY Acad Sci* 496:510–516, 1987.
47. Friedman H, Klein T, Specter S, et al: Drugs of abuse and virus susceptibility. *Adv Biochem Psychopharm* 44:125–137, (1988).
48. Khansari N, Whitten HD, Fudenberg HH: Phencyclidine induced immunodepression. *Science* 225:76–78, 1984.
49. Jerrell TR, Maretta CA, Bone G, et al: Ethanol associated immunosuppression. *Adv Biochem Psychopharm* 44:173–185, (1988).
50. Verma DS, Spitzer G, Gutterman JU, et al: Human leukocyte interferon-mediated granulopoietic differentiation arrest and its abrogation by lithium. *Am J Hematol* 12:39–46, 1982.
51. Fernandez LA, Fox RA: Perturbation of the immune system by lithium. *Clin Exp Immunol* 41:527–532, 1980.
52. Libikowa H: Psychopharmaca and ECT in relation to interferon. *Arch Immunol Ther Exp* 25:641–649, 1977.
53. Shaskan EG, Lovett EJ: Effects of haloperidol, a dopamine receptor antagonist, on a delayed type hypersensitivity reaction to 1-chloro, -2, 4-dinitrobenzene in mice. Res Common Psychiat. and Behav. 5:241–254, (1980).
54. Roszman TL, Jackson JC, Cross RJ, et al: Neuroanatomic and neurotransmitter influences on immune function. *J Immunol* 135:769s–772s, 1985.
55. Stanisz AJ, Befus D, Bienenstock J: Differential effects of vasoactive intestinial peptide, substance P, and somatostatin on immunoglobin synthesis and proliferations by lymphocytes from Peyer's patches, mesenteric lymph nodes, and spleen. *J Immunol* 136:152–156, 1986.
56. Hall NR, Suria A, Goldstein AL: *Lymphokine Res* 4:339–341, 1985.
57. Ader R, Cohen N: Behaviorally conditioned immunosuppression. *Psychosom Med* 37:333–340, 1975.
58. Kiecolt-Glaser JK, Garner W, Speicher C, et al: Psychosocial modifiers of immunocompetence. *Psychosom Med* 46:7–11, 1984.
59. Stein M, Keller SE, Schleifer SJ: Stress and immunomodulation: The role of depression and neuroendocrine function. *J Immunol* 135:827s–833s, 1985.
60. Yarchoan R, Brouwers P, Spitzer AR, et al: Response of HIV associated neurological disease to 3′-Azido-3′-deoxythymidine. *Lancet* 1:132–135, 1987.
61. Price RW, Brew B, Sidtis J, et al: The brain in AIDS: Central nervous system HIV-1 infection and AIDS dementia complex. *Science* 239:586–592, 1988.
62. Solomon GF: Psychoneuroimmunology: Interactions between central nervous system and immune system. *J Neurosci Res* 18:1–9, 1987.

Index